NANDA International
NURSING DIAGNOSES:
DEFINITIONS & CLASSIFICATION
2012–2014

NANDA International
NURSING DIAGNOSES:
DEFINITIONS & CLASSIFICATION
2012–2014

Edited by

T. Heather Herdman, PhD, RN

WILEY-BLACKWELL

A John Wiley & Sons, Ltd., Publication

Correct Citation (American Psychological Association):

Herdman, T.H. (2012) (Ed.). NANDA International Nursing Diagnoses: Definitions & Classification, 2012–2014. Oxford: Wiley-Blackwell.

Contents

Visit the supporting companion website for this book: www.wiley.com/go/ nursingdiagnoses

NANDA International Guidelines for Copyright Permission

The materials presented in this book are copyrighted and all copyright laws apply.

For any usage other than reading or consulting the book in the English language, a licence is required from Blackwell Publishing Ltd (a company of John Wiley & Sons Inc).

Examples of such reuse include, but are not restricted to:

1. A publishing house, other organization, or individual wishing to translate the entire book, or parts thereof.
2. An author or publishing house wishing to use the entire nursing diagnosis taxonomy, or parts thereof, in a commercially available textbook or nursing manual.
3. An author or company wishing to use the nursing diagnosis taxonomy in audio-visual materials.
4. A software developer or computer-based patient record vendor wishing to use the nursing diagnosis taxonomy in English in a software program or application (for example, an electronic health record or an electronic application for a smart phone/personal digital assistant [PDA]).
5. A nursing school, researcher, professional organization, or healthcare organization wishing to use the nursing diagnosis taxonomy in an educational program.
6. A hospital wishing to integrate the nursing diagnosis taxonomy into their own electronic health records.
7. Any of the usages outlined above in a language other than English.

Please send all requests by e-mail to: nanda@wiley.com, or by post to:

NANDA International Copyright Requests
Global Rights Department
John Wiley & Sons Ltd.
The Atrium
Southern Gate
Chichester
West Sussex
PO19 8SQ
UK

Translations Terms and Conditions

The full terms and conditions for translations will be as follows (this includes those already agreed and implemented for the current edition):

- There will be no buy-back by Wiley-Blackwell or NANDA-I of unsold copies of any translations at the time that the next edition is released.

- Publishers cannot add or remove any content from the original version provided by Wiley-Blackwell. This includes the addition of forwards, new prefaces or comments by translators or other parties. The only exception to this is the addition, under the name of the editor, of the translators of each version, who should be identified as translators (not as authors or editors).
- We will require publishers to submit the name, qualifications and résumé of the chief translator for approval prior to commencing any translation work.
- Publishers must also submit both the cover design and the manuscript of the translation to Wiley-Blackwell for approval by NANDA-I prior to printing the translation. NANDA-I requires up to 12 weeks to complete this approval process, so it should be built into your production schedule.
- Any and all changes requested by NANDA-I must be included in the translation, and publishers shall be required to submit page proofs for a final check before printing the translation.
- Publishers will be required to include an advertisement for NANDA-I membership in the translation.
- Publishers will be expected to allow digital licensees, predominantly software developers, to use their translation in their products upon a mutually agreed fee. To this end, the following Clause will be included in all translation licenses:

The Proprietor licenses the exclusive rights specified in clause 1 (a) (i) to the Publisher on the condition that the Publisher shall provide electronic files of the Translation to any third parties who have entered into a valid digital licence agreement with the Proprietor ("Digital Products Licensees"), following notification from the Proprietor of such licences. The electronic files provided by the Publisher to the Digital Products Licensees will be for use only in digital products such as software applications, smart phone applications, online learning courses and other digital products now existing or to be invented in the future ("Digital Products") solely in the Territory, but for the avoidance of doubt shall not include e-books (unabridged verbatim electronic copies of the print Translation). The Publisher may charge a reasonable fee for providing the electronic files to the above-mentioned Digital Products Licensees, such fee to be retained in full by the Publisher. The Proprietor's Digital Products Licensees shall credit the Publisher as the publisher of the Translation, and shall cooperate with the Publisher to promote the print Translation in all Digital Products made available in the Territory. It is understood and agreed that the Publisher shall have the first option to license the right to publish the Translation in e-book format, on terms to be agreed.

Preface

The 2012–2014 edition of NANDA International's classic text *Nursing Diagnoses: Definitions & Classification* builds on the success of the well-received "new look and feel" of the 2009–2011 edition. This latest edition includes 16 new and ten revised diagnoses together with several new or refreshed opening chapters. These essays in best practice in the development, testing, and use of Nursing Diagnoses have been written by some of the most accomplished scholars in the field, and I commend them to you. The aim of including these outstanding contributions is to ensure that we all use Nursing Diagnoses safely and consistently in our practice worldwide.

NANDA International is a not-for-profit membership organization. This means that, with the exception of our business management and administration functions, all of our work is done by volunteers. Indeed, some of the world's most talented nurse scientists and scholars are or have been NANDA International volunteers. So, contrary to popular belief, there is not an office block somewhere in the United States with rows of nurse researchers working on Nursing Diagnoses. Our volunteers are people like you and me who give their time and expertise to NANDA International because of their strongly held beliefs about the primacy of patient care and the contribution that nursing and nurses can make.

With the publication of each new edition of our work come more and more translations. I am proud that the work is now published in numerous languages, as befits an international membership organization dedicated to patient safety and high-quality, evidence-based nursing care. Our highly effective relationship with our publishing partner, Wiley-Blackwell, has become embedded during the last 2 years. One of the stated aims of this arrangement is to ensure that each and every translation is accurate and exact. Together with our publishers, we now have a robust quality assurance mechanism in place to ensure the accuracy of each translation. The source document for each translation is always this, the American English version. Whilst this might appear dogmatic, we are deeply committed to ensuring the integrity of our work worldwide and invite you to support us in this quest in order to improve patient safety and the consistency of care. As a not-for-profit organization, we obviously need a modest income to run the organization and this comes from the licenses we sell for publishing and the use of our work in electronic form.

Every year, I receive a number of questions from nurses at all levels about the cultural applicability of our work in their own countries or jurisdictions. As an international organization, we truly value cultural diversity and practice difference. However, as the provider of the world's most successful standardized nursing diagnostic language, we have a duty to provide you with exactly that – a standardized nursing diagnostic language. We do not support changing diagnoses at the request of translators or clinical specialists in just one edition in a particular language, even if the diagnosis in question lacks applicability in that particular culture. This is not only because we are deeply committed to realizing the clinical benefits of standardized language, but also because we do not believe that we should be supporting the censorship of the clinical information you can find in this text. As a registered nurse* you are accountable for the use of the diagnoses you choose to use in your practice. Clearly, it would be inappropriate for all of us to use all of the diagnoses in this edition as none of us could claim competence in every sphere of nursing practice simultaneously. Clinically safe nurses are reflective practitioners, and central to being safe is to thoroughly understand one's own clinical competence. It is highly likely that there are numerous diagnoses in this edition that you will never use in your own practice; others you may use daily. This links to the issue of cultural applicability because if, when studying this edition, you find a diagnosis that is not applicable to your practice or culture, it is within your gift simply not to use it. However, based on my own varied clinical experience as a registered nurse, I would implore you not to completely ignore those diagnoses that may at first seem culturally awkward. We live in a transcultural and highly mobile society, and exploring those diagnoses that might at first seem unusual can challenge your thinking and open up new possibilities and understanding. This is all part of being a reflective and life-long learning practitioner.

Each diagnosis has been the product of one of our many NANDA International volunteers, and most have a defined evidence-base. Each and every new and revised diagnosis will have been refined and debated by our Diagnosis Development Committee before finally being submitted to the members of NANDA International to be voted upon. Only if our members vote positively for the inclusion of a new or refined diagnosis does the work "make it" into the edition. When I first joined NANDA International, I was attracted to this level of democracy, and I am pleased that we have never departed from those founding values. However, if you feel that a particular diagnosis is incorrect and requires revision, we welcome your views. You should contact the Chair of our Diagnosis Development Committee through our website. Please provide as much evidence as possible to support your views. By working in this way, rather than changing just one translation or edition, we can ensure the continued integrity and consistency of our language, and that all benefit from the wisdom and work of individual scholars. We would, of course, also welcome your submissions of new diagnoses. Submission guidelines can be found in this edition and on our website.

One of the key membership developments in the past few years has been the inauguration of our Membership Network Groups. These groups of NANDA International members coming together to pursue scholarly activity and to promote Nursing Diagnosis have been an enormous success. We currently have groups in Brazil, Peru, Ecuador, Nigeria–Ghana, and a German language group. We would welcome applications to form further groups; further information can be found at our website www.nanda.org

I want to commend the work of all NANDA International volunteers, committee members, chairs, and the Board of Directors for their time, commitment, and enthusiasm, and indeed for their support. I also want to thank our staff, led by our former President, Dr. Heather Herdman, who is now our Executive Director. The development of our publishing partnership with Wiley-Blackwell is just one of the many developments we have put into place in the last few years. These developments will ensure that we remain a responsive, modern, and well-run organization.

---

*Our expectation is that nursing students are supervised in developing their diagnostic skills by a registered nurse, who remains accountable.

My special thanks to the members of the Diagnosis Development Committee and especially to the Chairs, Dr. Geralyn Meyers (until 2010) and Dr. Shigemi Kamitsuru (from 2010). This committee is the "power house" of NANDA International, and I am always deeply humbled and impressed by the extraordinary work of these volunteers.

Finally, when I first joined NANDA International nearly 20 years ago, I did not ever imagine that I would be elected President. I have been the first non-American President and the first male President! It has truly been an honor to serve as President. As long as we remain concerned about ensuring high-quality, evidence-based, safe patient care, NANDA International has a role. Indeed, our work is core to the future of nursing.

Professor Dickon Weir-Hughes
President, NANDA International

Introduction

This book is divided into four parts.

- *Part 1* provides the introduction to the NANDA International Taxonomy of Nursing Diagnoses. Taxonomy II organizes the diagnoses into domains and classes, and uses a multiaxial structure for the development of diagnostic concept foci.
- *Part 2* provides chapters on assessment and clinical judgment, nursing diagnosis in education, electronic health records, research, administration, and criteria for evaluation of nursing classifications. These chapters are written for students, clinicians, and educators. The accompanying website includes educational materials designed to support students and faculty in understanding and teaching this material.
- *Part 3* provides the traditional contents of the *NANDA International Nursing Diagnoses: Definitions & Classification* books: the diagnoses themselves, including definitions, defining characteristics, risk factors, and related factors, as appropriate. The diagnoses are listed by Domain first, and then Class, and then alphabetically (in the English language) by diagnostic foci within each class. We recommend that all translations maintain this order to facilitate ease of discussion between interlanguage groups. Information is provided on diagnoses that were removed from the Taxonomy during the past two review cycles.
- *Part 4* includes information that relates specifically to NANDA International. The results of an International Think Tank meeting are provided, along with two position statements regarding assessment frameworks and the structure of nursing diagnosis statements. A revised chapter details the process for submission of a new or revised nursing diagnosis to NANDA International's Diagnosis Development Committee (DDC). Processes and procedures related to review of NANDA International diagnoses, the submission process, and level of evidence criteria are provided. A glossary of terms is given. Finally, committee members within NANDA International are recognized, and information specific to the organization and the benefits of membership are outlined.

How to Use This Book

As noted above, the nursing diagnoses are listed by Domain first, and then Class, and then alphabetically (in the English language) by diagnostic foci within each class. For example, *Insufficient Breast Milk* is listed under Domain 2 (Nutrition), Class 1 (Ingestion):

Domain 2: Nutrition

Class 1: Ingestion
*Insufficient **Breast Milk*** (00216)

I hope that the organization of *NANDA-I Nursing Diagnoses: Definitions & Classification 2012–2014* will make it efficient and effective to use. I welcome your feedback. If you have suggestions, please send them by email to: execdir@nanda.org

Frequently Asked Questions

1) **When I reviewed the informatics codes provided in the book, I notice that there are some codes missing – does that mean that there are missing diagnoses?**

   No, the missing codes represent codes that were not assigned, or diagnoses that have been retired, or removed, from the Taxonomy over time. Please refer to Part 1, Introduction, Table I.1 to see those codes that were never assigned or that no longer appear in the Taxonomy. Codes are not reused, but rather are retired along with the diagnosis. Likewise, unassigned codes are never assigned later, out of sequence, but simply remain permanently unassigned.

2) **When a diagnosis is revised, how do we know what was changed? I noticed changes to some diagnoses, but they are not listed as revisions – why?**

   We are including a table that highlights changes considered by DDC to be revisions that were made, beginning with the previous edition (definition revised, defining characteristics added/removed, etc.). However the best way to see each individual change is to compare the current edition with the previous one. We do *not* consider minor editing of the diagnoses to be revisions. For example, if a defining characteristic is noted to have two separate foci, these may be divided into two separate characteristics. However, because the content has not changed, but merely the presentation of that content, this is not considered a revision. These revisions may be made to facilitate coding of component parts of the diagnoses (defining characteristics, related or risk factors) within electronic health records, or to standardize terms used for the component parts of the diagnoses. In these cases, there is no formal revision and therefore no revision date is identified. An example is shown below of an editorial change to defining characteristics:

Risk for Electrolyte Imbalance (00195)

2009–2011 edition	2012–2014 edition
Fluid imbalance (e.g., dehydration, water intoxication)	Deficient fluid volume
	Excess fluid volume

3) **Why don't all of the diagnoses show a level of evidence (LOE)?**

   NANDA International did not begin using LOE criteria until 2002; therefore diagnoses that were entered into the Taxonomy prior to that time do not show a

LOE criteria because none was identified when the diagnoses were submitted. All diagnoses that existed in the Taxonomy in 2002 were "grandfathered" into the Taxonomy, with those clearly not meeting criteria (e.g., no identified related factors, multiple diagnostic foci in the label, etc.) targeted for revision or removal over the next few editions. The last of these diagnoses is being removed in this edition.

4) **Some of the diagnoses have references, but not all of them do. Why doesn't NANDA-I print all of the references used for all of the diagnoses?**

NANDA-I did not begin publishing references until recently. We began by asking submitters to identify their three most important references, and those are what were published. Only in our last edition (2009–2011) did we begin to publish the full list of references, due to the large number of requests we receive from individuals regarding the literature reviewed for different diagnoses. Obviously, as the diagnoses age, so too will the references unless the diagnoses are revised. It is probable that we will stop publishing the references after two or three cycles, but will then maintain them on the Members Only section in the NANDA International website for researchers and others who want to access this information.

Acknowledgments

Changes have been made in this edition based on feedback from users, both to address the needs of students and clinicians, as well as to provide additional support to educators in clinical, administrative, research, and informatics courses. Some of the chapters have had significant revision, while others are completely new for this edition. Many of these chapters have corresponding PowerPoint presentations available for teachers and students that augment the information found within the chapters; icons appear in chapters that have these accompanying support tools.

It goes without saying that the dedication of several individuals to the work of NANDA International is evident in their donation of time and work to the improvement of this text. This text is a culmination of the tireless volunteer work of a group of very dedicated, extremely talented individuals. I would like to take the opportunity to acknowledge and personally thank the following individuals for their contributions to this text.

Chapter Authors

- Contributors to the NANDA-I Taxonomy (new) – Betty Ackley, MSN, RN
- The NANDA-I Taxonomy II – T. Heather Herdman, PhD, RN and Gunn Von Krogh, MNSc, RN (revision)
- Nursing assessment, clinical judgment, and nursing diagnoses: How to determine accurate diagnoses (revision) – Margaret Lunney, PhD, RN
- Nursing diagnosis in education (new) – Barbara Krainovich-Miller EdD, RN, PMHCNS-BC, ANEF, FAAN; Fritz Frauenfelder, MNS, EdN, RN; Maria Müller-Staub, PhD, RN
- Nursing diagnosis and research (new) – Margaret Lunney, PhD, RN and Maria Müller-Staub, PhD, RN
- The value of nursing diagnoses in electronic health records (new) – Jane M. Brokel, PhD, RN, Kay C. Avant, PhD, RN, FAAN, and Matthais Odenbreit, MNS, RN
- Clinical judgment and nursing diagnoses in nursing administration (new) – T. Heather Herdman, PhD, RN and Marcelo Chanes, PhD(c), RN
- Nursing classifications: Criteria and evaluation (new) – Matthias Odenbreit, MNS, RN, Maria Müller-Staub, PhD, RN, Jane M. Brokel, PhD, RN, Kay C. Avant, PhD, RN, FAAN, and Gail Keenan, PhD, RN
- The process for development of an approved NANDA-I nursing diagnosis (revision) – Leann Scroggins, MS, CRRN-A, APRN-BC, RN

Chapter Reviewers

- NANDA-I DDC Review Process – Shigemi Kamitsuru, PhD, RN
- The process for development of an approved NANDA-I nursing diagnosis – Gunn Von Krogh, MNSc, RN

That said, any errors that may be found in the book are mine and mine alone. Please contact me at execdir@nanda.org if you have questions on any of the content or if you do find errors, so that I may correct these for future publication and translation.

T. Heather Herdman, PhD, RN
Editor
Executive Director
NANDA International

New Nursing Diagnoses, 2012–2014

A significant body of work representing new and revised nursing diagnoses was provided to the NANDA International membership this review cycle for consideration. NANDA International would like to take this opportunity to congratulate those submitters who successfully met the level of evidence criteria with their submissions and/or revisions. Diagnoses are listed here in alphabetical order, based on diagnostic focus.

Approved diagnosis (new)	Submitter(s)
Risk for Ineffective **Activity Planning**	Diagnosis Development Committee
Risk for **Adverse Reaction to Iodinated Contrast Media**	Beatriz Cavalcanti Juchem, MSc, RN
Risk for **Allergy Response**	Judy Carlson, EdD, RN, BCIA
Insufficient **Breast Milk**	Iane Nogueira Vale, PhD, RN
Ineffective **Childbearing Process**	Diagnosis Development Committee, based on the work in 2009–2011 by: Yasuko Aoki, RMW, RN; Mitsuko Katayama, PhD, RMW, RN; Atsuko Kikuchi, RMW, RN; Minayo Kumazawa, MEd, RMW, RN; Atsuko Koyama, RMW, RN; Masuko Saito, DrMS, RMW, RN; Toyo Yamazaki, RMW, RN; Mayumi Hamasaki, MPH, RMW, RN; Shigemi Kamitsuru, PhD, RN
Risk for Ineffective **Childbearing Process**	Diagnosis Development Committee, based on the work in 2009–2011 by: Yasuko Aoki, RMW, RN; Mitsuko Katayama, PhD, RMW, RN; Atsuko Kikuchi, RMW, RN; Minayo Kumazawa, MEd, RMW, RN; Atsuko Koyama, RMW, RN; Masuko Saito, DrMS, RMW, RN; Toyo Yamazaki, RMW, RN; Mayumi Hamasaki, MPH, RMW, RN; Shigemi Kamitsuru, PhD, RN
Risk for **Dry Eye**	Elem Kocaçal Güler, MSc, RN; Ismet Eşer, PhD, RN
Deficient Community **Health**	Judy Carlson, EdD, RN, BCIA
Ineffective **Impulse Control**	Akira Nagata, MSN, RN
Risk for Neonatal **Jaundice**	Diagnosis Development Committee, based on the work in 2009–2011 by: David Wilson, MS, RNC

Approved diagnosis (new)	Submitter(s)
*Risk for Disturbed **Personal Identity***	Diagnosis Development Committee
*Ineffective **Relationship***	Diagnosis Development Committee, based on the work in 2009–2011 by: Yasuko Aoki, RMW, RN; Mitsuko Katayama, PhD, RMW, RN; Atsuko Kikuchi, RMW, RN; Minayo Kumazawa, MEd, RMW, RN; Atsuko Koyama, RMW, RN; Masuko Saito, DrMS, RMW, RN; Toyo Yamazaki, RMW, RN; Mayumi Hamasaki, MPH, RMW, RN; Shigemi Kamitsuru, PhD, RN
*Risk for Ineffective **Relationship***	Diagnosis Development Committee, based on the work in 2009–2011 by: Yasuko Aoki, RMW, RN; Mitsuko Katayama, PhD, RMW, RN; Atsuko Kikuchi, RMW, RN; Minayo Kumazawa, MEd, RMW, RN; Atsuko Koyama, RMW, RN; Masuko Saito, DrMS, RMW, RN; Toyo Yamazaki, RMW, RN; Mayumi Hamasaki, MPH, RMW, RN; Shigemi Kamitsuru, PhD, RN
*Risk for Chronic Low **Self-Esteem***	Diagnosis Development Committee
*Risk for **Thermal Injury***	Geralyn Meyer, PhD, RN
*Risk for Ineffective Peripheral **Tissue Perfusion***	Rita de Cassia Gengo e Silva, PhD, RN; Dina de Almeida Lopes Monteiro da Cruz, PhD, RN; Fernanda Marciano Consolim-Colombo, PhD, RN

Revised Nursing Diagnoses, 2012–2014

Approved diagnosis (revised)	Revision	Submitter(s)
*Readiness for Enhanced **Breastfeeding*** (Formerly *Effective Breastfeeding*)	Change in diagnostic label and definition to reflect change in focus from wellness to health promotion	Diagnosis Development Committee
*Ineffective **Breathing Pattern***	Removal of two related factors, addition of one related factor	Agueda Maria Ruiz Zimmer Cavalcante, MS, RN
*Impaired **Comfort***	Definition revised, defining characteristics revised: this was due to an error in the previous edition, which did not include these as they were accepted	Diagnosis Development Committee

Continued

Approved diagnosis (revised)	Revision	Submitter(s)
Risk for **Infection**	Revision of risk factors	Mark R. Hunter, CRNI, VA-BC, RN
Neonatal **Jaundice**	Removal of one defining characteristic, addition of one defining characteristic	Diagnosis Development Committee
Nausea	Definition revised, included references from the current and 2002 revisions	Gilmaikon Roela Pereira, RN, MSc, and Lilian Guardian, RN
Powerlessness	Definition revised, Addition of 5 defining characteristics	Tracy LaRock, D.O.M., RN
Risk for **Powerlessness**	Removal of one risk factor; addition of 8 risk factors	Tracy LaRock, D.O.M., RN
Readiness for enhanced **Self Health Management**	Addition of 2 defining characteristics	Diagnosis Development Committee
Risk for Impaired **Skin Integrity**	Change in definition to clarify meaning	Diagnosis Development Committee
Ineffective Peripheral **Tissue Perfusion**	Addition of 5 defining characteristics	Rita de Cassia Gengo e Silva, PhD, RN; Dina de Almeida Lopes Monteiro da Cruz, PhD, RN; Fernanda Marciano Consolim-Colombo, PhD, MD

Retired Nursing Diagnosis, 2012–2014

■ *Disturbed Sensory Perception* (Specify: Visual, Auditory, Kinesthetic, Gustatory, Tactile, Olfactory) (00122)

This diagnosis can be found in Part 3 of this text, and the Diagnosis Development Committee encourages members and users of nursing diagnoses to work on this and other retired diagnoses and submit them for re-entry into the taxonomy.

Changes to Slotting of Current Diagnoses within the NANDA International Taxonomy II, 2012–2014

A review of the current taxonomic structure and slotting of diagnoses within that structure led to some changes in the way some diagnoses are now classified within the NANDA-I Taxonomy. There have been 20 diagnoses reslotted within the NANDA International Taxonomy; these are noted in the table below, with their previous and new places in the Taxonomy noted.

Nursing diagnosis	Previously slotted		New slotting	
	Domain	Class	Domain	Class
Ineffective **Activity Planning**	Perception/ Cognition	Cognition	Coping/Stress Tolerance	Coping responses
Risk for **Bleeding**	Activity/Rest	Cardiovascular/ Pulmonary	Safety/ Protection	Physical Injury
Ineffective **Breastfeeding**	Role Relationship	Role Performance	Role Relationship	Caregiving Roles
Interrupted **Breastfeeding**	Role Relationship	Role Performance	Role Relationship	Caregiving Roles
Readiness for Enhanced **Breastfeeding**	Role Relationship	Role Performance	Role Relationship	Caregiving Roles
Readiness for Enhanced **Decision-Making**	Perception/ Cognition	Cognition	Life Principles	Value/Belief/ Action Congruence
Deficient **Diversional Activity**	Activity/Rest	Activity/ Exercise	Health Promotion	Health Awareness
Adult **Failure to Thrive**	Growth/ Development	Growth	Coping/Stress Tolerance	Coping Responses
Risk-Prone **Health Behavior**	Coping/Stress Tolerance	Coping Responses	Health Promotion	Health Management
Impaired **Home Maintenance**	Health Promotion	Health Management	Activity/Rest	Self-Care
Sedentary **Lifestyle**	Activity/Rest	Activity/ Exercise	Health Promotion	Health Awareness
Readiness for Enhanced **Nutrition**	Health Promotion	Health Management	Nutrition	Ingestion
Readiness for Enhanced **Power**	Self-Perception	Self-concept	Coping/Stress Tolerance	Coping Responses
Powerlessness	Self-Perception	Self-Concept	Coping/Stress Tolerance	Coping Responses
Risk for **Powerlessness**	Self-Perception	Self-Concept	Coping/Stress Tolerance	Coping Responses
Ineffective **Protection**	Safety/ Protection	Physical Injury	Health Promotion	Health Management
Self Neglect	Health Promotion	Health Management	Activity/Rest	Self-Care
Risk for **Shock**	Activity/Rest	Cardiovascular/ Pulmonary	Safety/ Protection	Physical Injury
Delayed **Surgical Recovery**	Activity/Rest	Activity/ Exercise	Safety/ Protection	Physical Injury
Wandering	Perception/ Cognition	Orientation	Activity/Rest	Energy Balance

Changes to Slotting of Current Diagnoses within the NANDA-I/NIC/NOC Taxonomy

A review of the current taxonomic structure and slotting of diagnoses within that structure led to changes in the way some diagnoses are now classified within the NANDA-I/NIC/NOC (NNN) Taxonomy. Seven diagnoses have been reslotted within the NNN taxonomy; these are noted in the table below, with their previous and new places in the Taxonomy noted.

Nursing diagnosis	Previously slotted		New slotting	
	Domain	Class	Domain	Class
Readiness for Enhanced **Breastfeeding**	Functional	Nutrition	Psychosocial	Roles/ Relationships
Ineffective **Breastfeeding**	Functional	Nutrition	Psychosocial	Roles/ Relationships
Interrupted **Breastfeeding**	Functional	Nutrition	Psychosocial	Roles/ Relationships
Adult **Failure to Thrive**	Functional	Growth and Development	Psychosocial	Coping
Risk-Prone **Health Behavior**	Psychosocial	Coping	Psychosocial	Behavior
Risk for Disturbed **Maternal- Fetal Dyad**	Psychosocial	Reproduction	Psychosocial	Roles/ Relationships
Wandering	Functional	Neurocognition	Functional	Activity/ Exercise

Revisions to Diagnoses within the NANDA International Taxonomy 2009–2011

Finally, based upon requests that were received after the previous edition was published, the following presents an explanation of changes that were made in the 2009–2011 edition. One diagnosis was removed from the taxonomy that was omitted from the list of retired diagnoses on p. xxi and from the chapter showing the retired diagnoses (pp. 403-408). This diagnosis, *Health-seeking behaviors*, is provided in this edition along with the one diagnosis being retired during this cycle (see, Part 3: *Nursing Diagnoses Retired from the NANDA-I Taxonomy 2009–2014*).

2009–2011 Approved diagnosis (REVISED)	2009–2011 revision	2009–2011 submitter(s)
Risk for Impaired **Attachment**	Label was changed from *Risk for Impaired Parent/Child Attachment* to *Risk for Impaired Attachment* because the definition clarifies the subjects of the diagnosis	Diagnosis Development Committee

2009–2011 Approved diagnosis (REVISED)	2009–2011 revision	2009–2011 submitter(s)
Risk-Prone **Health Behavior**	Definition slightly modified; two defining characteristics added	Diagnosis Development Committee
Defensive **Coping**	One defining characteristic added; related factors added (diagnosis was slotted for removal from the Taxonomy due to lack of related factors)	Céline Larouche
Dysfunctional **Family Processes**	Label was changed from *Dysfunctional Family Processes: Alcoholism* to current label because the definition and defining characteristics were found to be broader than solely alcoholism-focused	Diagnosis Development Committee
Risk for Imbalanced **Fluid Volume**	One risk factor removed, eight risk factors added	Louise Ritchie, MSc, RN; Geralyn Meyer, PhD, RN
Risk for Impaired **Liver Function**	Diagnosis was updated with literature review; references were added	Diagnosis Development Committee
Disturbed **Personal Identity**	Definition slightly modified; defining characteristics and related factors added (diagnosis was slotted for removal from the Taxonomy due to lack of defining characteristics and related factors)	Heidi Bjorge, MNSc, RN; Céline Larouche; Francine Fiset, MA, RN
Bathing **Self-Care** Deficit	Diagnosis formerly held the label, *Bathing/Hygiene Self-care Deficit*, which included two diagnostic foci in one label. Review of the defining characteristics showed a focus on bathing; therefore the label was changed to reflect the content of the diagnosis	Diagnosis Development Committee
Dressing **Self-Care** Deficit	Diagnosis formerly held the label, *Dressing/Grooming Self-care Deficit*, which included two diagnostic foci in one label. Review of the defining characteristics showed a focus on dressing; therefore the label was changed to reflect the content of the diagnosis	Diagnosis Development Committee
Chronic Low **Self-Esteem**	Related factors added (diagnosis was slotted for removal from the Taxonomy due to lack of related factors)	Céline Larouche

Continued

2009–2011 Approved diagnosis (REVISED)	2009–2011 revision	2009–2011 submitter(s)
Ineffective **Self-Health Management**	Label was changed from *Ineffective Therapeutic Regimen Management* to *Ineffective Self-Health Management*; references added	Margaret Lunney, PhD, RN
Ineffective **Tissue Perfusion** (specify type: renal, cerebral, cardiopulmonary, gastrointestinal, peripheral)	Diagnosis was revised by separating the diagnostic foci into five separate diagnoses: *Risk for Ineffective Gastrointestinal Perfusion, Risk for Decreased Cardiac Tissue Perfusion, Risk for Ineffective Cerebral Tissue Perfusion, Ineffective Peripheral Tissue Perfusion, Risk for Impaired Renal Perfusion*	Jennifer Hafner, BSN, RN

Part 1
The NANDA International Taxonomy

NANDA International Nursing Diagnoses: Definitions & Classification 2012–2014, First Edition.
Edited by T. Heather Herdman.
© 2012 NANDA International. Published 2012 by Blackwell Publishing Ltd.

Introduction

T. Heather Herdman

In this section, we provide what is currently known about the submitters and/or revisers of NANDA International (NANDA-I) diagnoses since the beginning of the taxonomy (Table I.1), based on the dedicated work of Betty Ackley, MSN, RN. We encourage individuals to help us to fill in the history of this work so that we can acknowledge the effort of nurses around the world who have and who continue to build and strengthen the knowledge of nursing. Information is also presented on the history of the NANDA-I taxonomy, and how it is currently structured. The multiaxial system for construction of nursing diagnostic concepts (through the process of diagnosis submission to the Diagnosis Development Committee) is discussed within the NANDA-I structure. Each axis is described and defined. The diagnostic concepts are provided, and each nursing diagnosis is shown as it fits within the NANDA-I Taxonomy and the NANDA-Nursing Interventions Classification (NIC)-Nursing Outcomes Classification (NOC), or NNN, Taxonomy. Considerations are provided about further, ongoing development of the NANDA-I Taxonomy. A clear link is made between the use of standardized nursing language that permits diagnostic accuracy and the aspect of patient safety; point-of-care "creation" of terms to describe clinical reasoning is strongly discouraged due to the lack of standardization, which can lead to inappropriate plans of care, poor outcomes, and the inability to accurately research or demonstrate the impact of nursing care on human responses.

Table I.2 provides all of the nursing diagnoses that are found within the NANDA-I Taxonomy, their five-digit codes, and their placement within the taxonomy's 13 domains and 47 classes. Table I.3 provides the nursing diagnoses as they are placed within the NNN Taxonomy of Nursing Practice.

Contributors to the NANDA-I Nursing Diagnosis Taxonomy

Frequently, NANDA-I receives requests for information on the name(s) of the submitter(s) of new diagnoses, or of the individual(s) who have revised diagnoses. Historically, NANDA-I did not track this information in any type of a systematic manner, although much of this resides within the NANDA-I Archives at Boston College (Chestnut Hill, MA, USA).

Betty Ackley, a long-time NANDA International member, felt that this situation needed to be resolved, and she recommended that NANDA-I seek out information on who had submitted new and revised diagnoses. She then generously volunteered to try to uncover as much information as possible so that we could acknowledge the work of those who have been involved in the development of the taxonomy over time. Although she was able to find much of this information (see Table I.1), you will note that we still have missing pieces for the list of contributors. It is also possible that there are mistakes, as some of the information gathered was based on memory of former Diagnosis Development Committee (DDC) members and chairwomen. The editor acknowledges Betty Ackley for her recommendation for and work on this significant project. As we move forward, we will be able to maintain this information – and add to it in the upcoming years – in an organized database.

If anyone has additional information or corrections regarding the names of submitters or those who have revised diagnoses, please send this information to the NANDA-I Executive Director at execdir@nanda.org.

NANDA International Nursing Diagnoses: Definitions & Classification 2012–2014, First Edition.
Edited by T. Heather Herdman.
© 2012 NANDA International. Published 2012 by Blackwell Publishing Ltd.

Table I.1 *List of NANDA-I diagnoses, placement in the taxonomy, coding structure, and contributors*

Page	Code	Domain	Class	Label	Submitter	Year	Revision	Year	Revision	Year	Revision	Year
151	97	01 Health Promotion	1 Health Awareness	Deficient Diversional Activity		1980						
152	168	01 Health Promotion	1 Health Awareness	Sedentary Lifestyle	Josep Adolf Guirao-Goris, MSN, RN	2004						
153	215	01 Health Promotion	2 Health Management	Deficient Community Health	Judy Carlson, EdD, RN, BCIA	2010						
155	188	01 Health Promotion	2 Health Management	Risk-Prone Health Behavior (Formerly titled *Impaired adjustment*)		1986		1998	Micky Gonzales, MSN, NP-C, RN	2006	DDC	2008
157	99	01 Health Promotion	2 Health Management	Ineffective Health Maintenance		1982						
158	186	01 Health Promotion	2 Health Management	Readiness for Enhanced Immunization Status	Margaret Lunney, PhD, RN; Roberta Cavendish, RN, PhD; Barbara Kraynyak Luise, RN, EdD; Kathryn Richardson, RN, MS	2006						
160	43	01 Health Promotion	2 Health Management	Ineffective Protection	Group from MD Anderson Medical Center	1990						
161	78	01 Health Promotion	2 Health Management	Ineffective Self-Health Management		1994		2008	Margaret Lunney, PhD, RN			
164	162	01 Health Promotion	2 Health Management	Readiness for Enhanced Self-Health Management	Margaret Lunney, PhD, RN; Roberta Cavendish, RN, PhD; Barbara Kraynyak Luise, RN, EdD; Kathryn Richardson, RN, MS	2002		2010	DDC			

167	80	01 Health Promotion	2 Health Management	Ineffective Family Therapeutic Regimen Management	Margaret Lunney, PhD, RN	1992	
N/A	81	01 Health Promotion	2 Health Management	DIAGNOSIS RETIRED (2008) Ineffective Community Therapeutic Regimen Management			
N/A	82	01 Health Promotion	2 Health Management	DIAGNOSIS RETIRED (2008) Effective Therapeutic Regimen Management			
171	216	02 Nutrition	1 Ingestion	Insufficient breast milk	Iane Nogueira Vale, RN, PhD	2010	
173	107	02 Nutrition	1 Ingestion	Ineffective Infant Feeding Pattern	Mary A. Fuerst-Dewys, BSN, RN	1992	Lynda Juall Carpenito-Moyet, MSN, RN, CRNP 2006
174	2	02 Nutrition	1 Ingestion	Imbalanced Nutrition: Less Than Body Requirements		1975	2000
175	1	02 Nutrition	1 Ingestion	Imbalanced Nutrition: More Than Body Requirements		1975	2000
176	163	02 Nutrition	1 Ingestion	Readiness for Enhanced Nutrition	Margaret Lunney, PhD, RN; Roberta Cavendish, RN, PhD; Barbara Kraynyak Luise, RN, EdD; Kathryn Richardson, RN, MS	2002	
177	3	02 Nutrition	1 Ingestion	Risk for Imbalanced Nutrition: More Than Body Requirements		1980	2000

Continued

Table I.1 *Continued*

Page	Code	Domain	Class	Label	Submitter	Year	Revision	Year	Revision	Year	Revision	Year
178	103	02 Nutrition	1 Ingestion	Impaired Swallowing		1986		1998				
180	179	02 Nutrition	4 Metabolism	Risk for Unstable Blood Glucose Level	Janice Denehy, PhD, RN	2006						
181	194	02 Nutrition	4 Metabolism	Neonatal Jaundice	David Wilson, MS, RNC	2008	DDC	2010				
182	230	02 Nutrition	4 Metabolism	Risk for Neonatal Jaundice	Diagnosis Development Committee	2010						
183	178	02 Nutrition	4 Metabolism	Risk for Impaired Liver Function	Kathryn White, BSN, MT, RN	2006	DDC	2008				
184	195	02 Nutrition	5 Hydration	Risk for Electrolyte Imbalance	Jennifer Hafner, BSN, RN, PCCN, TNCC; Leah Mylrea Speltz, BSN, RNC, NNR; Kathy Weaver, RN	2008						
185	160	02 Nutrition	5 Hydration	Readiness for Enhanced Fluid Balance	Margaret Lunney, PhD, RN; Roberta Cavendish, RN, PhD; Barbara Kraynyak Luise, RN, EdD; Kathryn Richardson, RN, MS	2002						
186	27	02 Nutrition	5 Hydration	Deficient Fluid Volume		1978		1996				
187	26	02 Nutrition	5 Hydration	Excess Fluid Volume		1982		1996				
188	28	02 Nutrition	5 Hydration	Risk for Deficient Fluid Volume		1978						
189	25	02 Nutrition	5 Hydration	Risk for Imbalanced Fluid Volume	Louise Ritchie, MSN, Bnur, RN; Geralyn Meyer, PhD, RN	1998		2008				
193	20	03 Elimination/ Exchange	1 Urinary Function	Functional Urinary Incontinence		1986		1998				
194	176	03 Elimination/ Exchange	1 Urinary Function	Overflow Urinary Incontinence	Geralyn Meyer, PhD, RN	2006						
195	18	03 Elimination/ Exchange	1 Urinary Function	Reflex Urinary Incontinence		1986		1998				

Page	Code	Domain	Class	Diagnosis	Year	Author	Year
196	17	03 Elimination/Exchange	1 Urinary Function	Stress Urinary Incontinence	1986	Geralyn Meyer, PhD, RN	2006
198	19	03 Elimination/Exchange	1 Urinary Function	Urge Urinary Incontinence	1986	Geralyn Meyer, PhD, RN	2006
199	22	03 Elimination/Exchange	1 Urinary Function	Risk for Urge Urinary Incontinence	1998		
200	16	03 Elimination/Exchange	1 Urinary Function	Impaired Urinary Elimination	1973	Lynda Juall Carpenito-Moyet, MSN, RN, CRNP	2006
201	166	03 Elimination/Exchange	1 Urinary Function	Readiness for Enhanced Urinary Elimination	2002	Margaret Lunney, PhD, RN; Roberta Cavendish, RN, PhD; Barbara Kraynyak Luise, RN, EdD; Kathryn Richardson, RN, MS	
202	23	03 Elimination/Exchange	1 Urinary Function	Urinary Retention	1986		
N/A	21	03 Elimination/Exchange	1 Urinary Function	DIAGNOSIS RETIRED (2009–2011) Total Urinary Incontinence	1986		
203	11	03 Elimination/Exchange	2 Gastrointestinal Function	Constipation	1975	Audrey M. McLane, RN, PhD & Ruth E. McShane, RN, PhD	1998
205	12	03 Elimination/Exchange	2 Gastrointestinal Function	Perceived Constipation	1988	Audrey M. McLane, RN, PhD	
206	15	03 Elimination/Exchange	2 Gastrointestinal Function	Risk for Constipation	1998	Audrey M. McLane, RN, PhD	
208	13	03 Elimination/Exchange	2 Gastrointestinal Function	Diarrhea	1975	Audrey M. McLane, RN, PhD	1998
209	196	03 Elimination/Exchange	2 Gastrointestinal Function	Dysfunctional Gastrointestinal Motility	2008	Joan Klehr, RNC, MPH	

Continued

Table I.1 *Continued*

Page	Code	Domain	Class	Label	Submitter	Year	Revision	Year	Revision	Year	Revision	Year
211	197	03 Elimination/Exchange	2 Gastrointestinal Function	Risk for Dysfunctional Gastrointestinal Motility	Joan Klehr, RNC, MPH	2008						
213	14	03 Elimination/Exchange	2 Gastrointestinal Function	Bowel Incontinence	Audrey M. McLane, RN, PhD	1975		1998				
214	30	03 Elimination/Exchange	4 Respiratory Function	Impaired Gas Exchange		1980		1996		1998		
217	95	04 Activity/Rest	1 Sleep/Rest	Insomnia	Aleita White, MSN, RN	2006						
219	96	04 Activity/Rest	1 Sleep/Rest	Sleep Deprivation		1998						
220	165	04 Activity/Rest	1 Sleep/Rest	Readiness for Enhanced Sleep	Margaret Lunney, PhD, RN; Roberta Cavendish, RN, PhD; Barbara Kraynyak Luise, RN, EdD; Kathryn Richardson, RN, MS	2002						
221	198	04 Activity/Rest	1 Sleep/Rest	Disturbed Sleep Pattern		1980		1998	DDC	2006		
222	40	04 Activity/Rest	2 Activity/Exercise	Risk for Disuse Syndrome	Kathy Tracey; Ann McCourt, MS, RN	1988						
223	91	04 Activity/Rest	2 Activity/Exercise	Impaired Bed Mobility	Brenda Emick-Herring, MSN, RN	1998	Meridean Maas, PhD, RN, FAAN	2006				
224	85	04 Activity/Rest	2 Activity/Exercise	Impaired Physical Mobility	ARN Rehab Association, Skokie, Ill	1973		1998				
225	89	04 Activity/Rest	2 Activity/Exercise	Impaired Wheelchair Mobility	Brenda Emick-Herring, MSN, RN	1998	Meridean Maas, PhD, RN, FAAN	2006				
226	90	04 Activity/Rest	2 Activity/Exercise	Impaired Transfer Ability	Brenda Emick-Herring, MSN, RN	1998	Meridean Maas, PhD, RN, FAAN	2006				

227	88	04 Activity/Rest	2 Activity/Exercise	Impaired Walking	Brenda Emick-Herring, MSN, RN	1998	Meridean Maas, PhD, RN, FAAN	2006				
228	50	04 Activity/Rest	3 Energy Balance	Disturbed Energy Field		1994	Rebecca Good, MA, RNC, ACRN, LPC	2004				
229	93	04 Activity/Rest	3 Energy Balance	Fatigue		1988		1998				
230	154	04 Activity/Rest	3 Energy Balance	Wandering	Meridean Maas, PhD, RN, FAAN	2000						
231	92	04 Activity/Rest	4 Cardiovascular/Pulmonary Responses	Activity Intolerance		1982						
232	94	04 Activity/Rest	4 Cardiovascular/Pulmonary Responses	Risk for Activity Intolerance		1982						
233	32	04 Activity/Rest	4 Cardiovascular/Pulmonary Responses	Ineffective Breathing Pattern		1980		1996		1998	Agueda Maria Ruiz Zimmer Cavalcante, MS, RN	2012
235	29	04 Activity/Rest	4 Cardiovascular/Pulmonary Responses	Decreased Cardiac Output		1975		1996		2000		
237	202	04 Activity/Rest	4 Cardiovascular/Pulmonary Responses	Risk for Ineffective Gastrointestinal Perfusion	Jennifer Hafner, RN, BSN, PCCN, TNCC	2008						
238	203	04 Activity/Rest	4 Cardiovascular/Pulmonary Responses	Risk for Ineffective Renal Perfusion	Jennifer Hafner, RN, BSN, PCCN, TNCC	2008						
239	33	04 Activity/Rest	4 Cardiovascular/Pulmonary Responses	Impaired Spontaneous Ventilation		1992						
240	204	04 Activity/Rest	4 Cardiovascular/Pulmonary Responses	Ineffective Peripheral Tissue Perfusion	Jennifer Hafner, RN, BSN, PCCN, TNCC; Leah Mylrea Speltz, BSN, RNC, NNR; Kathy Weaver, RN	2008	Rita de Cassia Gengo e Silva, PhD, RN; Dina de Almeida Lopes Monteiro da Cruz, PhD, RN; Fernanda Marciano Consolim-Colombo, PhD, MD	2010				

Continued

Table I.1 Continued

Page	Code	Domain	Class	Label	Submitter	Year	Revision	Year	Revision	Year	Revision	Year	Revision	Year
242	200	04 Activity/Rest	4 Cardiovascular/Pulmonary Responses	Risk for Decreased Cardiac Tissue Perfusion	Jennifer Hafner, RN, BSN, PCCN, TNCC	2008								
243	201	04 Activity/Rest	4 Cardiovascular/Pulmonary Responses	Risk for Ineffective Cerebral Tissue Perfusion	Jennifer Hafner, RN, BSN, PCCN, TNCC	2008								
244	228	04 Activity/Rest	4 Cardiovascular/Pulmonary Responses	Risk for Ineffective Peripheral Tissue Perfusion	Rita de Cassia Gengo e Silva, PhD, RN; Dina de Almeida Lopes Monteiro da Cruz, PhD, RN; Fernanda Marciano Consolim-Colombo, PhD, MD	2010								
246	34	04 Activity/Rest	4 Cardiovascular/Pulmonary Responses	Dysfunctional Ventilatory Weaning Response	Jean Jenny, co-author	1992								
N/A	24	04 Activity/Rest	4 Cardiovascular/Pulmonary Responses	DIAGNOSIS RETIRED (2009–2011) Ineffective tissue perfusion (specify type: renal, cerebral, cardiopulmonary, gastrointestinal, peripheral)		1980		1998						
248	98	04 Activity/Rest	5 Self-Care	Impaired Home Maintenance		1980								

249	182	04 Activity/Rest	5 Self-Care	Readiness for Enhanced Self-Care	Margaret Lunney PhD, RN; Roberta Cavendish, RN, PhD; Barbara Kraynyak Luise, RN, EdD; Kathryn Richardson, RN, MS	2006			
250	108	04 Activity/Rest	5 Self-Care	LABEL CHANGED 2008 Bathing Self-Care Deficit (Formerly Bathing/Hygiene Self-care Deficit)	Ann E. McCourt, MS, RN	1980	1998	DDC	2008
251	109	04 Activity/Rest	5 Self-Care	LABEL CHANGED 2008 Dressing Self-Care Deficit (Formerly Dressing/Grooming Self-Care Deficit)	Ann E. McCourt, MS, RN	1980	1998	DDC	2008
252	102	04 Activity/Rest	5 Self-Care	Feeding Self-Care Deficit	Ann E. McCourt, MS, RN	1980	1998		
253	110	04 Activity/Rest	5 Self-Care	Toileting Self-Care Deficit	Ann E. McCourt, MS, RN	1980	1998		
254	193	04 Activity/Rest	5 Self-Care	Self-Neglect	Susanne Gibons, C-GNP, RN	2008			
259	123	05 Perception/Cognition	1 Attention	Unilateral Neglect	Ibtihal Almakhzoomy, MSN, RN; Lina Rahal, MEd, RN; Danielle Schmouth, Med, RN; Genevieve Lefrancois, MSN, RN	1986	2006		
261	127	05 Perception/Cognition	2 Orientation	Impaired Environmental Interpretation Syndrome	Judith W. Harmer, RN, MSN, Nancy English, PhD, RN	1994			

Continued

Table I.1 *Continued*

Page	Code	Domain	Class	Label	Submitter	Year	Revision	Year	Revision	Year	Revision	Year
490	122	05 Perception/ Cognition	3 Sensation/ Perception	DIAGNOSIS RETIRED (2012–2014) Disturbed Sensory Perception (Specify: Visual, Auditory, Kinesthetic, Gustatory, Tactile, Olfactory)		1978		1980		1998		
262	128	05 Perception/ Cognition	4 Cognition	Acute Confusion	Elizabeth Kelchner Gerety, MS, RN, CS; Karen Inaba-Roland, MS, RN, CS	1994	DDC	2006				
265	129	05 Perception/ Cognition	4 Cognition	Chronic Confusion		1994						
266	173	05 Perception/ Cognition	4 Cognition	Risk for Acute Confusion	Peggy Stimpert, MSN, RN	2006						
269	222	05 Perception/ Cognition	4 Cognition	Ineffective Impulse Control	Akira Nagata, MSN, RN	2010						
271	126	05 Perception/ Cognition	4 Cognition	Deficient Knowledge		1980						
272	161	05 Perception/ Cognition	4 Cognition	Readiness for Enhanced Knowledge	Margaret Lunney, PhD, RN; Roberta Cavendish, RN, PhD; Barbara Kraynyak Luise, RN, EdD; Kathryn Richardson, RN, MS	2002						
273	131	05 Perception/ Cognition	4 Cognition	Impaired Memory	Linda S. Baas, PhD, RN	1994						

	No.	Category	Subcategory	Diagnosis	Author			
N/A	130	05 Perception/Cognition	4 Cognition	DIAGNOSIS RETIRED (2009–2011) Disturbed Thought Process		1973	1996	
274	157	05 Perception/Cognition	5 Communication	Readiness for Enhanced Communication	Margaret Lunney, PhD, RN; Roberta Cavendish, RN, PhD; Barbara Kraynyak Luise, RN, EdD; Kathryn Richardson, RN, MS	2002		
275	51	05 Perception/Cognition	5 Communication	Impaired Verbal Communication		1983	1996	1998
279	124	06 Self-Perception	1 Self-Concept	Hopelessness		1986		
280	174	06 Self-Perception	1 Self-Concept	Risk for Compromised Human Dignity	Susan Rosenberg, MSN, RN, CNRN, CHI	2006		
281	54	06 Self-Perception	1 Self-Concept	Risk for Loneliness	Charlotte Profitt, Med, MSNRN; Marjorie Byrn MEd, MS, RN	1994	2006	
282	121	06 Self-Perception	1 Self-Concept	Disturbed Personal Identity	Heidi Bjorge, MNSc, RN; Celine Larouche, RN; Francine Fiset, MA, BSN, RN	1978	2008	
283	225	06 Self-Perception	1 Self-Concept	Risk for Disturbed Personal Identity	Diagnosis Development Committee (Based on the work of Heidi Bjorge, MNSc, RN; Celine Larouche, RN; Francine Fiset, MA, RN)	2010		

Continued

Table I.1 *Continued*

Page	Code	Domain	Class	Label	Submitter	Year	Revision	Year	Revision	Year	Revision	Year
284	167	06 Self-Perception	1 Self-Concept	Readiness for Enhanced Self-Concept	Margaret Lunney, PhD, RN; Roberta Cavendish, RN, PhD; Barbara Kraynyak Luise, RN, EdD; Kathryn Richardson, RN, MS	2006						
285	119	06 Self-Perception	2 Self-Esteem	Chronic Low Self-Esteem		1988		1996	Celine Larouche, RN	2008		
287	120	06 Self-Perception	2 Self-Esteem	Situational Low Self-Esteem		1988		1996		2000		
288	224	06 Self-Perception	2 Self-Esteem	Risk for Chronic Low Self-Esteem	Diagnosis Development Committee (Based on the work of Celine Larouche, RN)	2010						
290	153	06 Self-Perception	2 Self-Esteem	Risk for Situational Low Self-Esteem		2000						
291	118	06 Self-Perception	3 Body image	Disturbed Body Image		1973		1998				
295	104	07 Role Relationships	1 Caregiving Roles	Ineffective Breastfeeding		1988						
296	105	07 Role Relationships	1 Caregiving Roles	Interrupted Breastfeeding		1992						

297	106	07 Role Relationships	1 Caregiving Roles	LABEL CHANGED 2010 Readiness for Enhanced Breastfeeding (Formerly Effective Breastfeeding)	Mary L. Henrikson, MN, RNC, ARNP; Ginna Hall, MN, RN; Doa Lethbridge, PhD, RN; Vicki E. McClurg, MN, RN	1990	DDC	2010	2000
298	61	07 Role Relationships	1 Caregiving Roles	Caregiver Role Strain		1992		1998	
301	62	07 Role Relationships	1 Caregiving Roles	Risk for Caregiver Role Strain		1992			
302	56	07 Role Relationships	1 Caregiving Roles	Impaired Parenting		1978		1998	
304	164	07 Role Relationships	1 Caregiving Roles	Readiness for Enhanced Parenting	Margaret Lunney, PhD, RN; Roberta Cavendish, RN, PhD; Barbara Kraynyak Luise, RN, EdD; Kathryn Richardson, RN, MS	2002			
305	57	07 Role Relationships	1 Caregiving Roles	Risk for Impaired Parenting		1978		1998	
307	58	07 Role Relationships	2 Family Relationships	Risk for Impaired Attachment	Kathy Wyngarden, MSN, RN	1994	DDC	2008	
308	63	07 Role Relationships	2 Family Relationships	LABEL CHANGED 2008 Dysfunctional Family Processes (Formerly Dysfunctional family processes: Alcoholism)		1994	DDC	2008	
311	60	07 Role Relationships	2 Family Relationships	Interrupted Family Processes		1982		1998	

Continued

Table I.1 *Continued*

Page	Code	Domain	Class	Label	Submitter	Year	Revision	Year	Revision	Year	Revision	Year	Revision	Year
312	159	07 Role Relationships	2 Family Relationships	Readiness for Enhanced Family Processes	Margaret Lunney, PhD, RN; Roberta Cavendish, RN, PhD; Barbara Kraynyak Luise, RN, EdD; Kathryn Richardson, RN, MS	2002								
313	223	07 Role Relationships	3 Role Performance	Ineffective Relationship	Diagnosis Development Committee, based on the work in 2009–2011 by: Yasuko Aoki, RN, RMW; Mitsuko Katayama, RN, RMW, PhD; Atsuko Kikuchi, RN, RMW; Minayo Kumazawa, RN, RMW, MEd; Atsuko Koyama, RN, RMW; Masuko Saito, RN, RMW, DrMS; Toyo Yamazaki, RN, RMW; Mayumi Hamasaki, RN, RMW, MPH; Shigemi Kamitsuru, RN, PhD	2010								

315	207	07 Role Relationships	3	Role Performance	Readiness for Enhanced Relationship		2006		
316	229	07 Role Relationships	3	Role Performance	Risk for Ineffective Relationship	Diagnosis Development Committee, based on the work in 2009–2011 by: Yasuko Aoki, RN, RMW; Mitsuko Katayama, RN, RMW, PhD; Atsuko Kikuchi, RN, RMW; Minayo Kumazawa, RN, RMW, MEd; Atsuko Koyama, RN, RMW; Masuko Saito, RN, RMW, DrMS; Toyo Yamazaki, RN, RMW; Mayumi Hamasaki, RN, RMW, MPH; Shigemi Kamitsuru, RN, PhD	2010		
317	64	07 Role Relationships	3	Role Performance	Parental Role Conflict		1988		
318	55	07 Role Relationships	3	Role Performance	Ineffective Role Performance		1978	1996	1998
320	52	07 Role Relationships	3	Role Performance	Impaired Social Interaction		1986		

Continued

Table I.1 Continued

Page	Code	Domain	Class	Label	Submitter	Year	Revision	Year	Revision	Year	Revision	Year
323	59	08 Sexuality	2 Sexual Function	Sexual Dysfunction		1980	Alexandra Souza Melo, PhD, RN; Emilia Campos de Carvalho, PhD, RN; Nilza Tereza Rotter Pelá, PhD, RN	2006				
325	65	08 Sexuality	2 Sexual Function	Ineffective Sexuality Pattern		1986	Alexandra Souza Melo, PhD, RN; Emilia Campos de Carvalho, PhD, RN; Nilza Tereza Rotter Pelá, PhD, RN	2006				
326	221	08 Sexuality	3 Reproduction	Ineffective Childbearing Process	DDC (based on work of Yasuko Aoki, RN, RMS; Mitsuko Katayama, RN, RMW, PhD; Atsuko Kikuchi, RN, RMW; Minayo Kumazawa, RN, RMW, Med; Atsuko Koyama, RN, RMW; Masuko Saito, RN, RMW, DrMS; Toyo Yamazaki, RN, RMW; Mayumi Hamasake, RN, RMW, MPH; Shigemi Kamitsuru, RN, PhD)	2010					

| 328 | 208 | 08 Sexuality | 3 Reproduction | Readiness for Enhanced Childbearing Process | 2008 | Yasuko Aoki, RN, RMS; Mitsuko Katayama, RN, RMW, PhD; Atsuko Kikuchi, RN, RMW; Minayo Kumazawa, RN, RMW, Med; Atsuko Koyama, RN, RMW; Masuko Saito, RN, RMW, DrMS; Toyo Yamazaki, RN, RMW; Mayumi Hamasake, RN, RMW, MPH; Shigemi Kamitsuru, RN, PhD |
| 330 | 227 | 08 Sexuality | 3 Reproduction | Risk for Ineffective Childbearing Process | 2010 | DDC (based on work of Yasuko Aoki, RN, RMS; Mitsuko Katayama, RN, RMW, PhD; Atsuko Kikuchi, RN, RMW; Minayo Kumazawa, RN, RMW, Med; Atsuko Koyama, RN, RMW; Masuko Saito, RN, RMW, DrMS; Toyo Yamazaki, RN, RMW; Mayumi Hamasake, RN, RMW, MPH; Shigemi Kamitsuru, RN, PhD) |

Table I.1 Continued

Page	Code	Domain	Class	Label	Submitter	Year	Revision	Year	Revision	Year	Revision	Year
331	209	08 Sexuality	3 Reproduction	Risk for Disturbed Maternal–Fetal Dyad	Sheri Holmes, MSN, APRN, BC	2008						
335	141	09 Coping/ Stress Tolerance	1 Post-Trauma Responses	Post-Trauma Syndrome		1986			1998			
336	145	09 Coping/ Stress Tolerance	1 Post-Trauma Responses	Risk for Post-Trauma Syndrome		1998						
337	142	09 Coping/ Stress Tolerance	1 Post-Trauma Responses	Rape-Trauma Syndrome	Penny Burgus	1980			1998			
338	114	09 Coping/ Stress Tolerance	1 Post-Trauma Responses	Relocation Stress Syndrome		1992			2000			
339	149	09 Coping/ Stress Tolerance	1 Post-Trauma Responses	Risk for Relocation Stress Syndrome		2000						
N/A	143	09 Coping/ Stress Tolerance	1 Post-Trauma Responses	DIAGNOSIS RETIRED (2009–2011) Rape-Trauma Syndrome: Compound Reaction		1980						
N/A	144	09 Coping/ Stress Tolerance	1 Post-Trauma Responses	DIAGNOSIS RETIRED (2009–2011) Rape-Trauma Syndrome: Silent Reaction		1980						
340	199	09 Coping/ Stress Tolerance	2 Coping Responses	Ineffective Activity Planning	France Maltais, BSc, Med	2008						
342	226	09 Coping/ Stress Tolerance	2 Coping Responses	Risk for Ineffective Activity Planning	Diagnosis Development Committee (based on the work of France Maltais, BSc, Med)	2010						

Continued

344	146	09 Coping/Stress Tolerance	2 Coping Responses	Anxiety	1973		1982	1998
346	71	09 Coping/Stress Tolerance	2 Coping Responses	Defensive Coping	1988	Celine Larouche, RN	2008	
348	69	09 Coping/Stress Tolerance	2 Coping Responses	Ineffective Coping	1978		1998	
349	158	09 Coping/Stress Tolerance	2 Coping Responses	Readiness for Enhanced Coping	2002	Margaret Lunney, PhD, RN; Roberta Cavendish, RN, PhD; Barbara Kraynyak Luise, RN, EdD; Kathryn Richardson, RN, MS		
350	77	09 Coping/Stress Tolerance	2 Coping Responses	Ineffective Community Coping	1994	Margaret Lunney, PhD, RN	1998	
351	76	09 Coping/Stress Tolerance	2 Coping Responses	Readiness for Enhanced Community Coping	1994	Margaret Lunney, PhD, RN		
352	74	09 Coping/Stress Tolerance	2 Coping Responses	Compromised Family Coping	1980		1996	
354	73	09 Coping/Stress Tolerance	2 Coping Responses	Disabled Family Coping	1980		1996	2008
355	75	09 Coping/Stress Tolerance	2 Coping Responses	Readiness for Enhanced Family Coping	1980	Margaret Lunney, PhD, RN; Roberta Cavendish, RN, PhD; Barbara Kraynyak Luise, RN, EdD; Kathryn Richardson, RN, MS		

Table I.1 *Continued*

Page	Code	Domain	Class	Label	Submitter	Year	Revision	Year	Revision	Year	Revision	Year
356	147	09 Coping/Stress Tolerance	2 Coping Responses	Death Anxiety		1998	Amor Aradilla, MS, RN; Lidia Fernandez, MS, RN; Pilar Fernandez, MS, RN; Joaquin Tomas, PhD, RN	2006				
358	72	09 Coping/Stress Tolerance	2 Coping Responses	Ineffective Denial		1988	Lina Rahal, Med, RN; Vivianne Saba, MSN, RN	2006				
360	101	09 Coping/Stress Tolerance	2 Coping Responses	Adult Failure to Thrive		1998						
361	148	09 Coping/Stress Tolerance	2 Coping Responses	Fear		1980		1996		2000		
363	136	09 Coping/Stress Tolerance	2 Coping Responses	Grieving		1980		1996	T. Heather Herdman, RN, PhD	2006		
365	135	09 Coping/Stress Tolerance	2 Coping Responses	Complicated Grieving		1980	Mary Ann Lavin, ScD, RN, BC, ANP, FAAN	2004	T. Heather Herdman, RN, PhD	2006		
367	172	09 Coping/Stress Tolerance	2 Coping Responses	Risk for Complicated Grieving	Mary Ann Lavin, ScD, RN, BC, ANP, FAAN	2004			T. Heather Herdman, RN, PhD	2006		
368	187	09 Coping/Stress Tolerance	2 Coping Responses	Readiness for Enhanced Power	Margaret Lunney, PhD, RN; Roberta Cavendish, RN, PhD; Barbara Kraynyak Luise, RN, EdD; Kathryn Richardson, RN, MS	2006						
370	125	09 Coping/Stress Tolerance	2 Coping Responses	Powerlessness	Judith F. Miller	1982					Tracy LaRock, D.O.M., RN	2012
372	152	09 Coping/Stress Tolerance	2 Coping Responses	Risk for Powerlessness		2000					Tracy LaRock, D.O.M., RN	2012

Page	Code	Domain	Class	Diagnosis	Author	Year	Year
374	210	09 Coping/Stress Tolerance	2 Coping Responses	Impaired Individual Resilience	Angela Oldenburg, BA, RN; Shelly Eisbach, PhDc, MSN, RN; Melissa Lehan-Mackin, RN, BSN	2008	
376	212	09 Coping/Stress Tolerance	2 Coping Responses	Readiness for Enhanced Resilience	Angela Oldenburg, BA, RN; Shelly Eisbach, PhDc, MSN, RN; Melissa Lehan-Mackin, RN, BSN	2008	
378	211	09 Coping/Stress Tolerance	2 Coping Responses	Risk for Compromised Resilience	Angela Oldenburg, BA, RN; Shelly Eisbach, PhDc, MSN, RN; Melissa Lehan-Mackin, RN, BSN	2008	
379	137	09 Coping/Stress Tolerance	2 Coping Responses	Chronic Sorrow		1998	
380	177	09 Coping/Stress Tolerance	2 Coping Responses	Stress Overload	Margaret Lunney, PhD, RN	2006	
N/A	70	09 Coping/Stress Tolerance	2 Coping Responses	DIAGNOSIS RETIRED (2007–2008) Impaired adjustment		1986	1988
383	9	09 Coping/Stress Tolerance	3 Neurobehavioral Stress	Autonomic Dysreflexia		1988	
384	10	09 Coping/Stress Tolerance	3 Neurobehavioral Stress	Risk for Autonomic Dysreflexia		1998	2000

Continued

Table I.1 *Continued*

Page	Code	Domain	Class	Label	Submitter	Year	Revision	Year	Revision	Year	Revision	Year
386	116	09 Coping/Stress Tolerance	3 Neurobehavioral Stress	Disorganized Infant Behavior	Mary A. Fuerst-Dewys, BSN, RN	1994		1998				
388	117	09 Coping/Stress Tolerance	3 Neurobehavioral Stress	Readiness for Enhanced Organized Infant Behavior	Mary A. Fuerst-Dewys, BSN, RN	1994						
389	115	09 Coping/Stress Tolerance	3 Neurobehavioral Stress	Risk for Disorganized Infant Behavior	Mary A. Fuerst-Dewys, BSN, RN	1994						
390	49	09 Coping/Stress Tolerance	3 Neurobehavioral Stress	Decreased Intracranial Adaptive Capacity	Pamela H. Mitchell, PhD, RN	1994						
393	185	10 Life Principles	1 Values	Readiness for Enhanced Hope	Margaret Lunney PhD, RN; Roberta Cavendish, RN, PhD; Barbara Kraynyak Luise, RN, EdD; Kathryn Richardson, RN, MS	2006						
394	68	10 Life Principles	2 Beliefs	Readiness for Enhanced Spiritual Well-Being	Noreen Frisch, PhD, RN; Barbara Dossey, MS, RN; Margaret Burkhart, PhD, RN; Cathie Guzzetta, PhD, RN	1994	Lisa Burkhart, PhD, RN	2002				
395	184	10 Life Principles	3 Value/Belief/Action Congruence	Readiness for Enhanced Decision-Making	Margaret Lunney, PhD, RN; Roberta Cavendish, RN, PhD; Barbara Kraynyak Luise, RN, EdD; Kathryn Richardson, RN, MS	2006						

No.	ID	Domain	Class	Diagnosis	Author	Year	Author	Year	Year
396	83	10 Life Principles	3 Value/Belief/Action Congruence	Decisional Conflict	Elizabeth Hiltunen	1988	Lisa Burkhart, PhD, RN; Beverly Kopala, PhD, RN	2006	
398	175	10 Life Principles	3 Value/Belief/Action Congruence	Moral Distress	Lisa Burkhart, PhD, RN; Beverly Kopala, PhD, RN	2006			
400	79	10 Life Principles	3 Value/Belief/Action Congruence	Noncompliance		1973		1996	1998
402	169	10 Life Principles	3 Value/Belief/Action Congruence	Impaired Religiosity	Lisa Burkhart, Phd, RN	2004			
405	171	10 Life Principles	3 Value/Belief/Action Congruence	Readiness for Enhanced Religiosity	Lisa Burkhart, PhD, RN	2004			
407	170	10 Life Principles	3 Value/Belief/Action Congruence	Risk for Impaired Religiosity	Lisa Burkhart, PhD, RN	2004			
410	66	10 Life Principles	3 Value/Belief/Action Congruence	Spiritual Distress	Roberta Cavendish, RN, PhD	1978	Lisa Burkhart, PhD, RN	2002	
412	67	10 Life Principles	3 Value/Belief/Action Congruence	Risk for Spiritual Distress	Roberta Cavendish, RN, PhD	1998		2004	
417	4	11 Safety/Protection	1 Infection	Risk for Infection	Mark R. Hunter, CRNI, VA-BC, RN	1986		2011	
421	31	11 Safety/Protection	2 Physical Injury	Ineffective Airway Clearance	Regina M. Maibusch, MS, RN	1980		1996	1998
422	39	11 Safety/Protection	2 Physical Injury	Risk for Aspiration	Judy Wooldrige, MNEd, RN	1988			
423	206	11 Safety/Protection	2 Physical Injury	Risk for Bleeding	Sheri Holmes, MSN, APRN, BC	2008			
425	48	11 Safety/Protection	2 Physical Injury	Impaired Dentition		1998			
426	219	11 Safety/Protection	2 Physical Injury	Risk for Dry Eye	Elem Kocacal Güler; Ismet Eser	2010			

Continued

Table I.1 Continued

Page	Code	Domain	Class	Label	Submitter	Year	Revision	Year	Revision	Year	Revision	Year
428	155	11 Safety/ Protection	2 Physical Injury	Risk for Falls		2000						
430	35	11 Safety/ Protection	2 Physical Injury	Risk for Injury		1978						
431	45	11 Safety/ Protection	2 Physical Injury	Impaired Oral Mucous Membrane		1982		1998				
433	87	11 Safety/ Protection	2 Physical Injury	Risk for Perioperative Positioning Injury	AORN	1994	Susan Kleinbeck, PhD, RN, CNOR	2006				
434	86	11 Safety/ Protection	2 Physical Injury	Risk for Peripheral Neurovascular Dysfunction		1992						
435	205	11 Safety/ Protection	2 Physical Injury	Risk for Shock	Jennifer Hafner, RN, BSN, PCCN, TNCC	2008						
436	46	11 Safety/ Protection	2 Physical Injury	Impaired Skin Integrity		1975		1998				
437	47	11 Safety/ Protection	2 Physical Injury	Risk for Impaired Skin Integrity		1975		1998	DDC	2012		
438	156	11 Safety/ Protection	2 Physical Injury	Risk for Sudden Infant Death Syndrome	Kathleen Arthur, RN	2002						
439	36	11 Safety/ Protection	2 Physical Injury	Risk for Suffocation		1980						
440	100	11 Safety/ Protection	2 Physical Injury	Delayed Surgical Recovery		1998	Susan Kleinbeck, PhD, RN, CNOR	2006				
442	220	11 Safety/ Protection	2 Physical Injury	Risk for Thermal Injury	Geralyn Meyer, PhD, RN	2010						
443	44	11 Safety/ Protection	2 Physical Injury	Impaired Tissue Integrity		1986		1998				
444	38	11 Safety/ Protection	2 Physical Injury	Risk for Trauma		1980						
446	213	11 Safety/ Protection	2 Physical Injury	Risk for Vascular Trauma	Cristina Arreguy- Senna, PhD, RN; Emilia Campos de Carvalho, PhD, RN	2008						

Continued

Table I.1 *Continued*

Page	Code	Domain	Class	Label	Submitter	Year	Revision	Year	Revision	Year	Revision	Year
470	8	11 Safety/Protection	6 Thermoregulation	Ineffective Thermoregulation		1986						
473	214	12 Comfort	1 Physical Comfort	Impaired Comfort	Mary Killeen, PhD, RN; Kathy Kolcaba, PhD, RN	2008	DDC	2010				
475	183	12 Comfort	1 Physical Comfort	Readiness for Enhanced Comfort	Margaret Lunney, PhD, RN; Roberta Cavendish, RN, PhD; Barbara Kraynyak Luise, RN, EdD; Kathryn Richardson, RN, MS	2006						
476	134	12 Comfort	1 Physical Comfort	Nausea	Hsiao Chen Jane Tang, MSN, RN (NDEC)	1998		2002	Gilmaikon Roela Pereira, MSc, RN & Lilian Guardian, RN	2012		
478	132	12 Comfort	1 Physical Comfort	Acute Pain		1996						
479	133	12 Comfort	1 Physical Comfort	Chronic Pain		1986		1996				
480	53	12 Comfort	3 Social Comfort	Social Isolation		1982						
483	113	13 Growth/Development	1 Growth	Risk for Disproportionate Growth		1998						
484	111	13 Growth/Development	1 Growth	Delayed Growth and Development		1986						
485	112	13 Growth/Development	2 Development	Risk for Delayed Development		1998						
	189	NOT ASSIGNED	NOT ASSIGNED	NOT ASSIGNED								
	190	NOT ASSIGNED	NOT ASSIGNED	NOT ASSIGNED								
	191	NOT ASSIGNED	NOT ASSIGNED	NOT ASSIGNED								
	192	NOT ASSIGNED	NOT ASSIGNED	NOT ASSIGNED								

Table I.2 *Taxonomy II: domains, classes, and diagnoses*

DOMAIN 1 HEALTH PROMOTION
The awareness of well-being or normality of function and the strategies used to maintain control of and enhance that well-being or normality of function

Class 1 Health Awareness Recognition of normal function and well-being

Approved Diagnoses
00097 Deficient **diversional activity**
00168 Sedentary **lifestyle**

Class 2 Health Management Identifying, controlling, performing, and integrating activities to maintain health and well-being

Approved Diagnoses
00215 Deficient community **health**
00188 Risk-prone **health behavior**
00099 Ineffective **health maintenance**
00186 Readiness for enhanced **immunization status**
00043 Ineffective **protection**
00078 Ineffective **self-health management**
00162 Readiness for enhanced **self-health management**
00080 Ineffective family **therapeutic regimen management**

DOMAIN 2 NUTRITION
The activities of taking in, assimilating, and using nutrients for the purposes of tissue maintenance, tissue repair, and the production of energy

Class 1 Ingestion Taking food or nutrients into the body

Approved Diagnoses
00216 Insufficient **breast milk**
00107 Ineffective infant **feeding pattern**
00002 Imbalanced **nutrition**: *less than body requirements*
00001 Imbalanced **nutrition**: *more than body requirements*
00003 Risk for imbalanced **nutrition**: *more than body requirements*
00163 Readiness for enhanced **nutrition**
00103 Impaired **swallowing**

Class 2 Digestion The physical and chemical activities that convert foodstuffs into substances suitable for absorption and assimilation

Approved Diagnoses
None at present time

Class 3 Absorption The act of taking up nutrients through body tissues

Approved Diagnoses
None at present time

Continued

Table I.2 *Continued*

Class 4   Metabolism The chemical and physical processes occurring in living organisms and cells for the development and use of protoplasm, the production of waste and energy, with the release of energy for all vital processes

Approved Diagnoses
00179   *Risk for unstable **blood glucose level***
00194   *Neonatal **jaundice***
00230   *Risk for neonatal **jaundice***
00178   *Risk for impaired **liver function***

Class 5   Hydration The taking in and absorption of fluids and electrolytes

Approved Diagnoses
00195   *Risk for **electrolyte imbalance***
00160   *Readiness for enhanced **fluid balance***
00027   *Deficient **fluid volume***
00026   *Excess **fluid volume***
00028   *Risk for deficient **fluid volume***
00025   *Risk for imbalanced **fluid volume***

DOMAIN 3   ELIMINATION AND EXCHANGE
Secretion and excretion of waste products from the body

Class 1   Urinary Function The process of secretion, reabsorption, and excretion of urine

Approved Diagnoses
00020   *Functional urinary **incontinence***
00176   *Overflow urinary **incontinence***
00018   *Reflex urinary **incontinence***
00017   *Stress urinary **incontinence***
00019   *Urge urinary **incontinence***
00022   *Risk for urge urinary **incontinence***
00016   *Impaired **urinary elimination***
00166   *Readiness for enhanced **urinary elimination***
00023   ***Urinary retention***

Class 2   Gastrointestinal Function The process of absorption and excretion of the end products of digestion

Approved Diagnoses
00011   ***Constipation***
00012   *Perceived **constipation***
00015   *Risk for **constipation***
00013   ***Diarrhea***
00196   *Dysfunctional **gastrointestinal motility***
00197   *Risk for dysfunctional **gastrointestinal motility***
00014   *Bowel **incontinence***

Class 3   Integumentary Function The process of secretion and excretion through the skin

Approved Diagnoses
None at present time

Table I.2 *Continued*

Class 4 **Respiratory Function** The process of exchange of gases and removal of the end products of metabolism

Approved Diagnoses
00030 Impaired **gas exchange**

DOMAIN 4 ACTIVITY/REST
The production, conservation, expenditure, or balance of energy resources

Class 1 **Sleep/Rest** Slumber, repose, ease, relaxation, or inactivity

Approved Diagnoses
00095 **Insomnia**
00096 **Sleep** *deprivation*
00165 *Readiness for enhanced* **sleep**
00198 *Disturbed* **sleep pattern**

Class 2 **Activity/Exercise** Moving parts of the body (mobility), doing work, or performing actions often (but not always) against resistance

Approved Diagnoses
00040 *Risk for* **disuse syndrome**
00091 *Impaired bed* **mobility**
00085 *Impaired physical* **mobility**
00089 *Impaired wheelchair* **mobility**
00090 *Impaired* **transfer ability**
00088 *Impaired* **walking**

Class 3 **Energy Balance** A dynamic state of harmony between intake and expenditure of resources

Approved Diagnoses
00050 *Disturbed* **energy field**
00093 **Fatigue**
00154 **Wandering**

Class 4 **Cardiovascular/Pulmonary Responses** Cardiopulmonary mechanisms that support activity/rest

Approved Diagnoses
00092 **Activity intolerance**
00094 *Risk for* **activity intolerance**
00032 *Ineffective* **breathing pattern**
00029 *Decreased* **cardiac output**
00202 *Risk for ineffective* **gastrointestinal perfusion**
00203 *Risk for ineffective* **renal perfusion**
00033 *Impaired* **spontaneous ventilation**
00204 *Ineffective peripheral* **tissue perfusion**
00200 *Risk for decreased cardiac* **tissue perfusion**
00201 *Risk for ineffective cerebral* **tissue perfusion**
00228 *Risk for ineffective peripheral* **tissue perfusion**
00034 *Dysfunctional* **ventilatory weaning response**

Continued

Table I.2 *Continued*

Class 5 *Self-care* Ability to perform activities to care for one's body and bodily functions

Approved Diagnoses
*00098 Impaired **home maintenance***
*00182 Readiness for enhanced **self-care***
*00108 Bathing **self-care** deficit*
*00109 Dressing **self-care** deficit*
*00102 Feeding **self-care** deficit*
*00110 Toileting **self-care** deficit*
*00193 **Self-neglect***

DOMAIN 5 PERCEPTION/COGNITION
The human information processing system including attention, orientation, sensation, perception, cognition, and communication

Class 1 *Attention* Mental readiness to notice or observe

Approved Diagnoses
*00123 **Unilateral neglect***

Class 2 *Orientation* Awareness of time, place, and person

Approved Diagnoses
*00127 Impaired **environmental interpretation syndrome***

Class 3 *Sensation/Perception* Receiving information through the senses of touch, taste, smell, vision, hearing, and kinesthesia, and the comprehension of sensory data resulting in naming, associating, and/or pattern recognition

Approved Diagnoses
None at this time

Class 4 *Cognition* Use of memory, learning, thinking, problem-solving, abstraction, judgment, insight, intellectual capacity, calculation, and language

Approved Diagnoses
*00128 Acute **confusion***
*00129 Chronic **confusion***
*00173 Risk for acute **confusion***
*00222 Ineffective **impulse control***
*00126 Deficient **knowledge***
*00161 Readiness for enhanced **knowledge***
*00131 Impaired **memory***

Class 5 *Communication* Sending and receiving verbal and nonverbal information

Approved Diagnoses
*00157 Readiness for enhanced **communication***
*00051 Impaired **verbal communication***

Table I.2 *Continued*

DOMAIN 6 SELF-PERCEPTION
Awareness about the self

Class 1 Self-concept The perception(s) about the total self

Approved Diagnoses
*00124 **Hopelessness***
*00174 Risk for compromised **human dignity***
*00054 Risk for **loneliness***
*00121 Disturbed **personal identity***
*00225 Risk for disturbed **personal identity***
*00167 Readiness for enhanced **self-concept***

Class 2 Self-esteem Assessment of one's own worth, capability, significance, and success

Approved Diagnoses
*00119 Chronic low **self-esteem***
*00224 Risk for chronic low **self-esteem***
*00153 Risk for situational low **self-esteem***
*00120 Situational low **self-esteem***

Class 3 Body Image A mental image of one's own body

Approved Diagnoses
*00118 Disturbed **body image***

DOMAIN 7 ROLE RELATIONSHIPS
The positive and negative connections or associations between people or groups of people and the means by which those connections are demonstrated

Class 1 Caregiving Roles Socially expected behavior patterns by people providing care who are not healthcare professionals

Approved Diagnoses
*00104 Ineffective **breastfeeding***
*00105 Interrupted **breastfeeding***
*00106 Readiness for enhanced **breastfeeding***
*00061 **Caregiver role strain***
*00062 Risk for **caregiver role strain***
*00056 Impaired **parenting***
*00164 Readiness for enhanced **parenting***   .
*00057 Risk for impaired **parenting***

Class 2 Family Relationships Associations of people who are biologically related or related by choice

Approved Diagnoses
*00058 Risk for impaired **attachment***
*00063 Dysfunctional **family processes***
*00060 Interrupted **family processes***
*00159 Readiness for enhanced **family processes***

Continued

Table I.2 *Continued*

Class 3 Role Performance Quality of functioning in socially expected behavior patterns

Approved Diagnoses
*00223 Ineffective **relationship***
*00207 Readiness for enhanced **relationship***
*00229 Risk for ineffective **relationship***
*00064 Parental **role conflict***
*00055 Ineffective **role performance***
*00052 Impaired **social interaction***

DOMAIN 8 SEXUALITY

Sexual identity, sexual function, and reproduction

Class 1 Sexual Identity The state of being a specific person in regard to sexuality and/or gender

Approved Diagnoses
None at present time

Class 2 Sexual Function The capacity or ability to participate in sexual activities

Approved Diagnoses
*00059 **Sexual dysfunction***
*00065 Ineffective **sexuality pattern***

Class 3 Reproduction Any process by which human beings are produced

Approved Diagnoses
*00221 Ineffective **childbearing process***
*00208 Readiness for enhanced **childbearing process***
*00227 Risk for ineffective **childbearing process***
*00209 Risk for disturbed **maternal–fetal dyad***

DOMAIN 9 COPING/STRESS TOLERANCE
Contending with life events/life processes

Class 1 Post-trauma Responses Reactions occurring after physical or psychological trauma

Approved Diagnoses
*00141 **Post-trauma syndrome***
*00145 Risk for **post-trauma syndrome***
*00142 **Rape-trauma syndrome***
*00114 **Relocation stress syndrome***
*00149 Risk for **relocation stress syndrome***

Table I.2 *Continued*

Class 2 **Coping Responses** The process of managing environmental stress

Approved Diagnoses
*00199 Ineffective **activity planning***
*00226 Risk for ineffective **activity planning***
*00146 **Anxiety***
*00074 Compromised family **coping***
*00071 Defensive **coping***
*00073 Disabled family **coping***
*00069 Ineffective **coping***
*00077 Ineffective community **coping***
*00158 Readiness for enhanced **coping***
*00076 Readiness for enhanced community **coping***
*00075 Readiness for enhanced family **coping***
*00147 **Death anxiety***
*00072 Ineffective **denial***
*00101 Adult **failure to thrive***
*00148 **Fear***
*00136 **Grieving***
*00135 Complicated **grieving***
*00172 Risk for complicated **grieving***
*00187 Readiness for enhanced **power***
*00125 **Powerlessness***
*00152 Risk for **powerlessness***
*00210 Impaired individual **resilience***
*00212 Readiness for enhanced **resilience***
*00211 Risk for compromised **resilience***
*00137 Chronic **sorrow***
*00177 **Stress** overload*

Class 3 **Neurobehavioral Stress** Behavioral responses reflecting nerve and brain function

Approved Diagnoses
*00115 Risk for disorganized infant **behavior***
*00009 **Autonomic dysreflexia***
*00010 Risk for **autonomic dysreflexia***
*00116 Disorganized infant **behavior***
*00117 Readiness for enhanced organized infant **behavior***
*00049 Decreased **intracranial adaptive capacity***

DOMAIN 10 LIFE PRINCIPLES
Principles underlying conduct, thought, and behavior about acts, customs, or institutions viewed as being true or having intrinsic worth

Class 1 **Values** The identification and ranking of preferred modes of conduct or end states

Approved Diagnoses
*00185 Readiness for enhanced **hope***

Continued

Table I.2 *Continued*

Class 2 Beliefs Opinions, expectations, or judgments about acts, customs, or institutions viewed as being true or having intrinsic worth

Approved Diagnoses
00185 *Readiness for enhanced* **hope**
00068 *Readiness for enhanced* **spiritual well-being**

Class 3 Value/Belief/Action Congruence The correspondence or balance achieved among values, beliefs, and actions

Approved Diagnoses
00184 *Readiness for enhanced* **decision-making**
00083 **Decisional conflict**
00175 **Moral distress**
00079 **Noncompliance**
00169 *Impaired* **religiosity**
00171 *Readiness for enhanced* **religiosity**
00170 *Risk for impaired* **religiosity**
00066 **Spiritual distress**
00067 *Risk for* **spiritual distress**

DOMAIN 11 SAFETY/PROTECTION
Freedom from danger, physical injury, or immune system damage; preservation from loss; and protection of safety and security

Class 1 Infection Host responses following pathogenic invasion

Approved Diagnoses
00004 *Risk for* **infection**

Class 2 Physical Injury Bodily harm or hurt

Approved Diagnoses
00031 *Ineffective* **airway clearance**
00039 *Risk for* **aspiration**
00206 *Risk for* **bleeding**
00048 *Impaired* **dentition**
00219 *Risk for* **dry eye**
00155 *Risk for* **falls**
00035 *Risk for* **injury**
00045 *Impaired* **oral mucous membrane**
00087 *Risk for* **perioperative positioning injury**
00086 *Risk for* **peripheral neurovascular dysfunction**
00205 *Risk for* **shock**
00046 *Impaired* **skin integrity**
00047 *Risk for impaired* **skin integrity**
00156 *Risk for* **sudden infant death syndrome**
00036 *Risk for* **suffocation**
00100 *Delayed* **surgical recovery**
00220 *Risk for* **thermal injury**
00044 *Impaired* **tissue integrity**
00038 *Risk for* **trauma**
00213 *Risk for* **vascular trauma**

Table I.2 *Continued*

Class 3 Violence The exertion of excessive force or power so as to cause injury or abuse

Approved Diagnoses
*00138 Risk for **other-directed violence***
*00140 Risk for **self-directed violence***
*00151 **Self-mutilation***
*00139 Risk for **self-mutilation***
*00150 Risk for **suicide***

Class 4 Environmental Hazards Sources of danger in the surroundings

Approved Diagnoses
*00181 **Contamination***
*00180 Risk for **contamination***
*00037 Risk for **poisoning***

Class 5 Defensive Processes The processes by which the self protects itself from the nonself

Approved Diagnoses
*00218 Risk for **adverse reaction to iodinated contrast media***
*00217 Risk for **allergy response***
*00041 **Latex allergy response***
*00042 Risk for **latex allergy response***

Class 6 Thermoregulation The physiological process of regulating heat and energy within the body for purposes of protecting the organism

Approved Diagnoses
*00005 Risk for imbalanced **body temperature***
*00007 **Hyperthermia***
*00006 **Hypothermia***
*00008 Ineffective **thermoregulation***

DOMAIN 12 COMFORT
Sense of mental, physical, or social well-being or ease

Class 1 Physical Comfort Sense of well-being or ease and/or freedom from pain

Approved Diagnoses
*00214 Impaired **comfort***
*00183 Readiness for enhanced **comfort***
*00134 **Nausea***
*00132 Acute **pain***
*00133 Chronic **pain***

Continued

Table I.2 *Continued*

Class 2 **Environmental Comfort** Sense of well-being or ease in/with one's environment

Approved Diagnoses
00214 Impaired **comfort**
00183 Readiness for enhanced **comfort**

Class 3 **Social Comfort** Sense of well-being or ease with one's social situations

Approved Diagnoses
00214 Impaired **comfort**
00053 **Social isolation**

DOMAIN 13 GROWTH/DEVELOPMENT
Age-appropriate increases in physical dimensions, maturation of organ systems, and/or progression through the developmental milestones

Class 1 **Growth** Increases in physical dimensions or maturity of organ systems

Approved Diagnoses
00113 Risk for disproportionate **growth**
00111 Delayed **growth and development**

Class 2 **Development** Progression or regression through a sequence of recognized milestones in life

Approved Diagnoses
00112 Risk for delayed **development**
00111 Delayed **growth and development**

Table I.3 *NNN Taxonomy of Nursing Practice: Placement of Nursing Diagnoses[1]*

Domains	Classes	Diagnoses, outcomes and interventions	NANDA-I nursing diagnoses
I. Functional Includes diagnoses, outcomes, and interventions to promote basic needs	**Activity/ Exercise**	Physical activity, including energy conservation and expenditure	Activity intolerance Risk for activity intolerance Risk for disuse syndrome Risk for falls Fatigue Impaired bed mobility Impaired physical mobility Impaired wheelchair mobility Sedentary lifestyle Impaired transfer ability Impaired walking Wandering
	Comfort	A sense of emotional, physical, and spiritual well-being and relative freedom from distress	Impaired comfort Readiness for enhanced comfort Disturbed energy field Nausea Acute pain Chronic pain
	Growth and Development	Physical, emotional, and social growth and development milestones	Readiness for enhanced childbearing process Risk for delayed development Delayed growth and development Risk for disproportionate growth Disorganized infant behavior Readiness for enhanced organized infant behavior Risk for disorganized infant behavior

Continued

Table I.3 *Continued*

Domains	Classes	Diagnoses, outcomes and interventions	NANDA-I nursing diagnoses
	Nutrition	Processes related to taking in, assimilating, and using nutrients	*Insufficient breast milk* *Ineffective infant feeding pattern* *Imbalanced nutrition: less than body requirements* *Imbalanced nutrition: more than body requirements* *Readiness for enhanced nutrition* *Risk for imbalanced nutrition: more than body requirements* *Impaired swallowing*
	Self-care	Ability to accomplish basic and instrumental activities of daily living	*Readiness for enhanced self-care* *Bathing self-care deficit* *Dressing self-care deficit* *Feeding self-care deficit* *Toileting self-care deficit* *Self-neglect*
	Sexuality	Maintenance or modification of sexual identity and patterns	*Sexual dysfunction* *Ineffective sexuality patterns*
	Sleep/Rest	The quantity and quality of sleep, rest, and relaxation patterns	*Insomnia* *Readiness for enhanced sleep* *Sleep deprivation* *Disturbed sleep pattern*
	Values/Beliefs	Ideas, goals, perceptions, spiritual, and other beliefs that influence choices or decisions	*Moral distress* *Impaired religiosity* *Readiness for enhanced religiosity* *Risk for impaired religiosity* *Spiritual distress* *Readiness for enhanced spiritual well-being* *Risk for spiritual distress*

II. Physiological Includes diagnoses, outcomes, and interventions to promote optimal biophysical health	**Cardiac Function** Cardiac mechanisms used to maintain tissue perfusion	*Decreased cardiac output* *Ineffective peripheral tissue perfusion* *Risk for ineffective peripheral tissue perfusion* *Risk for shock* *Ineffective tissue perfusion* *Risk for decreased cardiac tissue perfusion* *Risk for ineffective cerebral tissue perfusion* *Risk for ineffective gastrointestinal perfusion* *Risk for ineffective renal perfusion*
	Elimination Processes related to secretion and excretion of body wastes	*Constipation* *Perceived constipation* *Risk for constipation* *Diarrhea* *Bowel incontinence* *Functional urinary incontinence* *Overflow urinary incontinence* *Reflex urinary incontinence* *Stress urinary incontinence* *Urge urinary incontinence* *Risk for urge urinary incontinence* *Neonatal jaundice* *Risk for neonatal jaundice* *Dysfunctional gastrointestinal motility* *Risk for dysfunctional gastrointestinal motility* *Impaired urinary elimination* *Urinary retention* *Readiness for enhanced urinary elimination*
	Fluid and Electrolyte Regulation of fluids/electrolytes and acid–base balance	*Risk for bleeding* *Risk for electrolyte imbalance* *Readiness for enhanced fluid balance* *Deficient fluid volume* *Excess fluid volume* *Risk for deficient fluid volume*

Continued

Table I.3 *Continued*

Domains	*Classes*	*Diagnoses, outcomes and interventions*	*NANDA-I nursing diagnoses*
	Neurocognition	Mechanisms related to the nervous system and neurocognitive functioning, including memory, thinking, and judgment	*Ineffective activity planning* *Risk for ineffective activity planning* *Autonomic dysreflexia* *Risk for autonomic dysreflexia* *Acute confusion* *Chronic confusion* *Risk for acute confusion* *Impaired environmental interpretation syndrome* *Ineffective impulse control* *Decreased intracranial adaptive capacity* *Impaired memory* *Unilateral neglect*
	Pharmacological Function	Effects (therapeutic and adverse) of medications or drugs and other pharmacologically active products	*Risk for adverse reaction to iodinated contrast media*
	Physical Regulation	Body temperature, endocrine, and immune system responses to regulate cellular processes	*Risk for allergy response* *Latex allergy response* *Risk for latex allergy response* *Risk for unstable blood glucose level* *Risk for imbalanced body temperature* *Hyperthermia* *Hypothermia* *Risk for infection* *Risk for impaired liver function* *Risk for peripheral neurovascular dysfunction* *Ineffective protection* *Ineffective thermoregulation*

Reproduction	Processes related to human procreation and birth	*Ineffective childbearing process* *Risk for ineffective childbearing process*
Respiratory Function	Ventilation adequate to maintain arterial blood gases within normal limits	*Ineffective airway clearance* *Risk for aspiration* *Ineffective breathing pattern* *Impaired gas exchange* *Impaired spontaneous ventilation* *Risk for suffocation* *Dysfunctional ventilatory weaning response*
Sensation/ Perception	Intake and interpretation of information through the senses, including seeing, hearing, touching, tasting, and smelling	*Disturbed sensory perception*
Tissue Integrity	Skin and mucous membrane protection to support secretion, excretion, and healing	*Impaired dentition* *Risk for dry eye* *Impaired oral mucous membrane* *Impaired skin integrity* *Risk for impaired skin integrity* *Impaired tissue integrity*
Behavior	Actions that promote, maintain, or restore health	*Risk-prone health behavior* *Ineffective health maintenance* *Health-seeking behaviors* *Noncompliance* *Ineffective self-health management* *Readiness for enhanced self-health management* *Self-neglect* *Ineffective family therapeutic regimen management*
III. Psychosocial Includes diagnoses, outcomes, and interventions to promote optimal mental and emotional health and social functioning		

Continued

Table I.3 *Continued*

Domains	Classes	Diagnoses, outcomes and interventions	NANDA-I nursing diagnoses
	Communication	Receiving, interpreting, and expressing spoken, written, and nonverbal messages	Readiness for enhanced communication Impaired verbal communication
	Coping	Adjusting or adapting to stressful events	Decisional conflict Ineffective coping Ineffective community coping Readiness for enhanced community coping Readiness for enhanced coping Readiness for enhanced decision-making Defensive coping Compromised family coping Disabled family coping Readiness for enhanced family coping Ineffective denial Adult failure to thrive Grieving Complicated grieving Risk for complicated grieving Post-trauma syndrome Risk for post-trauma syndrome Rape-trauma syndrome Relocation stress syndrome Risk for relocation stress syndrome Risk for compromised resilience Readiness for enhanced resilience Impaired individual resilience Risk for self-directed violence Self-mutilation Risk for self-mutilation Risk for suicide Stress overload

Category	Definition	Diagnoses
Emotional	A mental state or feeling that may influence perceptions of the world	*Anxiety* *Death anxiety* *Fear* *Readiness for enhanced hope* *Hopelessness* *Chronic sorrow*
Knowledge	Understanding and skill in applying information to promote, maintain, and restore health	*Deficient knowledge* *Readiness for enhanced knowledge*
Roles/ Relationships	Maintenance and/or modification of expected social behaviors and emotional connectedness with others	*Risk for impaired attachment* *Effective breastfeeding* *Ineffective breastfeeding* *Interrupted breastfeeding* *Caregiver role strain* *Risk for caregiver role strain* *Dysfunctional family processes* *Interrupted family processes* *Readiness for enhanced family processes* *Risk for disturbed maternal–fetal dyad* *Parental role conflict* *Impaired parenting* *Readiness for enhanced parenting* *Risk for impaired parenting* *Ineffective relationship* *Readiness for enhanced relationship* *Risk for ineffective relationship* *Ineffective role performance* *Impaired social interaction* *Social isolation* *Risk for other-directed violence*

Table I.3 *Continued*

Domains	Classes	Diagnoses, outcomes and interventions	NANDA-I nursing diagnoses
	Self-perception	Awareness of one's body and personal identity	Disturbed body image Risk for compromised human dignity Risk for loneliness Disturbed personal identity Chronic low self-esteem Risk for chronic low self-esteem Situational low self-esteem Risk for situational low self-esteem Risk for disturbed personal identity Readiness for enhanced self-concept Readiness for enhanced power Powerlessness Risk for powerlessness
IV. Environmental Includes diagnoses, outcomes, and interventions to promote and protect the environmental health and safety of individuals, systems, and communities	**Healthcare System**	Social, political, and economic structures and processes for the delivery of healthcare services	Deficient community health

| Populations | Aggregates of individuals or communities having characteristics in common | |
| Risk Management | Avoidance of identifiable health threats | *Contamination*
Risk for contamination
Impaired home maintenance
Readiness for enhanced immunization
Risk for injury
Risk for perioperative positioning injury
Risk for poisoning
Risk for sudden infant death syndrome
Risk for thermal injury
Risk for trauma
Risk for vascular trauma |

[1]The taxonomy shown in columns 1–3 is in the public domain and can be freely used without permission: neither this taxonomy nor a modification can be copyrighted by any person, group or organization: any use of the taxonomy should acknowledge the source.
Taxonomy from: Dochterman, J., & Jones, D. (eds) (2003) *Unifying nursing languages: The harmonization of NANDA, NIC, and NOC.* Washington, DC: American Nurses Publishing.

Chapter 1

The NANDA International Taxonomy II 2012–2014

T. Heather Herdman, Gunn von Krogh

History of the Development of Taxonomy II

The history of the development of Taxonomy I and II can be found in detail on the NANDA-I website (www.nanda.org). A brief summary of the history of Taxonomy II, the current structure for NANDA-I, is provided here. In 1994, the NANDA Taxonomy Committee submitted a Q-sort methodology using four different potential taxonomic frameworks to the NANDA Board of Directors. None of these frameworks was entirely satisfactory, although Gordon's (1998) Functional Health Pattern framework was felt to be the best fit. With Gordon's permission, the Taxonomy Committee modified this framework to create a fifth framework.

One domain of the Functional Health Pattern framework was divided into two to reduce the number of classes and diagnoses falling within it. A separate domain was added for growth and development because the original framework did not contain that domain. Several other domains were renamed to better reflect the content of the diagnoses within them. The final taxonomic structure is much less like Gordon's original, but the changes have reduced misclassification errors and redundancies to nearly zero, which is a much-desired state in a taxonomic structure. This new structure was presented to, and accepted by, the NANDA membership in April 1998, at the 13th biennial conference in St. Louis, Missouri (USA).

Definitions were developed for all the domains and classes within the structure. The definition of each diagnosis was then compared with that of the class and the domain in which it was placed. Revisions and modifications in the diagnosis placements were made to ensure maximum match among domain, class, and diagnosis.

In January 2003, the Taxonomy Committee made further refinements to the terminology in Taxonomy II. Additionally, to foster its international focus, the axes in Taxonomy II were reviewed and compared with the International Standards Organization (ISO) Reference Terminology Model for a Nursing Diagnosis.

As with any expanding taxonomy, work continues as NANDA-I develops more terms to represent nursing knowledge. In 2007, the Taxonomy Committee again began a review of the current taxonomic structure, under the leadership of its chairperson, Gunn von Krogh. Concerns regarding the current taxonomic structure were presented at the NANDA-I conference in Miami (2008) and published in the NANDA-I journal (von Krogh, 2008). A draft of a new knowledge- and ontology-based taxonomy was presented at the 2010 Asociación Española de Nomenclatura,

NANDA International Nursing Diagnoses: Definitions & Classification 2012–2014, First Edition.
Edited by T. Heather Herdman.
© 2012 NANDA International. Published 2012 by Blackwell Publishing Ltd.

Taxonomía y Diagnósticos de Enfermería (AENTDE)/NANDA-I International Congress in Madrid, Spain, in 2010. A taxonomy workgroup was formed to develop this draft further and to establish rules for ontological review of nursing diagnoses. A revised draft of this work was presented at the 2011 NANDA-I Latin American Symposium (São Paulo, Brazil). Development of these proposed changes is still ongoing at the date of publication of this text, so Taxonomy II will be maintained throughout the life cycle of this edition.

For the 2012–2014 edition of the taxonomy, the nursing diagnoses and supporting materials that were approved by the Diagnosis Development Committee (DDC) were made available for voting to members on the NANDA-I website. This marks the second release of this text in which this method of approval was used for the ongoing expansion and revision of Taxonomy II. The Taxonomy Committee placed diagnoses within both the NANDA-I Taxonomy II and the NANDA-I, Nursing Interventions Classification (NIC), and Nursing Outcomes Classification (NOC) combined NNN Taxonomy of Nursing Practice, following approval of the nursing diagnoses by the DDC, NANDA-I membership and Board of Directors.

Structure of Taxonomy II

Clinicians are primarily concerned with the diagnoses within the taxonomy and may believe that they do not need to use the taxonomic structure itself. Familiarity with how a diagnosis is structured will, however, aid the clinician who needs to find information quickly, as well as those who wish to submit new diagnoses. A brief explanation of how the taxonomy is designed is therefore included here.

A taxonomy is defined as a "Classification: especially orderly classification of plants and animals according to their presumed natural relationships"; the word is derived from the root word, taxon – "the name applied to a taxonomic group in a formal system of nomenclature" (Merriam-Webster, 2009). We can adapt the definition for a nursing diagnosis taxonomy; specifically, we are concerned with the orderly classification of diagnostic foci of concern to nursing, according to their presumed natural relationships. Taxonomy II has three levels: domains, classes, and nursing diagnoses. Figure 1.1 depicts the organization of domains and classes in Taxonomy II; Table I.1 in the Introduction shows Taxonomy II with 13 domains, 47 classes, and numbers of diagnoses. A domain is "a sphere of knowledge, influence, or inquiry"; a class is "a group, set, or kind sharing common attributes" (Merriam-Webster, 2009).

The Taxonomy II code structure is a 32-bit integer (or if the user's database uses another notation, the code structure is a five-digit code). This structure provides for the stability, or growth and development, of the classification structure by avoiding the need to change codes when new diagnoses, refinements, and revisions are added. The Informatics Committee assigns new codes to newly submitted diagnoses that have been approved by the DDC and successfully voted upon by the NANDA-I membership and Board of Directors.

Taxonomy II has a code structure that is compliant with recommendations from the National Library of Medicine (NLM) concerning healthcare terminology codes. The NLM recommends that codes do not contain information about the classified concept, as did the Taxonomy I code structure, which included information about the location and the level of the diagnosis.

Figure 1.1 *Taxonomy II domains and classes*

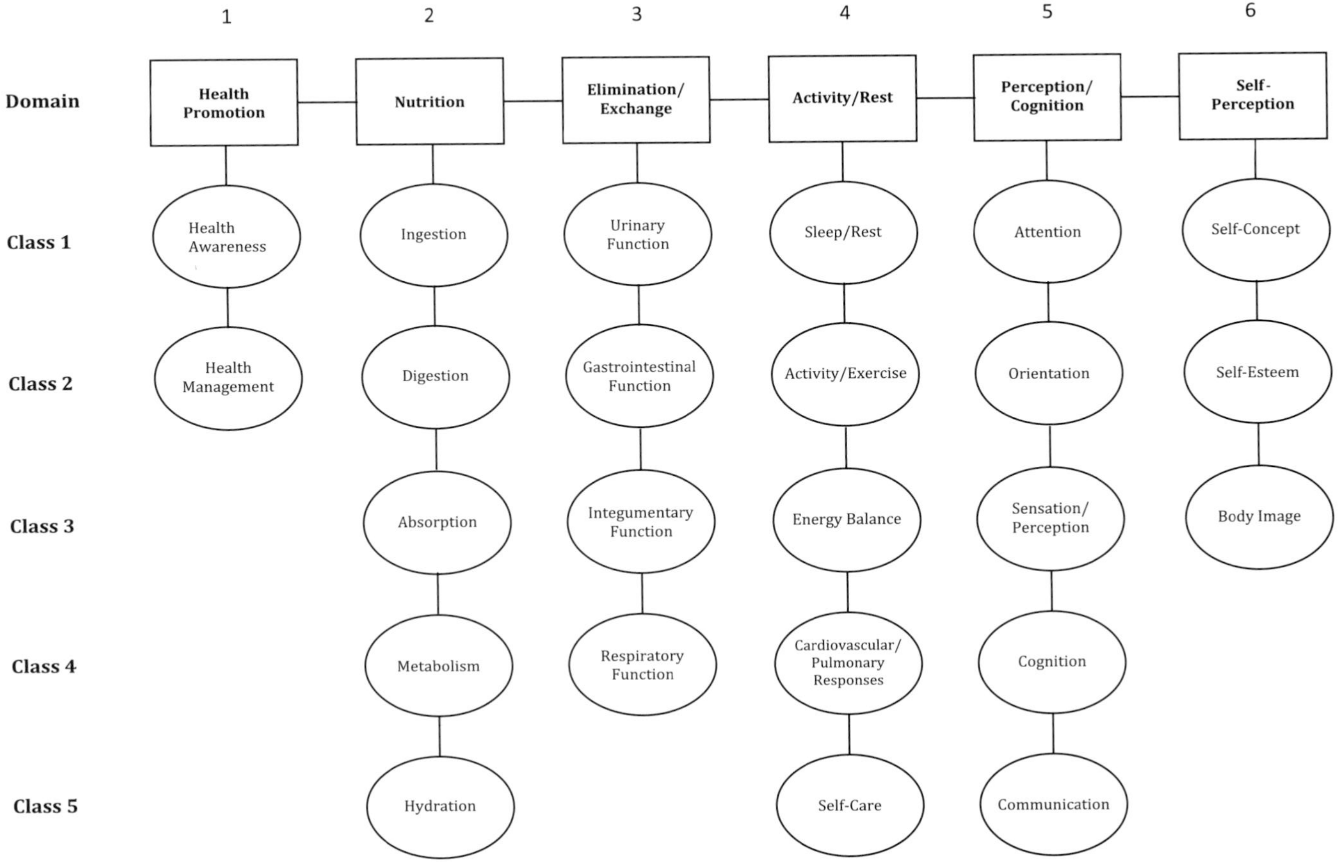

Figure 1.1 *Continued*

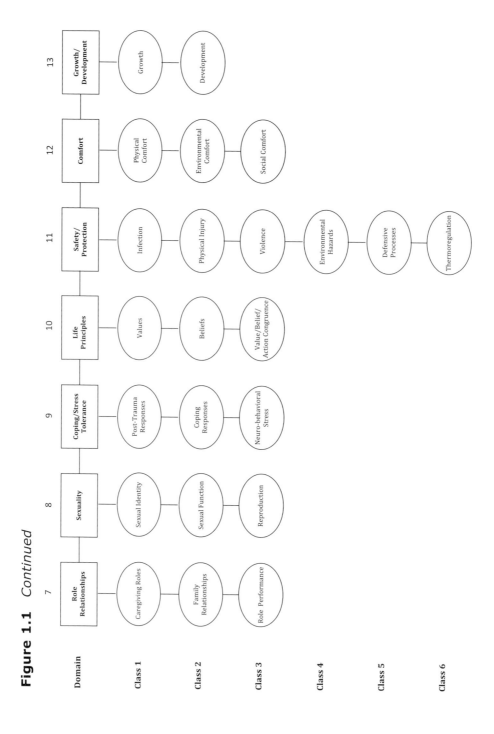

Domain

7	8	9	10	11	12	13
Role Relationships	Sexuality	Coping/Stress Tolerance	Life Principles	Safety/ Protection	Comfort	Growth/ Development

Class 1: Caregiving Roles | Sexual Identity | Post-Trauma Responses | Values | Infection | Physical Comfort | Growth

Class 2: Family Relationships | Sexual Function | Coping Responses | Beliefs | Physical Injury | Environmental Comfort | Development

Class 3: Role Performance | Reproduction | Neuro-behavioral Stress | Value/Belief/ Action Congruence | Violence | Social Comfort

Class 4: Environmental Hazards

Class 5: Defensive Processes

Class 6: Thermoregulation

The NANDA-I Taxonomy II is a recognized nursing language that meets the criteria established by the Committee for Nursing Practice Information Infrastructure of the American Nurses Association (ANA) (Lundberg, Warren, Brokel, Bulechek, Butcher, Dochterman, Johnson, et al., 2008). The benefit of a recognized nursing language is the indication that the classification system is accepted as supporting nursing practice by providing clinically useful terminology. The ANA recognition facilitates the inclusion of NANDA-I in the ANA Nursing Information and Data Set Evaluation Center criteria for clinical information systems (nursingworld.org/nidsec/index.htm) and the NLM's Unified Medical Language System (www.nlm.nih.gov/research/umls/umlsmain.html). NANDA-I diagnoses have been modeled into the Systematized Nomenclature of Medicine-Clinical Terms (SNOMED CT), which has been accepted as a terminology standard for the US Department of Health and Human Services, the US Consolidated Health Information Initiative, and the United Kingdom's National Health Service. A map of this modeling effort is available from SNOMED International (www.snomed.org). SNOMED CT "provides a consistent way of indexing, storing, retrieving and aggregating clinical data across specialties and sites of care" (Lundberg et al., 2008). NANDA-I nursing diagnoses are located within SNOMED CT under the top-level hierarchy of "clinical findings," which includes diagnoses, disorders, diseases that are necessarily abnormal, clinical observations, and signs and symptoms. The NANDA-I nursing diagnoses also comply with the ISO terminology model for a nursing diagnosis (Figure 1.2).

Figure 1.2 *The ISO reference terminology model for a nursing diagnosis*

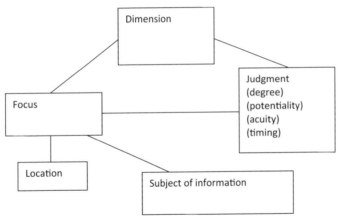

Finally, the taxonomy is registered with Health Level Seven International (www.HL7.org), a healthcare informatics standard, as a terminology to be used in identifying nursing diagnoses in electronic messages among clinical information systems.

A Multiaxial System for Constructing Diagnostic Concepts

The NANDA-I diagnoses are concepts constructed by means of a multiaxial system. This system consists of axes out of which components are combined to make the diagnoses substantially equal in form, and in coherence with the ISO model.

NANDA-I does not support the *random construction* of diagnostic concepts that would occur by simply matching terms from one axis to another to create a diagnosis label to represent judgments based on a patient assessment. Clinical problems/areas of nursing foci that are identified and that do not have a NANDA-I label should be carefully described in documentation to ensure accuracy of other nurses'/healthcare professionals' interpretation of the clinical judgment. Creating a diagnosis to be used in clinical documentation by matching terms from different axes, without development of the definition and other component parts of a diagnosis (defining characteristics, related factors, or risk factors) in an evidence-based manner, negates the purpose of a standardized language as a method to truly represent, inform, and direct clinical judgment and practice. This is a serious concern with regard to patient safety, because the lack of the knowledge inherent within the component diagnostic parts makes it impossible to ensure diagnostic accuracy. Nursing terms arbitrarily created at the point of care could result in misinterpretation of the clinical problem/area of focus, and subsequently lead to inappropriate outcome setting and intervention choice. It also makes it impossible to accurately research the incidence of nursing diagnoses, or to conduct outcome or intervention studies related to diagnoses since, without clear component diagnostic parts (definitions, defining characteristics, and related or risk factors), it is impossible to know if the concept being studied truly represents the same phenomena. Therefore, when discussing construction of diagnostic concepts in this chapter, the intent is to inform clinicians how diagnostic concepts are developed, and to provide clarity for individuals who are developing diagnoses for submission into the NANDA-I Taxonomy. It *should not* be interpreted to suggest that NANDA-I supports the creation of diagnosis labels by clinicians at the point of patient care.

An axis, for the purpose of the NANDA-I Taxonomy II, is operationally defined as a dimension of the human response that is considered in the diagnostic process. There are seven axes. The *NANDA-I Model of a Nursing Diagnosis* displays the seven axes and their relationship to each other (Figure 1.3). The ordering and some of the labels and definitions were changed after the 2005–2006 edition of this book in order to parallel the International Standards Reference Model for a Nursing Diagnosis:

- Axis 1: the diagnostic focus;
- Axis 2: subject of the diagnosis (individual, family, group, community);
- Axis 3: judgment (impaired, ineffective, etc.);
- Axis 4: location (bladder, auditory, cerebral, etc.);
- Axis 5: age (infant, child, adult, etc.);
- Axis 6: time (chronic, acute, intermittent);
- Axis 7: status of the diagnosis (actual, risk, health promotion).

The axes are represented in the labels of the nursing diagnoses through their values. In some cases, they are named explicitly, such as with the diagnoses *Ineffective Community Coping* and *Compromised Family Coping*, in which the subject of the diagnosis (in the first instance "community" and in the second instance "family") is named using the two values "community" and "family" taken from Axis 2 (subject of the diagnosis). "*Ineffective*" and "*compromised*" are two of the values contained in Axis 3 (judgment).

In some cases, the axis is implicit, as is the case with the diagnosis *Activity Intolerance*, in which the subject of the diagnosis (Axis 2) is always the patient. In

Figure 1.3 *The NANDA-I model of a nursing diagnosis*

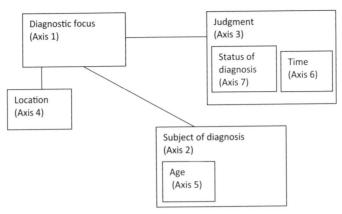

some instances, an axis may not be pertinent to a particular diagnosis and therefore is not part of the nursing diagnostic label. For example, the time axis may not be relevant to every diagnosis. In the case of diagnoses without explicit identification of the subject of the diagnosis, it may be helpful to remember that NANDA-I defines "patient" as "an individual, family, group or community."

Axis 1 (the diagnostic focus) and Axis 3 (judgment) are essential components of a nursing diagnosis. In some cases, however, the diagnostic focus contains the judgment (e.g., *Nausea*); in these cases, the judgment is not explicitly separated out in the diagnostic label. Axis 2 (subject of the diagnosis) is also essential, although, as described above, it may be implied and therefore not included in the label. The DDC requires these axes for submission; the other axes may be used where relevant for clarity.

Definitions of the Axes

Axis 1: The Diagnostic Focus

The diagnostic focus is the principal element or the fundamental and essential part, the root, of the diagnostic concept. It describes the "human response" or experience that is the core of the diagnosis.

The diagnostic focus may consist of one or more nouns. When more than one noun is used (e.g., *Activity Intolerance*), each one contributes a unique meaning to the diagnostic focus, as if the two were a single noun; the meaning of the combined term, however, is different from when the nouns are stated separately. Frequently, an adjective (*Spiritual*) may be used with a noun (*Distress*) to denote the diagnostic focus *Spiritual Distress*.

In some cases, the diagnostic focus and the diagnostic concept are one and the same, as is seen with the diagnosis of *Nausea*. This occurs when the nursing diagnosis is stated at its most clinically useful level and the separation of the diagnostic focus adds no meaningful level of abstraction. It can be very difficult to determine exactly what should be considered the diagnostic focus. For example, using the diagnoses of *Bowel Incontinence* and *Stress Urinary Incontinence*, the question becomes: Is the diagnostic focus *incontinence* alone, or are there two foci – *bowel incontinence* and *urinary incontinence*? In this instance, *incontinence* is the focus, and the location terms (Axis 4) of *bowel* and *urinary* provide more clarification about the focus. However, *incontinence* in and of itself is a judgment term that can stand alone, and so it becomes the diagnostic focus regardless of location.

In some cases, however, removing the location (Axis 4) from the diagnostic focus would prevent it from providing meaning to nursing practice. For example, if we look at the focus of the diagnosis *Risk for Imbalanced Body Temperature*, is the diagnostic focus *body temperature* or simply *temperature*? Or if you look at the diagnosis *Disturbed Personal Identity*, is the focus *identity* or *personal identity*?

Decisions about what constitutes the essence of the diagnostic focus, then, are made on the basis of what helps to identify the nursing practice implication, and whether or not the term indicates a human response. *Temperature* could mean environmental temperature, which is not a human response – so it is important to identify *body temperature* as the diagnostic concept. Similarly, *identity* can mean nothing more than one's gender, eye color, height, or age – again, these are characteristics but not human responses; *personal identity*, however indicates one's self-perception and is a human response. In some cases, the focus may seem similar, but is in fact quite distinct: *violence* and *self-directed violence* are two different human responses, and therefore must be identified separately in terms of diagnostic foci within Taxonomy II.

The diagnostic foci of the NANDA-I nursing diagnoses are:

- **A**ctivity intolerance
- Activity planning
- Adverse reaction to iodinated contrast media
- Airway clearance
- Allergy response
- Anxiety
- Aspiration
- Attachment
- Autonomic dysreflexia
- **B**ehavior
- Bleeding
- Blood glucose level
- Body image
- Body temperature
- Breast milk
- Breastfeeding
- Breathing pattern
- **C**ardiac output
- Caregiver role strain
- Childbearing process
- Comfort
- Communication
- Confusion
- Constipation
- Contamination

- Coping
- **D**eath anxiety
- Decisional conflict
- Decision-making
- Denial
- Dentition
- Development
- Diarrhea
- Disuse syndrome
- Diversional activity
- Dry eye
- **E**lectrolyte imbalance
- Energy field
- Environmental interpretation syndrome
- **F**ailure to thrive
- Falls
- Family processes
- Fatigue
- Fear
- Feeding pattern
- Fluid balance
- Fluid volume
- **G**as exchange
- Gastrointestinal motility
- Gastrointestinal perfusion
- Grieving
- Growth
- Growth and development
- **H**ealth
- Health behavior
- Health maintenance
- Home maintenance
- Hope
- Hopelessness
- Human dignity
- Hyperthermia
- Hypothermia
- **I**mmunization status
- Impulse control
- Incontinence
- Infection
- Injury
- Insomnia
- Intracranial adaptive capacity
- **J**aundice
- **K**nowledge
- **L**ifestyle
- Liver function
- Loneliness

- **M**aternal–fetal dyad
- Memory
- Mobility
- Moral distress
- **N**ausea
- Noncompliance
- Nutrition
- **O**ral mucous membrane
- Other-directed violence
- **P**ain
- Parenting
- Perioperative positioning injury
- Peripheral neurovascular dysfunction
- Personal identity
- Poisoning
- Post-trauma syndrome
- Power
- Powerlessness
- Protection
- **R**ape-trauma syndrome
- Relationship
- Religiosity
- Relocation stress syndrome
- Renal perfusion
- Resilience
- Role conflict
- Role performance
- **S**elf-care
- Self-concept
- Self-directed violence
- Self-esteem
- Self-health management
- Self-mutilation
- Self-neglect
- Sexual dysfunction
- Sexuality pattern
- Shock
- Skin integrity
- Sleep
- Sleep pattern
- Social interaction
- Social isolation
- Sorrow
- Spiritual distress
- Spiritual well-being
- Spontaneous ventilation
- Stress
- Sudden infant death syndrome
- Suffocation

- Suicide
- Surgical recovery
- Swallowing
- **T**herapeutic regimen management
- Thermal injury
- Thermoregulation
- Tissue integrity
- Tissue perfusion
- Transfer ability
- Trauma
- **U**nilateral neglect
- Urinary elimination
- Urinary retention
- **V**ascular trauma
- Ventilatory weaning response
- Verbal communication
- **W**alking
- Wandering.

Axis 2: Subject of the Diagnosis

The subject of the diagnosis is defined as the person(s) for whom a nursing diagnosis is determined. The values in Axis 2 are individual, family, group, and community, representing the NANDA-I definition of "patient":

- *Individual*: a single human being distinct from others, a person.
- *Family*: two or more people having continuous or sustained relationships, perceiving reciprocal obligations, sensing common meaning, and sharing certain obligations toward others; related by blood and/or choice.
- *Group*: a number of people with shared characteristics.
- *Community*: a group of people living in the same locale under the same governance. Examples include neighborhoods and cities.

When the subject of the diagnosis is not explicitly stated, it becomes the individual by default. However, it is perfectly appropriate to consider such diagnoses for the other subjects of the diagnosis as well. The diagnosis *Grieving* could be applied to an individual or family who has lost a loved one. It could also be appropriate for a community that has experienced a mass casualty or suffered the loss of an important community leader, devastation due to natural disasters, or even the loss of a symbolic structure within the community (a school, religious structure, historic building, etc.).

Axis 3: Judgment

A judgment is a descriptor or modifier that limits or specifies the meaning of the diagnostic focus. The diagnostic focus together with the nurse's judgment about it forms the diagnosis. The values in Axis 3 are:

Value	Definition
Complicated	Intricately involved, complex
Compromised	Damaged, made vulnerable
Decreased	Lessened (in size, amount, or degree)
Defensive	Used or intended to defend or protect
Deficient/deficit	Insufficient, inadequate
Delayed	Late, slow, or postponed
Disabled	Limited, handicapped
Disorganized	Not properly arranged or controlled
Disproportionate	Too large or too small in comparison with the norm
Disturbed	Agitated, interrupted, interfered with
Dysfunctional	Not operating normally
Effective	Producing the intended or desired effect
Enhanced	Improved in quality, value, or extent
Excess	Greater than necessary or desirable
Failure	Cessation of proper functioning or performance
Imbalanced	Out of proportion or balance
Impaired	Damaged, weakened
Ineffective	Not producing the intended or desired effect
Insufficient	Quantity or quality that is not able to fulfill a need or requirement
Interrupted	Having its continuity broken
Low	Below the norm
Organized	Properly arranged or controlled
Perceived	Observed through the senses
Readiness for	In a suitable state for an activity or situation
Risk for	Increased danger, probability, or vulnerability
Situational	Related to a particular circumstance.

Axis 4: Location

Location describes the parts/regions of the body and/or their related functions – all tissues, organs, anatomical sites, or structures. The values in Axis 4 are:

- Auditory
- Bladder
- Body
- Bowel
- Breast
- Cardiac
- Cardiopulmonary
- Cerebral
- Dentition
- Gastrointestinal
- Gustatory
- Intracranial
- Kinesthetic

- Liver
- Mucous membranes
- Neurovascular
- Olfactory
- Oral
- Peripheral
- Peripheral vascular
- Renal
- Skin
- Tactile
- Tissue
- Vascular
- Verbal
- Visual
- Urinary.

Axis 5: Age

Age refers to the age of the person who is the subject of the diagnosis (Axis 2). The values in Axis 5 are:

- Fetus
- Neonate
- Infant
- Toddler
- Preschool child
- School-age child
- Adolescent
- Adult
- Older adult.

Axis 6: Time

Time describes the duration of the diagnostic concept (Axis 1). The values in Axis 6 are:

- *acute:* lasting less than 6 months;
- *chronic:* lasting more than 6 months;
- *intermittent:* stopping or starting again at intervals, periodic, cyclic;
- *continuous:* uninterrupted, going on without stopping.

Axis 7: Status of the Diagnosis

The status of the diagnosis refers to the actuality or potentiality of the problem/ syndrome or to the categorization of the diagnosis as a health promotion diagnosis. The values in Axis 7 are as follows:

- *Actual:* existing in fact or reality, existing at the present time.
- *Health promotion:* behavior motivated by the desire to increase well-being and actualize human health potential (Pender, Murdaugh & Parsons, 2006).
- *Risk:* vulnerability, especially as a result of exposure to factors that increase the chance of injury or loss.
- *Syndrome:* clinical judgment describing a specific cluster of nursing diagnoses that occur together, and are best addressed together and through similar interventions.
- *Wellness: NANDA International no longer defines a category of nursing diagnosis as a "wellness diagnosis." It was determined at the NANDA-I Think Tank meeting (2009) that this area of concern was already encompassed within the health-promotion nursing diagnosis category. This diagnosis type and definition were eliminated from the NANDA International taxonomy, and any wellness diagnoses were converted to health-promotion diagnoses.*

Construction of a Nursing Diagnostic Concept

A nursing diagnosis is constructed by combining the values from Axis 1 (the diagnostic focus), Axis 2 (subject of the diagnosis), and Axis 3 (judgment) where needed, and adding values from the other axes for relevant clarity. Thus, you start with the diagnostic focus (Axis 1) and add the judgment (Axis 3) about it. Remember that these two axes are sometimes combined into a single diagnostic concept, as can be seen with the nursing diagnosis *Fatigue*. Next, you specify the subject of the diagnosis (Axis 2). If the subject is an "individual," you need not make it explicit (Figure 1.4). You can then use the remaining axes, if they are appropriate, to add more detail. Figures 1.5 and 1.6 illustrate other examples, using the "risk" diagnoses (Figure 1.5) and "readiness for enhanced" diagnoses (Figure 1.6).

Please see Chapter 8, *The Process for Development of an Approved NANDA-I Nursing Diagnosis,* for a detailed explanation on the diagnosis submission process for new

Figure 1.4 *A NANDA-I nursing diagnosis model: (Individual) Ineffective Coping*

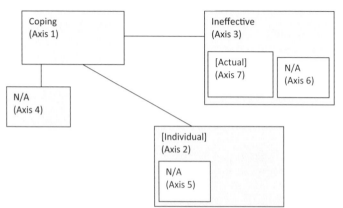

Figure 1.5 *A NANDA-I nursing diagnosis model: Risk for Disorganized Infant Behavior*

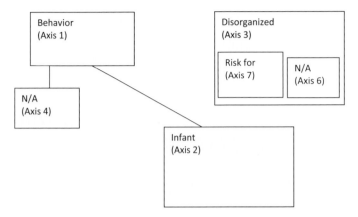

Figure 1.6 *A NANDA-I nursing diagnosis model: Readiness for Enhanced Family Coping*

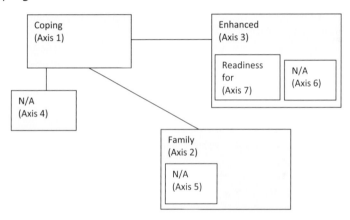

and revised diagnoses. It is also recommended that you review the submission guidelines posted on the NANDA-I website (www.nanda.org), as any updates that might be made to these guidelines after the publication of this text will be available at that location.

The NNN Taxonomy of Nursing Practice

The NANDA-I Taxonomy II appeared for the first time in *NANDA Nursing Diagnoses: Definitions and Classification, 2001–2002*. During this period, NANDA began to negotiate an alliance with the Classification Center at the College of Nursing, University of Iowa, Iowa City, Iowa (USA). As a part of that alliance, the possibility of developing a common taxonomic structure was explored. The purposes of a common structure are to make relationships among the three classifications – nursing diagnoses, nursing interventions, and nursing outcomes – visible, and to facilitate the linkage of the three systems. The possibilities were discussed among members of the NANDA Board of Directors and the leadership of the Classification Center.

Dr. Dorothy Jones, representing NANDA, and Dr. Joanne McCloskey, representing the Classification Center, developed a proposal to convene an invitational conference. The proposal was funded by the NLM, and a 3-day meeting was held in August 2001 at the Starved Rock Conference Center in Utica, Illinois. It was attended by 24 experts in standardized nursing language development, testing, and refinement. The goal was to develop a common taxonomic structure for nursing practice, including NANDA (nursing diagnoses), NIC (nursing interventions), and NOC (nursing outcomes), with the possibility of including other languages. A detailed account of the conference, as well as the history and development, can be found in *Unifying Nursing Languages: The Harmonization of NANDA, NIC, and NOC* (Dochterman and Jones, 2003).

The NANDA-I Taxonomy Committee met in January 2003 to place the nursing diagnoses from the *NANDA-I Nursing Diagnoses: Definitions and Classifications 2003–2004* into the NNN Taxonomy of Nursing Practice. The committee established rules governing the placement of the nursing diagnoses:

1. The nursing diagnosis definition, defining characteristics, or risk factors guide the placement of the nursing diagnosis.
2. When a nursing diagnosis bridges two or more domains, the Taxonomy Committee reviews the nursing diagnosis definition, defining characteristics, related factors or risk factors, and places it in the domain most clinically consistent with that information.
3. Upon review of the definition, defining characteristics or risk factors of a nursing diagnosis, if it is clinically consistent with two or more domains, the nursing diagnosis is placed where the practicing nurse would most expect to find it.
4. "Risk for" or "readiness for enhanced" nursing diagnoses are placed in the same domain and class as the actual nursing diagnosis, when one exists.

Table I.2 in the Introduction shows the placement of the 217 current nursing diagnosis approved by NANDA-I in the NNN Taxonomy of Nursing Practice.

Further Development of the NANDA-I Taxonomy

A taxonomy and a multiaxial framework for developing nursing diagnoses allows clinicians to see where gaps exist in the taxonomy, and provides the opportunity to develop clinically useful new diagnoses. If you construct a new diagnosis that is useful to your practice, please submit it to NANDA-I so that others can share in the discovery. Submission guidelines are found in Chapter 8, *The Process for Development of an Approved NANDA-I Nursing Diagnosis.* Submission forms and information can also be found on the NANDA-I website (www.nanda.org). The DDC will be glad to help you prepare the submission. For assistance and/or questions, contact the DDC committee chair through the NANDA-I website.

References

Dochterman, J.M., & Jones, D. (eds) (2003). *Unifying nursing languages: The harmonization of NANDA, NIC, and NOC*. Washington, DC: American Nurses Association.

Gordon, M. (1998). *Manual of nursing diagnosis*. St. Louis: Mosby.

Lundberg, C., Warren, J., Brokel, J., Bulechek, G., Butcher, H., Dochterman, J., Johnson, M., Maas, M., Martin, K., Moorhead, S., Spisla, C., Swanson, E., & Giarrizzo-Wilson, S. (2008). Selecting a standardized terminology for the electronic health record that reveals the impact of nursing on patient care. *Online Journal of Nursing Informatics, 12*(2). Available at http://ojni.org/12_2/lundberg.pdf.

Merriam-Webster (2009). *Merriam-Webster's collegiate dictionary* (11th ed.). Springfield, MA: Merriam-Webster.

NANDA (2001). *NANDA nursing diagnoses: Definitions and classifications 2001–2002*. Philadelphia: NANDA.

NANDA International (2003). *NANDA International Nursing Diagnoses: Definitions and Classifications 2003–2004*. Philadelphia: NANDA International.

Pender, N.J., Murdaugh, C.L., & Parsons, M.A. (2006). *Health promotion in nursing practice* (5th ed.). Upper Saddle River, NJ: Pearson Prentice-Hall.

Von Krogh, G. (2008). An examination of the NANDA International Taxonomy for domain completeness, ontological homogeneity, and clinical functionality. *International Journal of Nursing Terminologies and Classifications, 19*, 65–75.

Part 2

Education and Implementation of NANDA International Nursing Diagnoses within Practice, Administration, Research, Informatics and Education

NANDA International Nursing Diagnoses: Definitions & Classification 2012–2014, First Edition.
Edited by T. Heather Herdman.
© 2012 NANDA International. Published 2012 by Blackwell Publishing Ltd.

In this section, we present chapters that are written with three audiences in mind. Chapters address the needs of students, current nurses, and nurse educators. The accompanying text website features presentation materials to supplement the information provided in each chapter.

Chapter 2 Nursing Assessment, Clinical Judgment, and Nursing Diagnoses: How to Determine Accurate Diagnoses

Margaret Lunney

In this chapter, Dr. Lunney discusses the importance of competencies in clinical judgment and diagnostic reasoning, and the need for nurses to engage in reflective practice. The critical link between holistic nursing assessment and nursing diagnostic accuracy is made, as the need to work with patients and families throughout the nursing process is emphasized. Using the Functional Health Pattern assessment framework (Gordon, 2010), Lunney walks students, clinicians, and educators through a case study that focuses on data collection, hypothesis generation, diagnostic accuracy, and validation. Study tools are available to complement this chapter, including presentation materials and a video showing a real patient scenario with a nurse utilizing the Functional Health Pattern assessment framework to determine patient diagnosis. The video, with commentary throughout by an expert in critical thinking, is a wonderful tool to use with students as they are learning to do focused assessments to identify nursing diagnoses in their patients.

Chapter 3 Nursing Diagnosis in Education

Barbara Krainovich-Miller, Fritz Frauenfelder, Maria Müller-Staub

Written primarily for nurse educators, the authors build on the work in Chapter 2 and provide several teaching strategies for successful learning of the nursing process and specifically of nursing diagnostic reasoning and clinical judgment. The importance of prioritization of diagnoses is discussed, as is the linkage to nursing-sensitive patient outcomes and nursing interventions. Study tools are available to complement this chapter.

Chapter 4 The Value of Nursing Diagnoses in Electronic Health Records

Jane M. Brokel, Kay C. Avant, Matthias Odenbreit

This chapter discusses various ways in which the representations of nursing clinical judgments are integrated into electronic health records. Strategies are outlined for undergraduate and graduate students, educators, and nursing informatics clinical specialists. The realities of the variation in vendor solutions are discussed, along with methods to ensure that nursing content is included in the record. Study tools are available to complement this chapter.

Chapter 5 Nursing Diagnosis and Research

Margaret Lunney, Maria Müller-Staub

The authors discuss the need for ongoing research to improve the evidence base of the NANDA-I Taxonomy of nursing diagnoses. Research discussed includes concept analyses, content validation, construct-related, criterion-related, and consensus validation studies. Additionally, studies that establish the sensitivity, specificity, and predictive value of clinical indicators in specific populations, studies of accuracy of nurses' diagnoses, and implementation studies are reviewed. Study tools are available to complement this chapter.

Chapter 6 Clinical Judgment and Nursing Diagnoses in Nursing Administration

T. Heather Herdman, Marcelo Chanes

The authors discuss the implications of the use of data derived from standardized nursing terminologies in making administrative decisions within nursing. As the focus on patient safety – and nursing's role as a leader in that area – continues to sharpen, the authors argue that nurse administrators must understand the importance of proper use and implementation of nursing language that represents the clinical judgment of nurses in practice. Information that can be derived from data embedded within NANDA-I, NOC, and NIC classifications are discussed in light of the need to justify nursing salaries, and to support nursing models of care. The need for nurse executives and managers to support the implementation, utilization, and evaluation of care and of nurse practice is also discussed. Study tools are available to complement this chapter.

Chapter 7 Nursing Classifications: Criteria and Evaluation

Matthias Odenbreit, Maria Müller Staub, Jane C. Brokel, Kay M. Avant, Gail Keenan

The explosion of electronic health records into clinical settings worldwide is posing a variety of challenges to nurses in practice today. Critical among these challenges is the need to ensure the availability of nursing classification systems that support safe, point-of-care documentation of evidence-based clinical judgments. The authors review several classification schemes and review the literature to provide some key decision points for those who are faced with the challenge of determining which nursing classification terminologies will best meet the need of nurses providing clinical care. Often the individuals tasked with the decision-making do not have significant knowledge about the pros and cons of various classifications, and may only look at one or two criteria in making a selection. A broad range of criteria, supported in the nursing literature, is discussed, and systems are reviewed using a literature-based classification matrix.

Chapter 2

Nursing Assessment, Clinical Judgment, and Nursing Diagnoses: How to Determine Accurate Diagnoses

Margaret Lunney

The nursing process describes how nurses organize the care of individuals, families, groups, and communities. This process has been broadly accepted by nurses since 1967 (Yura & Walsh, 1967). Initially, the nursing process was described as having four components: assessment, planning, implementation, and evaluation. But soon after, nurse leaders recognized that the meaning of assessment data had to be identified before planning and interventions could occur. Currently, the nursing process is described as a five-part cyclical process that includes assessment, diagnosis, planning, implementation, and evaluation (American Nurses Association, 2010; Doenges & Moorhouse, 2008; Wilkinson, 2007).

Nurses identify the meaning of assessment data through the use of clinical judgment. Clinical judgment is defined as "an interpretation or conclusion about a patient's needs, concerns, or health problems, and/or the decision to take action (or not), use or modify standard approaches, or improvise new ones as deemed appropriate by the patient's response" (Tanner, 2006, p. 204). Nurses continuously use clinical judgment to make sense of assessment data as the basis for providing nursing interventions to achieve positive health outcomes.

In every instance of helping people to be healthy, nurses must interpret assessment data because all human beings, including nurses, have limited capacities in both short-term and working memory (Jarrold & Towse, 2006). Short-term memory is the "ability to store or maintain information over a limited time period" (p. 39). Working memory is the "ability to hold information in mind, while manipulating and integrating other information in the service of a cognitive goal" (p. 39). Cognitive goals in nursing include determining a patient's response to a health problem, or which interventions will be most helpful. A simple example to illustrate how quickly and easily people can mentally move from collecting data to data interpretation is interpreting whether a person is female or male. This interpretation is based on over 20 bits of data, for example hair and dress styles, body language, facial structure, name, and voice. We do not remember the bits of data; we only remember the interpretation – male or female.

If a nurse decides to assist a patient to move from a bed to a chair, this is based on an interpretation of data indicating that the patient wants or needs to be out of bed and needs assistance with moving from bed to chair. Some of the data that a nurse might use for this interpretation are that the patient is one day post-operative abdominal surgery, the patient has reported pain, and the patient has said that she or he feels

NANDA International Nursing Diagnoses: Definitions & Classification 2012–2014, First Edition.
Edited by T. Heather Herdman.
© 2012 NANDA International. Published 2012 by Blackwell Publishing Ltd.

"shaky." Nursing diagnoses are scientific interpretations of assessment data that are used to guide nurses' planning, implementation, and evaluation. For example, nurses mentally replace data such as bluish skin color, high respiratory effort, and orthopnea with interpretations of the data, such as *Ineffective Breathing Pattern*.

Only six years after Yura and Walsh's description of the nursing process in 1967, two nurses from St. Louis, Missouri, USA – Mary Ann Lavin and Kristine Gebbie – organized the first invitational conference of 100 nurses from the United States and Canada to identify the interpretations of data that represent the phenomena of concern to nurses (Gebbie, 1998). This was the first conference on nursing diagnosis, out of which 80 nursing diagnoses were identified and defined. Since then, the list of approved diagnoses has been steadily refined and grown through regular meetings and the work of members of the nursing diagnosis association that sponsors this book, now known as NANDA International (NANDA-I). This chapter describes nurses as diagnosticians, identifies the competencies needed for the nursing process, the personal strengths of tolerance for ambiguity and reflective practice, and the relation of assessment and accurate nursing diagnoses. A case study illustrates application of assessment and clinical judgment, leading to accuracy in nursing diagnosis.

Nurses Are Diagnosticians

With use of the term "nursing diagnosis," it became apparent that nurses are diagnosticians. Prior to that time, the clinical judgment used in clinical practice to decide the focus of nursing care was invisible or not named. Today, in healthcare agencies where nurses do not use nursing diagnoses, or use them without a concern for accuracy, the invisibility of the nurses' role as a diagnostician may still exist. With the start of this formal classification of nursing diagnoses, however, it was broadly accepted that nurses are diagnosticians who need to use the diagnostic process and work in partnership with the people they serve to identify the best diagnoses to guide nursing care.

The diagnostic process in nursing differs from the diagnostic process in medicine in that, in a majority of situations, the person or persons who are the focus of nursing care should be intimately involved as partners with nurses in the assessment and diagnostic process. This is because the focus of nursing care is the whole person or persons' achievement of well-being and self-actualization. People's experiences and responses to heath problems and life processes have specific meanings to them, and these meanings are identified with the help of nurses (Hobbs, 2009; Stefancyk, 2009). It is also assumed that nurses do not make people healthy with their diagnoses and interventions; people make themselves healthy with their own behaviors. Thus, to achieve positive changes in behaviors that affect health, people and nurses together identify the most accurate diagnoses that have potential to guide nursing care for the achievement of positive health outcomes. Nursing interventions for diagnoses of human responses offer additional ways, besides treating medical problems, that the health of people can be promoted, protected, and restored.

The focus of nursing is the "health" of "human beings," two of the most complex scientific concerns, more complex, for example, than chemistry and astronomy. Health-related phenomena, such as sleep, comfort, or nutrition, are complex because they involve human experiences. We can never know for sure what other human beings are experiencing; yet nursing's goal is to identify people's experiences or responses in order to support them. With human responses, there is also a tremendous overlap of cues to diagnoses and many contextual factors such as culture that can change the perspective of "What is the diagnosis?" It has been verified that interpretations of clinical cases have the potential to be less accurate than is indicated by the data (Lunney, 2008).

With nursing diagnoses serving as the foundation of nursing care, nurses need to develop diagnostic competencies in order to become good diagnosticians. Diagnosticians are people who interpret data within their fields of expertise in order to provide needed services. For example, an automobile mechanic must be able to diagnose why the car will not start in order to be able to fix it. A key element of data interpretations is that they are subject to error. A good diagnostician must be mindful that there are always risks to the accuracy of data interpretations. Becoming a nurse diagnostician, therefore, requires the development of professional and personal skills and characteristics.

Two propositions are the basis for development of diagnostic competencies:

- Diagnosis in nursing requires competencies in intellectual, interpersonal, and technical domains.
- Diagnosis in nursing requires development of the personal strengths of tolerance for ambiguity and use of reflective practice.

Intellectual, Interpersonal, and Technical Competencies

Intellectual Competencies

Intellectual competencies are discussed first because this is an invisible aspect of nursing that is very important for becoming a diagnostician. Intellectual skills include both knowledge of nursing diagnoses and the mental processes for use of that knowledge. Nurses need to attain knowledge of diagnoses, their definitions, and defining characteristics, especially diagnoses that are common to the populations with which they work, the interventions to treat the diagnoses, and the diagnostic processes that are used to interpret patient data. This knowledge is extensive and complex, so nurses are not expected to memorize the available knowledge; rather, they need to know how to access the information they need, and the resources to obtain this knowledge should be available when needed.

Besides knowledge, thinking ability is the other important aspect of the intellectual domain. Even though, traditionally, thinking processes have not been emphasized in nursing, they are essential to the use of nursing diagnoses. The cognitive skills of analyzing, logical reasoning, and applying standards are just three of the thinking processes that are needed for accurate diagnosis in nursing (Scheffer & Rubenfeld, 2000; Tanner, 2006). These skills are developed, for example, through discussions of how data should be clustered to generate accurate diagnoses, the relation of data clusters to diagnoses, and comparisons of existing data to expected data based on research findings. Research findings in cognitive science and nursing show that adults at the same levels of education and experience vary in their thinking abilities (Jarrold & Towse, 2006; Lunney, 1992; Sternberg, 1997; Willingham, 2007).

Research findings from cognitive science and other disciplines also show that thinking processes can be improved (Sternberg, 1997; Willingham, 2007). In nursing, research studies have shown that critical thinking abilities vary widely, and that critical thinking and clinical judgment can be improved with education and effort (Tanner, 2006). This can be achieved through energy, focus, and support. To do this, students and nurses need to think about their thinking, referred to as *metacognition* (Kuiper & Pesut, 2004). This is done by using the concepts of thinking that are relevant to nursing practice. A Delphi study of nurse experts in critical thinking (Rubenfeld & Scheffer, 2010; Scheffer & Rubenfeld, 2000) generated seven cognitive skills and 10 habits of mind that were considered as highly relevant to nursing practice. These 17 concepts of thinking should be used by nurses to think about their thinking. In any nursing situation, two or more cognitive skills are probably being used. The habits of mind support the cognitive skills. The combinations of these critical thinking abilities that are needed for clinical situations are probably unique, so nurses need to cultivate all these critical thinking processes and not just focus on a few of them (Lunney, 2010).

Critical thinking abilities are essential to achieve accurate interpretations of patient data and appropriate selection of interventions and outcomes, so developing high-level thinking abilities is a high priority. To do this, nurses and nursing students can:

- use thinking processes, rather than just receiving knowledge from others;
- when learning, think about the concepts rather than just memorizing knowledge;
- seek support from others, including teachers, other nurses, and patients, to validate their thinking processes;
- develop confidence in their ability to think.

Interpersonal Competencies

Nursing diagnoses are best used by nurses who have exquisite interpersonal communication skills. Such skills are needed so that patients will trust nurses enough to tell them about their responses to health problems and life processes. Trust is enhanced through a mature ability to communicate with others.

Nurses must assume that they do not know other people (Munhall, 1993). The only way other people can be known is through interpersonal processes, especially listening. Nurses who assume that they know patients without listening to them will not achieve accuracy of diagnosis. The best use of nursing diagnoses is in partnership with patients, families, groups, and communities. Many case study examples of working in partnership with patients and families are provided in the book by Lunney and contributors (2009). To work in partnership, nurses need to speak to people with respect and care, listen effectively, respect the opinions and views of others, and know how to validate perceptions with patients and families. Learning these skills is a challenge, so the interpersonal aspects of nursing need to be an integral part of learning to use nursing diagnoses.

Technical Competencies

Another baseline competency is the technical skill of conducting a nursing assessment. Obtaining valid and reliable data is the backbone of using nursing diagnoses, so nurses' development of the ability to conduct comprehensive and focused health histories and physical examinations is essential. This technical skill is learned in courses on the topic and through the use of nursing textbooks that focus on health assessment within a nursing framework. For example, the diagnosis and treatment of pain requires sophisticated assessment knowledge, including ways to explore the types and locations of pain, the factors that make the pain worse or better, etc. The same is true of many of the diagnostic concepts such as *Disturbed Body Image*.

An assessment is a "nursing" assessment if it yields the data that are needed for nursing care. The assessment data that are generated by a biological systems review, which is carried out to yield medical diagnoses, are insufficient to yield the data needed for nursing diagnoses. Thus, other assessment frameworks, such as Functional Health Patterns (Gordon, 2007), are being used in healthcare systems where the accuracy of nurses' diagnoses is considered important. The Functional Health Patterns framework is used with the case study example at the end of the chapter to demonstrate how to generate nursing diagnoses from assessment data.

Personal Strengths: Tolerance for Ambiguity and Reflective Practice

The personal strengths of tolerance for ambiguity and reflective practice need to be developed because decisions are so complex in nursing and the use of clinical judgment needs to be an ongoing learning process. Each decision that nurses make is relative to the context of the situation and to the specific nature of the individual, family, group, or community with whom they are working. With experience, nurses become familiar with many types of contextual situations that can positively influence diagnostic abilities. Tolerance for ambiguity and reflective practice enables nurses to incorporate these contextual experiences to advance their professional development from novice to expert (Benner, 1984; Benner, Tanner & Chelsea, 1996, 2009).

Tolerance for Ambiguity

Tolerance for ambiguity is needed because there are numerous factors that influence clinical situations, such as agency policies, the nurses' job description, the nursing scope of practice or standards of care, and the availability of resources. Tolerance for ambiguity enables nurses to consider the broad range of influencing factors within the diagnostic process and to be able to focus on the most accurate diagnoses for quality-based services for individuals, families, and communities.

In addition, the human beings for whom nurses provide care are extremely complex and diverse, especially when the focus is the person's response or experience and not the illness itself. Ambiguity is expected, so nurses need to adjust to it. In studies of uncertainty, fear of negative evaluation by others has been identified as a cause of ambiguity aversion (Trautmann, Vieider & Wakker, 2008). Nurse leaders and teachers can help students and nurses to improve tolerance for ambiguity by decreasing the fear of negative evaluation by others, pointing out that ambiguity is the reality of being a nurse, and by role modeling tolerance for ambiguity.

Reflective Practice

Reflective practice is a process of re-examining feelings and behaviors in relation to clinical events for the purposes of planning for future events (Beam, O'Brien, & Neal, 2010). Reflective practice is a prerequisite for self-evaluation, and to accomplish it, we must to some extent expose ourselves, our frailties, and our mistakes. Reflective practice supports continuous development or growth in clinical judgment with the assumption that we benefit by thinking about our own behaviors, which includes diagnostic reasoning (Tanner, 2006).

Assessment and Nursing Diagnosis

Nursing assessments at all levels of analysis – individual, family, and community – consist of subjective data from the person or persons, and objective data from diagnostic tests and other sources. Assessments of individuals consist of a health history (subjective data) and a physical examination (objective data) (Weber & Kelley, 2009). Family assessments consist of obtaining specific information from the family members (subjective data) and observing family interactions (objective data) (Wright & Leahey, 2009). Assessments of communities consist of obtaining information from key informants within the community (subjective data) and statistical data (objective data) (Anderson & McFarlane, 2010).

There are two types of assessment that are carried out to generate accurate nursing diagnoses: comprehensive and focused. Comprehensive assessments cover all aspects of a nursing assessment framework such as the 11 Functional Health Patterns (Gordon, 2007) to determine the health status of the individual, family, group, or community. Comprehensive assessments of individuals are done, for example, when admitting a patient to a hospital or to home-care services. Focused assessments concentrate on a particular issue or concern, such as pain, sleep, or respiratory status. Focused assessments are done when specific symptoms need to be explored further, such as when a person says "I am having difficulty with breathing," or something generates an increased risk for a particular problem, such as when a person needs an anticoagulant medication, which leads to an increased risk of bleeding.

The goals for a nursing assessment are as follows:

- It focuses on the data needed to identify the human responses and experiences
- It is conducted in partnership with the individual, family, group or community
- The findings are based on research and other evidence.

Assessment Framework

For nursing, assessment frameworks need to be broad enough to yield data to guide nursing care for health promotion, health protection (primary, secondary, and tertiary prevention), and health restoration. Health promotion focuses on the positive aspects of increasing health or self-actualization (Pender, Murdaugh & Parsons, 2011). An example of a health-promotion diagnosis is *Readiness for Enhanced Sleep*. Health protection is a process of helping people to reduce risks to health and protect themselves from existing risk states (Pender, Murdaugh & Parsons, 2011). An example of a diagnosis in the realm of health protection is *Risk for Infection*. Health restoration, also referred to as illness management, is a process of helping people to manage health problems. The actual (problem) nursing diagnoses such as *Pain, Anxiety, Fear,* and *Ineffective Self-Health Management* are examples of diagnoses in the realm of health restoration.

A nursing assessment framework that is widely used to generate accurate nursing diagnoses is the Functional Health Patterns Framework (Gordon, 2007). This framework includes 11 patterns of individuals (see the Appendix), families, groups and communities.

Diagnostic Reasoning Associated with Nursing Assessment

The diagnostic reasoning associated with nursing assessment involves recognizing the existence of cues, mentally generating possible diagnoses, comparing cues to possible diagnoses, conducting a focused data collection, and validating diagnoses. The principles to include throughout the process are the following:

- The individual, family, group, or community is involved throughout the assessment and diagnostic processes.
- Diagnostic hypotheses are considered throughout the assessment process and are used along with a formal assessment guide to generate the data needed for diagnoses.
- In a comprehensive assessment, diagnoses are not finalized until completion of the assessment. Assessment of each pattern informs the nurse and patient about the diagnostic hypotheses.

Recognizing the Existence of Cues

Nurses *mentally recognize* cues early in the diagnostic process and continue to integrate cue recognition throughout the process. Cues are units of data (e.g., a person's rate of breathing) that a nurse collects during intentional or unintentional assessment. Intentional assessment involves deliberate collection of data as a foundation for nursing actions. Unintentional assessment involves noticing cues that are important without planning to do so. In clinical situations, nurses notice cues to diagnoses by thinking about what they see, hear, smell, touch, and taste. Information pertaining to the healthcare consumer is *thought about* in relation to the *nurse's knowledge* of the health state or life situation of the consumer. Nurses attend to information based on established ideas of what should occur in various situations. A nurse may not notice a person's rate of breathing, for example, unless it looks unusual in the context of a health problem (e.g., if the individual is one day postoperative abdominal surgery) or other aspects of the clinical situation (such as when the individual has just completed vigorous exercise). A nurse's recognition of a unit of data as a cue with special meaning is dependent on *knowledge stored in memory*. Knowledge bases in memory are used for the comparison of current data with expected data.

Mentally Generating Possible Diagnoses

The meaning that nurses assign to cues noticed early in the diagnostic process can only be understood if there are possible and plausible explanations for the cues within the context of the situation. This is an *active thinking process* whereby the nurse explores knowledge in memory for possible explanations of data. Often, there are many possible diagnoses or explanations that may be considered. Sometimes, there is only one plausible meaning for cues noticed early in the diagnostic process. For example, if a woman who is newly admitted to a hospital unit for a surgical procedure is rapidly asking the nurse many questions, and exhibits a fast rate of breathing, the cues are not specific enough to consider only one possible diagnosis. The nurse in this instance would consider a number of possible explanations for this set of cues, such as *Fear, Anxiety, Ineffective Breathing Pattern*, and others. A nurse diagnostician avoids deciding on a diagnosis prematurely, that is, before there are sufficient data to support a diagnostic judgment. Flexibility of thinking enables nurses to make a broad search of the mind for possible diagnoses. Logical reasoning in collaboration with the patient enables nurses to derive the most accurate diagnosis when the data are sufficient to do so.

Comparing Cues to Possible Diagnoses

Cues are analyzed in relation to possible diagnoses through a *mental process of evaluation*. Evaluation involves a process of mental matching wherein the existing cues are matched with the expected cues for the diagnoses being considered. Information about the expected cues to diagnoses is found in this book and current literature on specific phenomena such as *pain, coping,* and *fluid volume*. During the evaluation of cues and related diagnoses, nurses may decide that there is not enough evidence to make a diagnostic decision *or* that there is enough evidence for one likely diagnosis. If a nurse decides that there are not enough data to make a diagnosis, the next step involves a focused search for additional cues. If a nurse decides that there is enough supporting evidence, a diagnosis is made and then validated.

Conducting a Focused Data Collection

In order to confirm or rule out diagnoses that are under consideration, additional cues may be collected by focusing questions to obtain data for one or more diagnoses. With the preoperative patient mentioned above, for example, the nurse might ask the patient how she feels about the surgical procedure. The answer to a broad question such as this can yield data to support many possible diagnoses in the psychosocial realm. If the patient mentions fear of death or fear of anesthesia risks in relation to the surgery, the nurse can begin to confirm *Fear* as the diagnosis and eliminate some of the other possibilities such as *Anxiety*. When the nurse conducts a medical history and physical examination, biological reasons for the fast respiratory rate can also be confirmed or ruled out. A focused data collection concludes when the nurse synthesizes available data and selects one of the diagnoses being considered, rules out all of the diagnoses being considered, or revises the diagnoses being considered to incorporate new diagnoses. If a diagnosis under consideration is supported through focused data collection, the next step is to validate the diagnosis. If all of the diagnoses are ruled out or not confirmed, new diagnoses are considered or the nurse concludes that there is no diagnosis. If new diagnoses are considered, a focused data collection continues until the revised set of diagnoses are confirmed or ruled out through supporting evidence (cues).

Validating Diagnoses

Since human behavior is complex and nurses cannot truly "know" what other people are experiencing (Munhall, 1993), it is important that nurses' thinking and technical processes be accompanied by collaborative interpersonal processes with consumers and other providers. In most instances, nurses should validate diagnoses with healthcare consumers. For example, a nurse may say: "From the information you have just given me, it seems that you are experiencing *Fear* associated with surgery. Is that correct?" Based upon the patient's response, the nurse validates or refutes the diagnosis. In cases when patients are unable to collaborate with nurses because they are too sick, developmentally unable, or mentally incompetent, nurses can validate diagnoses with family members or other providers. For example, a nurse may say: "From the information you have given me about your son, it seems that he is having difficulty coping with the stress of the illness. Is that correct?" To validate with another provider, a nurse may say: "From my physical examination, I concluded that Mary's airway clearance is impaired. Do you agree?" Validation of diagnoses with others helps to ensure the accuracy of the diagnoses as the bases for subsequent stages of the nursing process. In order to save the time, energy, and costs associated with interventions for diagnoses, diagnoses should be validated as highly accurate.

Case Study Example

The following case study was developed by Maria Cruz, BS, RN, who was a bachelor's degree student at the College of Staten Island when she wrote this case study. The Functional Health Pattern Assessment tool in the Appendix was used to collect data.

CW is a 30-year-old male who currently works in the marketing department for a major credit card company in Manhattan. He attends a university part time in the evenings to complete his Master's degree in business administration.

CW believes he is in good general health, and being healthy is very important to him. The last time he was "sick" was last fall when he had a head cold. CW maintains his health status by trying to eat healthily, exercising at a gym, and maintaining good personal hygiene. He limits his intake of alcohol to social occasions and says he smokes "once in a blue moon."

He has psoriasis, a skin condition that he developed as a child. Currently, he has a large patch on his left shin that is dry, scaly, and very itchy. He stated that the last time he saw the dermatologist was two years ago and that he really should see him more often. He "put it off" because he knows the condition is chronic. CW is taking two medications on a regular basis, Pandel Cream, a class 5 steroid cream that he occasionally uses for the psoriasis, and minoxidil for his thinning hair. He uses the cream whenever the psoriasis "acts up," which temporarily relieves itching. He has expressed the possibility and desire to better manage flare-ups of the psoriasis.

CW has a family history of mental illness and of becoming overweight. Both his grandmothers were diagnosed with depression, and they are on many medications. His father is very heavy now, but when he was younger he was fit and healthy. CW fears that the same may happen to him.

CW has expressed concern about maintaining his health status, but he has not had a physical examination in over two years. He stated that if he feels well he sees no reason to go to a physician. Because psoriasis is a chronic condition, he sometimes feels that the lesions will occur no matter what he does. According to him, the cream is messy and stains everything, which are barriers to using the cream. With regards to self-efficacy, CW is capable of using the cream, but he has not committed to doing so. The fact that the cream is messy and stains creates a negative activity-related affect for CW.

CW tries to eat balanced meals but finds it difficult sometimes because of his hectic work and school schedule. He eats low-fat, low-sugar, and low-sodium foods, which are good sources of protein, and dairy products. A typical day's meals include vegetables and fruits, and CW has a "weakness" for sweets and desserts. He has a good appetite, and in order to maintain his weight he has been going to WeightWatchers for the past year. He has reached his goal weight for his height and needs to "stick to a plan" to stay there. He sometimes has difficulties making healthy choices at the supermarket because there are too many things to choose from, but he loves to cook and try new things. He bites his nails when he feels stressed.

CW's pattern of urine elimination is within normal limits, voiding light yellow urine about five times per day. He has no trouble moving his bowels, although he does have small hemorrhoids, which bother him from time to time.

CW has a daily routine of walking to the bus stop, which is about three blocks away, to go to work. He sits at a desk most of the day, but goes to the gym three times a week for a cardiovascular workout. He also enjoys taking his dog on walks. Three nights a week, he attends college classes. He loves going out to dinner with friends and family, going to the movies, or watching movies at home. He is a frequent traveler to local destinations such as Atlantic City, and he also likes going to travel internationally.

During the week, CW usually gets about eight hours of sleep each night, and, on the weekend, he sleeps longer. CW uses a sound machine that makes "white noise" to help him fall asleep. He started using this when he first moved to the city from a more rural part of New York, because all the night sounds in the city made it difficult for him to fall asleep. Even though he now lives in a quiet area, he says he cannot sleep without the soothing sounds the machine makes. Because of his schedule, CW does not find too much time to rest during the day, but he takes a nap on the bus while commuting.

CW's senses are within normal limits. CW has perfect ("20-20") vision, and his hearing is normal. He denies any problems with his sense of taste, touch, or smell, and denies having pain.

CW has a positive self-perception and moderate self-esteem. He describes himself as an extroverted, spontaneous, family-oriented person with an intimate social circle of friends and colleagues. His strengths include his determination and his "all or nothing" attitude. He is ambitious, although he feels he is also simple and modest. Sometimes, he says, "I spread myself too thin," trying to accomplish too many things at one time. This may add to his feelings of being easily distracted and having trouble focusing at work. His physical self is also somewhat positive. He is happy about his general appearance, height, and symmetrical body. He feels he has too much body hair, but not enough hair on his head, and tries to hide the patches of psoriasis: for example, he wears jeans, not shorts.

At work, CW assumes a leadership role when he leads his marketing team. As a student, he deals with responsibilities of going to class and doing assignments. He is proud of being a homeowner. He describes his relationships as loving, peaceful, supportive, open, and nonconflictual. He is the youngest of three children, and he has a close relationship with his mother and sisters. Overall, he is happy and satisfied with these aspects of his life, although he wishes he were closer to his dad. He gets a lot of support from family, friends, and his partner.

CW states he has no concerns regarding sexuality. He practices safe sex and is currently in a committed relationship.

Currently, CW has a long list of stressors. He has to balance the stress of school and work, and is in the process of selling his house and buying a new one before the end of the summer. He has shared that, like any relationship, he feels stressed about helping his partner with goals such as getting US citizenship, and passing the driver's license test. He feels that the daily routine of keeping up with the responsibilities of owning a house and going to work and school adds to his stress level, which he rates as moderate. In dealing with stress, he has one bad habit, biting his nails. On the positive side, he tries to get things done so work does not "pile up," and he takes frequent vacations. Despite all of these stressors, he feels that he thrives on them, not that they hold him back or have a negative impact on his health.

CW's cultural and family traditions promote a balance between hard work and rest. He is not very religious, and he is unsure how religion plays a role in his health. At this point in life, he feels his goals are being met and he is satisfied with his health status.

Analysis of Health Data: Nursing Diagnoses

There were several NANDA-I diagnoses that the nurse considered, including: *Impaired Skin Integrity, Ineffective Health Maintenance, Deficient Knowledge, Disturbed Body Image, Powerlessness, Readiness for Enhanced Coping*, and *Readiness for Enhanced Self-Health Management* (Herdman, 2009). *Impaired Skin Integrity* is not the best diagnosis to guide nursing care because the problem of psoriasis mostly requires medical interventions. *Ineffective Health Maintenance* was rejected because CW generally has a healthy lifestyle. Although *Deficient Knowledge* was considered as a diagnosis, it is more appropriate as a contributing factor to his management of therapeutic regimen for psoriasis, and there is not very much that the nurse can teach him that he does not already know. There are not enough data to support the diagnoses of *Disturbed Body Image* and *Powerlessness*, and, since CW perceives that he has no health problems, a health-promotion diagnosis is more appropriate. Even though CW admits to having a lot of stress, he includes many stress-management techniques in his daily routines, so there is less data support for *Readiness for Enhanced Coping* than *Readiness for Enhanced Self-Health Management*. This diagnosis, defined as "a pattern of regulating and integrating into daily living a program for treatment of illness and its sequelae that is sufficient for meeting health-related goals and can be strengthened," is the one that CW and I decided to address.

Defining characteristics for *Readiness for Enhanced Self-Health Management* are that CW expressed a desire to want to change how he manages his skin condition and an awareness that, perhaps, the number of flare-ups could be reduced. His sporadic pattern of treatment may not be the most effective, and there may be newer easier treatments for him to consider. In addition, CW already maintains his health in a number of ways, which reduces his risk for the condition to worsen.

Interpersonal influences that can have an impact on CW's behavior are his partner, his family, and his dermatologist (Pender et al., 2011). Perhaps his family and significant other could support and encourage him to use the cream daily by reminding him and reinforcing positive outcomes. One situational influence in this case is that since CW has not been to his physician in a long time, he may not be aware of other possible options available, which may be even more effective than his current treatment.

Nursing Outcomes Classification

Based on our discussion, we decided to use the Nursing Outcomes Classification outcome *Health-Promoting Behavior* (1602), defined as "Personal actions to sustain or increase wellness" (Moorhead, Johnson, Maas & Swanson, 2008, p. 384). The outcome scale is: 1 = never demonstrated, 2 = rarely demonstrated, 3 = sometimes demonstrated, 4 = often demonstrated, and 5 = consistently demonstrated. CW's score on the overall outcome is 3, and his goal is 5. For indicator 160207, "Performs healthy behaviors routinely," he is at level 3, and his goal is 5. For indicator 160213, "Obtains recommended health screenings," CW is currently at 2, and his goal is 5.

Nursing Interventions Classification

To achieve the desired outcome, we chose the Nursing Interventions Classification intervention of *Patient Contracting*, defined as "Negotiating an agreement with an individual that reinforces a specific behavior change" (Bulechek, Butcher & Dochterman, 2008, p. 541). The activities for this intervention that were used are to help CW to identify the health practice he wishes to change, that is, better management of his skin condition, and to identify the goals of care. For CW, one goal is to see his dermatologist on a regular basis and to find a way to treat his skin condition that he can routinely use. During our discussion, we learned that some barriers exist for CW to carry out his current plan, and perhaps developing a regimen with these barriers in mind will help to improve management. It is important for the nurse to assist CW in developing a plan to meet the goals, and to facilitate a written contract with all agreed-upon elements. Another activity is to assist CW in developing a flow chart, through use of a journal to record his skin condition and daily use of the cream. Perhaps this would help show him if continued use would have a better effect than sporadic use. Finally, we coordinated opportunities to review the contract and goals. This gives CW and me a chance to see his progress and whether or not his plan is working.

References

American Nurses Association. (2010). *Nursing: Scope and standards of practice* (2nd ed.). Washington, DC: Nurses Books.com.

Anderson, E.T., & McFarlane, J.A. (2010). *Community as partner: Theory and practice in nursing* (6th ed.). Philadelphia: Lippincott Williams & Wilkins.

Beam, R.J., O'Brien, R.A., & Neal, M. (2010). Reflective practice enhances public health nurse implementation of nurse-family partnership. *Public Health Nursing, 27*, 131–139.

Benner, P. (1984). *From novice to expert: Excellence and power in clinical nursing practice*. Menlo Park, CA: Addison-Wesley.

Benner P., Tanner C.A., & Chelsea C.A. (1996). *Expertise in nursing: caring, clinical judgment and ethics*. New York: Springer.

Benner, P., Tanner, C.A., & Chelsea, C.A. (2009). *Expertise in clinical practice: Caring, clinical judgment, and ethics* (2nd ed.). New York: Springer.

Bulechek, G.M., Butcher, H.K., & Dochterman, J.M. (2008). *Nursing interventions classification (NIC)* (5th ed.). St. Louis, MO: Mosby.

Doenges, M.E., & Moorhouse, M.F. (2008). *Application of nursing process and nursing diagnosis: An interactive text for diagnostic reasoning*. Philadelphia, PA: F.A. Davis.

Gebbie, K. (1998). Utilization of a classification of nursing diagnosis. *Nursing Diagnosis, 9*(2 Suppl.), 17–26.

Gordon, M. (2007). *Manual of nursing diagnosis* (11th ed.). Sudbury, MA: Jones & Bartlett.

Herdman, T.H. (ed.) (2009). *NANDA International Nursing Diagnoses: Definitions & Classification, 2009–2011*. Singapore: Wiley-Blackwell.

Hobbs, J.L. (2009). A dimensional analysis of patient-centered care. *Nursing Research, 58*, 52–62.

Jarrold, C., & Towse, J.N. (2006). Individual differences in working memory. *Neuroscience, 139*, 39–50.

Kuiper, R.A., & Pesut, D.I. (2004). Promoting cognitive and metacognitive reflective reasoning skills in nursing practice: Self-regulated learning theory. *Journal of Advanced Nursing, 45*, 381–391.

Lunney, M. (1992). Divergent productive thinking factors and accuracy of nursing diagnoses. *Research in Nursing and Health, 15*, 303–311.

Lunney, M. (2008). The critical need to address accuracy of nurses' diagnoses. *OJIN: Online Journal of Issues in Nursing*. Available at http://www.nursingworld.org/MainMenuCategories/ANAMarketplace/ANAPeriodicals/OJIN/TableofContents/vol132008/No1Jan08/ArticlePrevious Topic/AccuracyofNursesDiagnoses.aspx.

Lunney, M. (2009). *Critical thinking to achieve positive health outcomes*. Ames, IA: Wiley-Blackwell.

Lunney, M. (2010). Use of critical thinking in the diagnostic process. *International Journal of Nursing Terminologies and Classifications, 21*, 82–88.

Moorhead, S., Johnson, M., Maas, M.L., & Swanson, E. (2008). *Nursing Outcomes Classification (NOC)* (4th ed.). St. Louis, MO: Mosby.

Munhall, P.J. (1993). "Unknowing:" Toward another pattern of knowing in nursing. *Nursing Outlook, 41*, 125–128.

Pender, N.J., Murdaugh, C.L., & Parsons, M.A. (2011). *Health promotion in nursing practice* (6th ed.). Upper Saddle River, NJ: Prentice Hall.

Rubenfeld, G.M., & Scheffer, B.K. (2010). *Critical thinking TACTICS for nurses: Achieving the IOM competencies* (2nd ed.). Boston: Jones & Bartlett.

Scheffer, B.K., & Rubenfeld, M.G. (2000). A consensus statement on critical thinking. *Journal of Nursing Education, 39*, 352–359.

Stefancyk, A.L. (2009). Placing the patient at the center of care. *American Journal of Nursing, 109*, 27–28.

Sternberg, R.J. (1997). *Successful intelligence: How practical and creative intelligence determine success in life*. New York: Plume Books.

Tanner, C.A. (2006). Thinking like a nurse: A research-based model of clinical judgment in nursing. *Journal of Nursing Education, 45*(6), 204–211.

Trautmann, S.T., Vieider, F.M., & Wakker, P.P. (2008). Causes of ambiguity aversion: Known versus unknown preferences. *Journal of Risk Uncertainty, 36*, 225–243.

Weber, J.R., & Kelley, J. (2009). *Health assessment in nursing* (4th ed.). Philadelphia, PA: Lippincott.

Wilkinson, J.M. (2007). *Nursing process and critical thinking* (4th ed.). Upper Saddle River, NJ: Prentice Hall.

Willingham, D.T. (2007). *Cognition: The thinking animal* (3rd ed.). Upper Saddle River, NJ: Pearson Prentice Hall.

Wright, L.M., & Leahey, M. (2009). *Nurses and families: A guide to family assessment and interventions* (5th ed.). Philadelphia, PA: FA Davis.

Yura, H., & Walsh, M. (1967). *The nursing process*. Norwalk, CT: Appleton-Century-Croft.

Appendix: Functional Health Pattern Assessment Framework

Directions

1. The categories in the left-hand column provide guidance on the type of information that is included in the pattern description. The client's pattern should be described on the right. The description as written should be understandable by others, for example, *Correct:* no history of related physical and psychological problems; *Incorrect:* none.
2. Use interviewing techniques as described in the literature, including silence and statements, not just questions.
3. Since all of the data represent subjective data, quotation marks should not be used. Every sentence should represent the words of the individual and family, *or* their words can be paraphrased.
4. Since the subject of every sentence is "I" or "we," the subject should not be repeated throughout. The person's responses can be written as incomplete sentences; for example, the nurse can write "Attends church every day at 9 a.m." (the subject is assumed to be "I" or "We").
5. When people have long stories to tell in relation to an assessment category, the data can be shortened by paraphrasing, but be careful to retain the essence of their descriptions.
6. As much as possible, record your data in the form of cues, not inferences. Cues are units of sensory data. Inferences are the subjective meanings that persons apply to cues.
7. Avoid interjecting diagnoses into the database, for example *anxious* (a diagnosis) about a patient's relationship with her family. This statement should only be in the database if it is specifically stated by the patient.
8. Consider the assessment categories of this form as incomplete for any particular client. *Follow through on cues that are raised in the assessment.* For example, if Mary states she smokes one pack of cigarettes per day, identify whether she knows the dangers of smoking, how she feels about smoking, what is her motivation to quit, and whether smoking affects other aspects of her life; also note if there are other risk factors for heart and lung disease.

Date: _____ Nurse: _____

Client: _____ Age _____ Gender: _____ Occupation: _____
Physician(s): _____ Pharmacist: _____
Reason for Contact: _____

Health Perception–Health Management Pattern

Meaning of health	
Description of health status	
Health promotion: food and fluids, exercise, lifestyle and habits, stress management	
Health protection: screening programs, visits to primary health, exercise, stress management, rest, economic factors	
Self-examination of: breast and/or testicles, blood pressure, other	
Knowledge of self-examination	
Medical history, hospitalizations and surgery; family medical history	
Behaviors to manage health problems: diet, exercise, medications, treatments	
Names, dosage, and frequency of prescription and nonprescription drugs	
Risk factors related to health (family history, lifestyle and/or habits, low socioeconomic status)	
Relevant physical examination (PE) data: Complete.	

Nutrition–Metabolic Pattern

Usual number of meals and snacks	
Types and amounts – foods, fluids	
24-hour recall or 3-day diet history	
Shopping and cooking habits	
Satisfaction with weight	
Influences on food choices (religious, ethnic, cultural, economic)	
Perceptions of metabolic needs	
Related factors, (activity, illness, stress)	
Ingestion factors: appetite, discomfort, taste and smell, teeth, oral mucosa, nausea or vomiting, dietary restrictions, food allergies	
History of related physical and/or psychological problems	
Relevant PE data: General survey, skin, hair, nails, abdomen	

Elimination Pattern

Usual voiding pattern: frequency, amount, color, odor, discomfort, nocturia, control, any changes	
Usual defecation pattern: regularity, color, amount, consistency, discomfort, control, any changes	
Health/cultural beliefs	
Level of self-care: toileting, hygiene	
Aids for excretion: medications, enemas	
Actions to prevent cystitis	
History of related physical and/or psychological problems	
Relevant PE data: abdomen, genitals, prostate	

Activity–Exercise Pattern

Typical activities of daily living (ADLs)	
Exercise: type, frequency, duration, intensity	
Leisure activities	
Beliefs about exercise	
Ability for self-care: dressing (upper and lower), bathing, feeding, toileting	
Independent, dependent, or assistance needed	
Use of equipment, (cane, walker, etc.)	
Related factors (self-concept, etc.)	
History of related physical and/or psychological problems	
Relevant PE data: respiratory, cardiovascular, musculoskeletal, neurological	

Sleep–Rest Pattern

Usual sleep habits (number of hours, time of sleep and awakening, bedtime rituals, sleep environment, rested after sleep)	
Cultural beliefs	
Use of sleep aids (drugs, relaxation tapes, etc.)	
Scheduled rest and relaxation	
Symptoms of sleep pattern disturbance	
Related factors (pain, temperature, aging, etc.)	
History of related physical and/or psychological problems	
Relevant PE data: General survey	

Cognitive–Perceptual Pattern

Description of special senses: vision, hearing, taste, touch, smell	
Aids to senses, (glasses, hearing aids, etc.)	
Recent changes in senses	
Perception of comfort/pain	
Cultural beliefs regarding pain	
Aids to relieve discomfort	
Educational level	
Decision-making ability	
History of related physical, developmental, or psychological problems	
Relevant PE data: General survey, neurological	

Self-Perception–Self-Concept Pattern

Social self: occupation, family situation, social groups	
Personal identity: description of self, strengths and weaknesses	
Physical self: any concerns about body, likes/dislikes	
Self-esteem: feelings about self	
Threats to self-concept (illness, change in roles)	
History of related physical and/or psychological problems	
Relevant PE data: General survey	

Role–Relationship Pattern

Description of roles with family, friends, coworkers	
Role satisfaction/dissatisfaction	
Effect of health status	
Importance of family	
Family structure and support	
Family decision-making processes	
Family problems and/or concerns	
Child-rearing patterns	
Relationships with others	
Significant relationships	
History of related physical and/or psychological problems	
Relevant PE data: General survey	

Sexuality–Reproductive Pattern

Sexual concerns or problems	
Description of sexual behavior (safe sex practices, etc.)	
Knowledge related to sexuality and reproduction	
Effect of health status	
Menstrual and reproductive history	
History of related physical and/or psychological problems	
Relevant PE data: general survey, genitals, breasts, rectal	

Coping–Stress Tolerance Pattern

Nature of current stressors	
Perceived level of stress	
Description of overall and specific responses to stress	
Usual stress management strategies and their effectiveness	
Life changes and losses	
Coping strategies usually used	
Perceived control over events	
Knowledge and use of stress management techniques	
Relationship of stress management to family dynamics	
History of related physical and/or psychological problems	
Relevant PE data: General survey	

Value–Belief Pattern

Cultural/ethnic background	
Economic status, health behaviors that relate to cultural/ethnic group	
Goals in life	
What is important to client and family	
Importance of religion/spirituality	
Effect of health problems on spirituality	
Relevant PE data: General survey	

Analysis of Data, Nursing Diagnoses, Outcomes, and Interventions

- Record the key points of your discussion with the individual and family regarding *strengths* and *weaknesses*. Analyze *each* of the patterns *and* the relationships between and among the patterns. Incorporate physical examination data (normal and abnormal) for decision-making.
- State the highest priority nursing diagnosis(es) according to the individual/ family.
- Do you agree? If not, why not? Consider health promotion, risk states, and problem diagnoses.
- Record appropriate and realistic outcomes that were decided on with the patient. Explain what type of intervention(s) a nurse can use (stay within the domain of nursing) *to help* this person achieve the outcomes.

Chapter 3

Nursing Diagnosis in Education

Barbara Krainovich-Miller, Fritz Frauenfelder, Maria Müller-Staub

Significance for Nursing Education

Nursing's framework for professional practice is the nursing process. NANDA-I's Taxonomy II of nursing diagnoses is a hallmark of professional practice; it represents one of the most important components of the nursing process as it signifies that nurses have an independent role as well as a collaborative role with other healthcare providers. Further, nursing diagnoses are the basis for the daily professional work of nurses regardless of the setting.

Chapter 2, "Nursing Assessment, Clinical Judgment, and Nursing Diagnoses: How to Determine Accurate Diagnoses," presents a historical background as a theoretical framework for the nursing process and its relationship to the formulation of nursing diagnoses. Internationally, the generally accepted components of the nursing process framework are: Assessment, Diagnosis, Outcomes Identification, Planning, Implementation, and Evaluation (ANA, 2010). Although presented as steps, the nursing process is actually a dynamic interrelated process that requires the nurse to demonstrate critical thinking, critical reading, and professional communication skills. It is a process that requires the nurse to critically appraise and apply appropriate knowledge from the arts and sciences. Evaluation is viewed as a component of the process that must be clearly documented in relation to whether interventions of the plan were effective and whether outcomes were met. However, evaluation is also a continuous part of the nursing process used when collecting and clustering data, validating the diagnosis, choosing appropriate and realistic outcomes related to the diagnosis(es), as well as deriving the appropriate plan of interventions (nursing care plan) that will bring about the desired outcomes (Gordon, 2008; Lunney, 2012).

Nursing diagnosis, as a component of the nursing process, is central to professional nursing practice, and therefore to nursing education. The work of international nurse researchers on validating nursing diagnoses to improve the accuracy of formulating nursing diagnoses is critical to building nursing's science (Lunney, 2012). Using the nursing process requires that nurses critically analyze the available research to determine the best available evidence for use in practice. The NANDA-I Taxonomy of diagnoses is an example of one of the best available sources of nursing science categorized for use in practice. Within nursing education, faculty can use the Taxonomy as an example of nursing's body of knowledge that is focused on improving the health outcomes of individuals, families, and communities.

The era of evidence-based practice (EBP) and the mantra to include quality and safety in educating nurses (QSEN) reinforces the need to teach nursing students the

NANDA International Nursing Diagnoses: Definitions & Classification 2012–2014, First Edition.
Edited by T. Heather Herdman.
© 2012 NANDA International. Published 2012 by Blackwell Publishing Ltd.

NANDA-I Taxonomy. This calls for nurse educators to use an approved taxonomy of diagnoses that has gone through a rigorous review process. The NANDA-I Taxonomy is an approved taxonomy for EBP. It is equally important to inform students of two other evidence-based classification systems that will enable them to fully carry out the nursing process. These systems are the Nursing Outcomes Classification (NOC) (Moorhead, Johnson & Mass, 2008) and the Nursing Interventions Classification (NIC) (Bulechek, Butcher & Dochterman, 2008).

Teaching the Nursing Process Framework

In Chapter 2, Lunney presented the nursing process as a framework for practice. Teaching the nursing process to nursing students starts with helping them understand (1) why it is considered a framework for practice, and (2) why the nursing process is more than carrying out the steps of the process in a linear fashion. A typical example to give to students is that the assessment component requires collecting both objective and subjective data during a nurse's first encounter with an individual. Although the purpose of nursing students assessing (i.e., collecting data/information) individuals, families, groups, and communities is to identify the foci of nursing diagnosis; for beginning students, it is best to first focus on the individual, who in most cases is referred to as the patient.

Teaching the Assessment Phase of the Nursing Process

When beginning to teach about the nursing process, it is important to discuss synonyms for the "nursing process" that students might see in the literature, such as diagnostic reasoning, or clinical reasoning, as well as to compare and contrast the "problem-solving" process to the nursing process. Another strategy to help nursing students, especially beginning students, to comprehend the complexity of the nursing process is to have them focus on the individual rather than including the assessment of the family, group, or community. Students need concrete examples that demonstrate their use of critical thinking during the assessment phase of the nursing process. The main point is for them to understand that the point of conducting an assessment is to formulate a nursing diagnosis based on the clustering of specific assessment data.

As mentioned in Chapter 2, the nursing history and physical (H&P) assessment can be comprehensive or focused. Nursing education programs usually teach how to conduct a comprehensive assessment in a health assessment course taught as one of the first courses of a curriculum. This course may include an on-campus clinical simulation session traditionally referred to as a "lab." There is an expectation that what students learn in their health assessment course (didactic and simulation) will be transferred to their off-site clinical learning setting with actual patients. An overall teaching strategy to ensure the accuracy of the diagnostic concept(s) derived from a comprehensive H&P is to have students use, as noted in Chapter 2, Gordon's (2007) functional health patterns.

Nurse educators in the clinical courses need to reinforce the concepts related to health assessment and help students apply the assessment phase of the nursing process during their on-campus clinical simulation experiences as well as their off-campus clinical learning experiences. Students collect data during their nursing

H&P assessment. A synonym for objective data is "signs," and for subjective data it is "symptoms." NANDA-I refers to the combined objective and subjective data as "defining characteristics." From a nursing process and NANDA-I perspective, the purpose of the nursing H&P examination is to identify the defining characteristics and related factors of one or more nursing diagnoses.

It is also important to teach students about when a focused assessment of an individual is conducted versus a comprehensive H&P. Students actually need repeated explanations of when a focused assessment is a priority over a comprehensive H&P. Offering students a typical example of a comprehensive H&P can help them understand the difference. For instance, a typical example of when a nurse conducts a comprehensive nursing H&P is for a patient newly admitted to a unit of a health facility. A newly admitted patient requires that the nurse conduct a full nursing history and a "head-to-toe" systems assessment of the patient. If a patient has already been admitted to a unit or a person comes to an emergency room with a specific complaint, the focused assessment begins with where the person voices the complaint (e.g., "I have pain in my right wrist"); the nurse therefore begins a focused assessment of the right wrist. Another important teaching strategy is to let students know why they may not see staff nurses conducting a comprehensive assessment on all their patients, yet, as nursing students, their instructor may ask them to conduct a comprehensive assessment on an assigned patient who is not a newly admitted patient.

Students also need multiple examples of what are defining characteristics for a particular diagnostic concept. Defining characteristics, as previously noted, refer to objective and subjective data collected during the assessment phase of the nursing process. A nurse's observation of an individual's "facial grimace" is objective data ("signs"), as is obtaining a person's vital signs, and/or obtaining information from other documented sources such as the medical diagnosis or the results of diagnostic tests. Chapter 2 describes these "units of data" as "cues". What a patient tells the nurse – what the nurse hears the patient state – is subjective data ("symptoms"), for example, "my ribs hurt when I cough" (Weber & Kelley, 2009). A useful teaching strategy is for the instructor to choose one diagnostic concept and its defining characteristics. Ask half the group to make a determination of which are, as stated, objective versus subjective data, and the other half to identify which are signs and which are symptoms; then compare what the two groups have identified.

Important to the assessment phase of the nursing process is the nurse's effective communication skills, which literally activate the nursing process in relation to collecting direct data on an individual as well as other sources (e.g., family, significant others, and other health professionals). Emphasis needs to be placed on the importance of the nurse's nonverbal as well as verbal communication skills in order to be culturally sensitive and effective during the process. Students also need to be taught that the assessment process includes their critical reading and analysis of other data sources related to the individual. For example, they need to critically appraise research and other available online sources of evidence on the diagnosis, be it a life process or a health problem.

Faculty should not assume that the concept and implementation of the nursing process concept is easy for students to grasp, as it is a very complex way of processing information, especially for the beginning student. Faculty need to provide sufficient time for students to practice developing their nursing process skills. Students easily collect a lot of data on an individual when asked to do a comprehensive H&P

on an individual, yet they may have difficulty determining what data support a particular diagnosis. A simple yet overlooked strategy to decrease students' anxiety is to inform them that it takes time to learn how to conduct a comprehensive versus a focused H&P, cluster the data, make a preliminary nursing diagnosis or diagnoses, and verify the diagnosis to determine accuracy. As described in Chapter 2, the nurse is actually mentally generating possible diagnoses that can only "be understood if there are possible and plausible explanations for the cues within the context of the situation" (Lunney, 2012, pp. 77–78).

Student challenges include first learning what to detect during the physical assessment, what is normal, and then what is a deviation from normal for that individual. Students must at the same time apply their cultural competency knowledge during their data collection and interactions with the individual. What students find difficult is simultaneously clustering the data and drawing inferences in order to derive an appropriate diagnosis or to perform differential diagnosis. One effective strategy is to have students state what they are thinking as they are collecting the data. This is best accomplished in an on-campus simulation setting, which is a safe learning environment where students can practice without fear of hurting the patient or being embarrassed if they do not say the right thing. Using an appropriate faculty-developed or standardized case with a hi-fidelity patient simulator, with the faculty member playing the role of patient in terms of answering the student's questions, can be quite effective. In this type of setting, faculty during debriefing can give students feedback on whether: (1) their "verbalized" thinking demonstrated a logical and systematic method for data collection; (2) they demonstrated the use of a problem-solving focus while simultaneously "clustering the data"; and (3) their verbal and nonverbal communication was effective during the data collection process.

Teaching Nursing Diagnoses as a Component of the Nursing Process

Nursing diagnosis is defined as "a clinical judgment about individual, family, group, or community experiences/responses to actual or potential health problems/ life processes...[and] provides the basis for selection of nursing interventions to achieve outcomes for which the nurse has accountability" (see the Glossary of Terms for a full definition). Reviewing the concepts of accuracy and validity of nursing diagnoses can help students understand the fact that nurses are held accountable by their license and scope of practice for the nursing diagnoses they determine.

Determining defining characteristics of a nursing diagnosis requires that the nursing student collects and clusters the objective (signs) and subjective (symptoms) data as part of the diagnostic reasoning process. This means that, while collecting data, the nursing student simultaneously begins to cluster the data. The clustered data serve as cues or inferences of the manifestations of a nursing diagnosis – an actual problem or health-promotion state, or a potential risk state.

The key to teaching the formulation of accurate nursing diagnoses rests with helping students understand the importance of the assessment process. Taking the time to show students how to use Taxonomy II of NANDA-I for the validation process helps them understand the concept of how important the accuracy of a diagnosis is to implementing the nursing process. At the same time, it is an opportunity to emphasize and link improved health outcomes to the accuracy of the diagnosis. Lunney provides a clear explanation of the concept of accuracy in Chapter 2, and the authors of Chapter 5 discuss research related to diagnostic accuracy.

A beginning strategy is to provide students with a definition of a taxonomy and to explain the primary purpose of a taxonomy. A user-friendly explanation is that "a taxonomy is simply a scientific way to categorize and classify diagnoses," and that it provides clinicians with a way of communicating with each other. Explaining that the categorization and classification of medical diagnoses with etiologies and signs and symptoms is medicine's taxonomy for practice is also helpful. Part of helping students to use the NANDA-I taxonomy is by reviewing that it includes, at this time, 217 nursing diagnoses in this current edition. It is useful to discuss at least one diagnosis from each of the following 13 domains or categories of nursing practice: Health Promotion, Nutrition, Elimination and Exchange, Activity/Rest, Perception/Cognition, Self-Perception, Role Relationships, Sexuality, Coping/Stress Tolerance, Life Principles, Safety/Protection, Comfort, and Growth/Development. For example, the diagnosis of *Acute Pain* is listed in the practice domain of "Comfort" (Herdman, 2012).

Another important teaching strategy is to provide students with a format to use after collecting all data from an individual. For example, students should be asked to identify the data or cues that they have clustered to support a diagnosis, and then indicate if the data collected fit with the data presented for a diagnosis from a standardized evidence-based source such as the NANDA-I Taxonomy. The factors or variables influencing diagnoses are integrated with the history, patient records, and other evidence. These variables provide the context, the "related factors," that are combined with the defining characteristics to make nursing diagnoses. Related factors may be described as antecedent to, associated with, related to, contributing to, or supporting the diagnosis; they closely align with the concept of etiology. It is useful to explain to students that nurses treat, when possible, related factors with nursing interventions to prevent or reduce the impact of the related factor on the individual. For example, if a derived nursing diagnosis is *Impaired Skin Integrity* related to physical immobilization, the nurse would provide intervention to increase the patient's mobility. When it is not possible for nurses to treat a related factor, they treat the defining characteristics with selected evidence-based nursing interventions that will bring about the predetermined measurable health outcomes. For example, if the related factor for this diagnosis were "extremes of age," such as the patient being a frail, 96-year-old individual, the nurse would direct nursing interventions towards the defining characteristics such as destruction of tissue.

The Nursing Process. Exemplar – Nursing History/ Physical Assessment: Identifying Defining Characteristics and Related Factors

Linking the use of the nursing process to nurses performing a nursing H&P assessment on an individual is a usual teaching strategy for beginning students. It is important that the appropriate level patient case is presented so as not to overwhelm the student. It is helpful to students to let them know that the related factors of some diagnoses do not always become apparent during the history-taking or physical assessment phase. Often, the related factor(s) show up while reading through documentation, or prior to seeing the individual when getting the "hand-off report" from the nurse caring for the individual. Related factors provide the context for the defining characteristics; they show some type of patterned relationship with the nursing diagnosis. In other words, diagnostic reasoning requires that the nurse continuously evaluate and cluster data.

For example, while a nursing student is taking a nursing H&P assessment on Sarah, she states, "I am having bad pain in my right wrist" and "I can't sleep" (subjective data). The nursing student further observes that Sarah is crying and moaning, and that her pulse is 118 and regular (baseline 80 beats per minute and regular), her blood pressure is 130/80 (baseline 118/80 mmHg), her respirations are 24 and regular (baseline 18 per minute and regular), the cast on her right wrist is dry and intact, she can move her fingers, and there is no swelling of her fingers (objective data). The nurse asks Sarah to rate her pain level on a scale of 1 to 10. Sarah answers, "It's a 9" (subjective data). In reviewing Sarah's information, the nurse notes that she is 18 years old, and that it is her first time in the hospital. She had surgery late last evening on her right wrist for a fracture, and has a cast on her lower right leg also due to a fracture. Sarah's surgery becomes a related factor for the pain Sarah is experiencing; it is the most probable etiology of the pain she describes in her right wrist. Further assessment reveals that there is medication ordered every 4 hours for the postoperative pain at the surgery wrist site, and that her last dose was 5 hours ago. The nursing student clustered the defining characteristics (i.e., signs and symptoms or objective and subjective data), and her preliminary nursing diagnosis is *Acute Pain*. Next, the nursing student will review the diagnostic label's definition, defining characteristics, and related factors to determine whether assessment and clustering of data has supported or refuted the derived diagnosis, thus determining the accuracy of the diagnosis.

The Nursing Process. Exemplar – Accuracy of the Nursing Diagnosis Label

The diagnosis label conveys a combination of the definition, defining characteristics, and related factor(s), if available. From the perspective of both the nursing student and the nurse, the nursing diagnosis label(s) is first selected based on the initial clustering of H&P assessment data. This initial step is facilitated by students using the alphabetical list of diagnostic concepts in Taxonomy II. A teaching strategy is to have the students copy this list from the inside cover of this book, *Nursing Diagnosis: Definitions & Classification 2012–2014*, as this is easier to use in the clinical setting. A determination must be made as to whether the collected data best fit the data for the derived diagnoses as presented in the taxonomy. Accuracy is then determined by comparing the assessed data with the available defining characteristics and related factors. Therefore, it is very important that the student has access to the official NANDA-I book to verify the data before determining the final list of diagnoses.

In the case of Sarah, the definition of *Acute Pain* is "unpleasant sensory and emotional experience arising from actual or potential tissue damage or described in terms of such damage (International Association for the Study of Pain); sudden or slow onset of any intensity from mild to severe with an anticipated or predictable end and a duration of <6 months (see *Acute Pain* in Domain 12: Comfort)." In the example, Sarah stated, "I am having bad pain in my right wrist," and her heart rate had increased from baseline; she was restless and had a grimace on her face. She rated her pain as a 9 on a scale of 1 to 10, with 10 being the worst possible pain. The nursing student's data matched several of the defining characteristics as well as the stated related factor of physical injury. The key teaching point regarding identifying the appropriate nursing diagnosis is helping students to cluster data and verify this against the diagnostic label's defining characteristics and risk factors.

It is important that nurses communicate in their documentation the specific assessment data including the related factors used to support the diagnosis they make, so that others caring for the patient know why a diagnosis was selected.

Risk Diagnoses

Nurses have always been responsible for identifying individuals, families, groups, and communities at risk, and protecting them from this risk. A risk diagnosis is "a clinical judgment about human experiences/responses to health conditions/life processes that have a high probability of developing in a vulnerable individual, family, group or community". It is supported by risk factors that contribute to increased vulnerability (see Glossary of Terms). For example, the diagnosis of *Risk for Infection* is defined as "at increased risk for being invaded by pathogenic organisms," in the case of Sarah, the fact that she had had surgery, a type of "invasive procedures" – surgery being a "risk factor" identified by NANDA-I for this risk diagnosis (see Domain 11, Class 1). Risk diagnoses, like actual diagnoses, require selecting an appropriate outcome and that the plan have evidence-based interventions to achieve the identified outcome(s). Offering concrete examples of risk diagnoses that nurses commonly deal with, such as infection, falls, and pressure ulcers, helps students understand the important role of the nurse in providing quality improvement and addressing patient safety (QSEN).

Health-Promotion Diagnoses

Nurses have always been responsible for identifying health-promotion opportunities for individuals, families, groups, and communities since the time of Florence Nightingale. A health-promotion diagnosis is a "clinical judgment about a person's family's, group's or community's motivation and desire to increase well-being and actualize human health potential as expressed in the readiness to enhance specific health behaviors", such as nutrition and exercise. Health-promotion diagnoses can be used in any health state and do not require current levels of wellness. This readiness is supported by defining characteristics. Interventions are selected in concert with the individual/family/group/community to best ensure the ability to reach the stated outcomes" (see Glossary of Terms).

Prioritizing Diagnoses

The quality improvement and patient safety emphasis in nursing practice and education demonstrate the need to document in a standardized manner so that all health professionals can understand as well as implement and document that patients needs were addressed, in priority order. Therefore, prioritizing nursing diagnoses has become an equally important aspect of implementing the nursing process. Prioritizing the diagnoses with appropriate outcomes and plans of interventions is an indication to the instructor that nursing students are using critical thinking/clinical reasoning, in other words, demonstrating the nursing process.

Educators, in particular with beginning nursing students, need to explicitly ask for a prioritized list of nursing diagnoses rather than simply ask students to list their diagnoses. It is important to provide a rationale to the students as to why prioritizing is so important, and to link it to providing quality and safe patient care. A second strategy is to emphasize that prioritization should not be completed until students have verified their collected and clustered data with the NANDA-I taxonomy to determine the accuracy of the diagnoses. Priorities are established based on the needs of individuals, families, groups, and communities; again for the beginning student, start with the individual. Some faculty request that students choose a nursing diagnosis they can address during their particular clinical experience. This is not the same thing as prioritizing nursing diagnosis to reflect what needs to be carried out first. It is important to discuss with students when they are not able to directly address a priority diagnosis. For example, in the case of Sarah, if this were a beginning student and administering medications was not an expected clinical learning outcome, the faculty member would assist the student in reporting this diagnosis to the nurse who was responsible for the patient.

Linking Nursing Diagnoses to Outcomes and Interventions

In the case of Sarah, the nursing student used the NOC outcome of "decreased pain" (Moorhead et al., 2008) and used an applicable NIC nursing intervention of "pain management" (Bulechek et al., 2008). One of the NIC activities was "Select and implement pharmacological [based on medical order] and other non-pharmacological, and interpersonal measures, as appropriate to facilitate pain relief." As discussed above, although *Acute Pain* was a priority nursing diagnosis, the nursing student was not expected to carry out giving the medications, but instead to collaborate with her instructor and the staff nurse so that the patient would receive the appropriate intervention. However, the nursing student would be able to carry out other outcomes of this plan.

Accurate and valid nursing diagnoses determine the nurse-sensitive outcomes. These outcomes guide the selection of interventions that are likely to produce the desired treatment effects. Again, interventions will treat either related factors (or risk factors) or defining characteristics. Faculty members and their students can use the linkages to nursing diagnoses provided in the back of the NOC (Moorehead et al., 2008) and NIC (Bulechek et al., 2008) books, and in the linkage book (Johnson et al., 2006). Some faculty members suggest that students should come up with their own outcomes and interventions. However, in an EBP and QSEN era it is strongly recommended that students use established classification systems. Critical thinking can be enhanced by helping students adapt their NANDA-I diagnosis, NOC outcome, and NIC interventions to their individual patients. In addition, having students conduct electronic, data-based searches for studies focused on a particular diagnosis, outcome, or interventions for an outcome is another important strategy.

Once the studies have been retrieved, students can critically appraise this evidence, which requires critical thinking. Having students then compare their findings to what is presented in the NANDA-I, NOC, or NIC classifications is another way of demonstrating that they are using critical thinking, critical reading and appraisal skills. For students further along in their curriculum, another strategy is to have them write a paper for publication based on their critical appraisal, their synthesis of research literature, and their comparison of these findings to a particular diagnosis from NANDA-I or to a NOC outcome or NIC intervention.

References

American Nurses' Association. (2010). *Nursing: Scope and standards of practice* (2nd ed.). Silver Spring, MD: ANA.

Bulechek, G.M., Butcher, B.K., & Dochterman, J.M. (2008). *Nursing interventions classification (NIC)* (5th ed.). St. Louis, MO: Mosby.

Gordon, M. (2007). *Manual of nursing diagnosis* (11th ed.). Sudbury, MA: Jones & Bartlett.

Gordon M. (2008). *Assess Notes: Nursing assessment and diagnostic reasoning*. Philadelphia, PA: FA Davis.

Herdman, T.H. (ed.). (2012). *NANDA International nursing diagnoses: Definitions & classification 2012–2014*. Singapore: Wiley-Blackwell.

Johnson, M., Bulechek, G., Butcher, H., et al. (2006). *NANDA, NOC and NIC linkages: Nursing diagnoses, outcomes, and interventions* (2nd ed.). St. Louis, MO: Mosby.

Lunney, M. (2012). Assessment, clinical judgment, and nursing diagnoses. In T.H. Herdman (ed.), *NANDA International Nursing Diagnoses & Classification, 2012–2014*, 71–89.

Moorhead, S., Johnson, M., & Mass, M. (2008). *Nursing outcomes classification (NOC)* (4th ed.). St. Louis, MO: Mosby.

Weber, J.R., & Kelley, J. (2009). *Health assessment in nursing* (4th North American ed.). London: Lippincott Williams & Wilkins.

Chapter 4

The Value of Nursing Diagnoses in Electronic Health Records

Jane M. Brokel, Kay C. Avant, Matthias Odenbreit

The purpose of this chapter is to describe how nurses use nursing diagnoses within the electronic health record (EHR). We first explain features of the digital record, and then review the importance of nursing diagnoses, the use of nursing diagnoses, and documentation of the nursing diagnoses by students and practicing nurses. Next, we address the role of graduate students and informatics nurse specialists in nursing informatics engaging in roles to further develop and improve the functions, features, and information in an EHR. This section discusses how some EHRs guide nurses with the use of expert applications and knowledge content, which assist nurses in clinical decision-making. The last section is for faculty, who teach the use of nursing diagnosis with the use of EHRs.

Student Use of the Electronic Health Record (EHR)

Use of the EHR encompasses a variety of methods. This chapter describes a nurse's and a student's clinical experiences using a longitudinal EHR. The chapter begins with describing what an EHR is and how the longitudinal record is used, as well as the nurse's role using nursing diagnoses within the EHR.

Electronic Health Record

An EHR is an evolving concept (Barrett, 2000; Englebardt & Nelson, 2002). The EHR in its simplest form provides past, present, or future physical/mental or condition information on an individual (Murphy, Waters & Amatayakul, 1999). These data come from multiple sources. The compiled information is accurate and complete when those who collect the information validate what is in the record with the patient. The repository of information is organized into a very large database called a data warehouse.

An EHR comprises many computer applications such as documenting assessments, monitoring and administering medications, and care planning (Englebardt & Nelson, 2002). When a nurse uses the EHR, she or he enters, uploads, views, and retrieves the information throughout the day to make thoughtful decisions to diagnose and treat patients. Nurses make use of historical data collected by others (e.g., laboratory personnel or the primary care provider) and the newly collected

NANDA International Nursing Diagnoses: Definitions & Classification 2012–2014, First Edition.
Edited by T. Heather Herdman.
© 2012 NANDA International. Published 2012 by Blackwell Publishing Ltd.

information, including nursing assessments or biomedical device downloads, by using different EHR applications.

Longitudinal Use

The EHR serves the patient across multiple settings. Nurses and other professionals may access the EHR at the actual time of providing patient care, or in the future to reuse patient information. The patient data are in a digital format and stored in a well-organized table that is capable of being retrieved when needed, or shared across different healthcare settings. When nurses interact with patients, the demographic patient data, allergy list, immunization status, laboratory results, radiology images, and history of problems should be reused. For the most part, the information comes from the patient but is documented within the longitudinal health record by nurses, therapists, physicians, and others. Much of the information is captured from physical examinations, observations, medical devices attached to the patient, and the nurse's interviewing and screening of the patient. The reuse of existing information is encouraged, but a nurse should routinely ask the patient questions and make observations to determine "What is new?," in order to contribute to patient assessment, and add to and modify the record.

Importance of Nursing Diagnoses in EHRs

The documentation of nursing diagnoses is important for the patient and others providing care. In the EHR, students:

- view the patient's ongoing risks (*Risk for Aspiration*, *Risk for Falls*, etc.) and problems (*Impaired Gas Exchange*, *Bowel Incontinence*, etc.) that others have identified and documented;
- decide on and document new nursing diagnoses based on the patient assessment findings;
- facilitate communication of the patient's actual problems (*Urinary Retention*, *Impaired Skin Integrity*, etc.) with nurses and others on the care team;
- use the nursing diagnosis to make decisions about what mutual goals the patient desires (patient outcomes) and what can be done (nursing interventions);
- determine and document when the nursing diagnoses (risk, health promotion, or actual problem) are resolved.

The interdisciplinary team caring for the patient is able to view the patient's risks, health-promotion possibilities and actual long-term problems. When those risks are documented and the patient is scheduled to go to other departments in the hospital (such as the radiology department or physical therapy), those risks are viewed in the EHR (Figoski & Downey, 2006). For example, when a nurse identifies and documents the *Risk for Aspiration*, there are interventions added to the patient's plan of care for positioning the patient and teaching the patient. Other members of the team (including therapists, dietitians, and pharmacists) benefit from knowing that the patient has a *Risk for Aspiration*, which will lead to their reuse of positioning upright, and altering the medications or meal preparations to increase safety. If the *Risk for Aspiration* continues, this nursing diagnosis needs to be shared with others. Documenting the nursing diagnoses in the EHR will help the patient upon discharge to:

- provide the patient care information to the home-care, long-term care, or rehabilitation unit nurse who continues to care for the patient after he or she has been discharged from the hospital;
- share the patient's nursing diagnoses on the problem list through the health information exchange (HIE) record locator services, through the continuity of care document's problem list and plan of care.

When the patient is discharged and the risks remain, the nursing diagnoses are stored within a special data warehouse for others to access through the HIE. The nurse receiving the patient into home-care services is able to use a web portal to access the online record locator service to search for the patient's information and to look for the patient's problem list, plan of care, and laboratory results, as well as viewing the past care interventions and patient progress toward desired outcomes. It is through a record locator service that another facility such as a home-care service or nursing home can view the patient's problems during the hospital stay and understand what care was provided. For example, when the nurse diagnosed and documented a patient with *Risk for Falls* or *Risk for Aspiration*, the nurse would have added the risk diagnoses to the problem list and the fall prevention and aspiration precaution interventions within the care plan or computerized provider order entry. Patient outcomes would have been identified in the patient's plan of care, along with the patient's progress towards mutual goals. The problem list and plan of care are two components of the continuity of care document to share within the HIE.

Documenting Nursing Diagnoses in the EHR

The nursing diagnosis is documented in a couple of sections within the EHR. Nursing diagnoses can be long-lasting, or they can be resolved within the current setting. When the diagnosis is short term and resolved during the hospitalization or visit, the problem can be part of the interdisciplinary plan of care for ordering interventions and is not documented on the problem list. Risk diagnosis (*Risk for Aspiration*), health promotion (*Readiness for Enhanced Self-Care*), and the actual problem (*Unilateral Neglect*) are three examples of diagnoses that are likely to last beyond a patient's discharge and could be documented on the patient's problem list.

In the EHR, nurses and students need to share patient information among settings. One predominate way to share is by nurses documenting long-lasting nursing diagnoses within the "problem list." This problem list is generated from a pick-list of standardized clinical terms that include NANDA-I nursing diagnoses as well as medical diagnoses regarding diseases and syndromes. Diagnoses, diseases, or syndromes that are long-lasting for the patient should appear on the patient's problem list until resolved. Any short-term diagnosis, problem, or risk that has been resolved with treatments or procedures should not be displayed on the problem list.

The problem list should be a list of diagnoses, risks, chronic diseases, and syndromes that impact the future care of the patient. For example, *Risk for Aspiration*, *Unilateral Neglect*, diabetes mellitus, a cerebral syndrome, or *Risk for Falls* are likely to continue beyond the hospitalization for many patients. These problems reveal needs that require care across all settings. The documentation of the nursing diagnoses in the EHR's problem list communicates a known risk or unresolved problem or health-promotion opportunity to all healthcare professionals beyond the hospital stay or ambulatory clinic visit. The patient benefits when nursing care continues in long-term care facilities, and in the care provided by home-care, community, occupational, parish, and school nurses.

Differences Between EHRs

Students of nursing will use different EHR systems when having clinical experiences in different hospitals. The EHRs are not organized in the same manner, so the documentation for nursing assessments and for the risk nursing diagnoses, health-promotion diagnoses, and actual nursing diagnoses may vary with the different EHRs in various healthcare settings. A nurse is able to select the nursing diagnosis within the problem list within most EHRs. This application requires the nurse to search for the nursing diagnoses from a very large select list. Members of the professional interdisciplinary team that diagnose problems are able to add nursing diagnoses (*Risk for Aspiration*, for example) and medical diagnoses (such as diabetes mellitus) to the problem list. This type of EHR integrates the problems identified by the interdisciplinary team. The problem list may trigger a message to place an order for an intervention or care set of orders for the patient (plan of care) if this is not already present. In this situation, the care set for fall prevention and aspiration precautions is added to the patient's orders for all others to see.

Other types of EHRs allow nurses to document the nursing diagnosis within the care plan so that it is separate from the patient orders placed by the physician. In this situation, the physician and other members of the team need to look in a second place to find the fall prevention and aspiration precaution orders for the plan of care. In this situation, the team is using the same EHR, but there are two distinct applications in use. In this type of application, the nurse searches a shorter list to find the nursing diagnoses in the care plan. Other nursing units (a medical-surgical patient care unit, for example) and departments (such as the physical therapy department) who are later involved with the patient are able to view the nursing diagnoses and see the nursing orders, but may have to look in the care plan for the patient care orders that are separate from the physician orders.

Both methods, although different, need to be used by nurses to provide a list of the nursing diagnoses and to communicate follow-up interventions and reassessments for these problems, health-promotion opportunities, and risks. In a few EHRs, the nurse receives a message during or after the documentation of the assessments. In these systems, patient assessment data are linked directly to potential diagnoses through the documentation of defining characteristics and related and/or risk factors during assessment. This message could provide an even shorter list of appropriate nursing diagnoses to consider. A pre-designed list is often supported by evidence and supports the nurse's decision.

Clinical decision support (CDS) messages can remind the nurse to order care interventions or to document later in the day according to the patient's plan of care. These reminders may be placed on a navigator list or task list to remind the nurse of the need for targeted reassessments of the patient, and to document any changes in condition. Each EHR varies in its design and technical capabilities. Students working in multiple facilities will see these differences. It is important to first look for the diagnoses that other nurses have identified for the patient, and to make additions and updates as necessary.

Documenting Defining Characteristics, Related Factors, and Risk Factors in the EHR

The accurate documentation of nursing diagnoses should be supported by defining characteristics, risk factors, and/or related factors. These components of the patient assessments are documented within the EHR. The accuracy of a nursing diagnosis can be validated when a nurse links the documented nursing diagnoses to patient assessments. Box 4.1 gives an example of supporting a selected diagnosis with a related factor and defining characteristics. The documentation of nursing diagnoses and the rationale for a nurse's decision supports patient hand-offs to others.

Box 4.1 *Documentation of a Nursing Diagnosis*

Impaired swallowing (nursing diagnosis) related to esophageal defect (related factor), as evidenced by abnormality in esophageal phase by swallow study, repetitive swallowing and vomiting (defining characteristics)

There are several CDS tools within some EHRs to help students and new nurses. Some EHRs provide the definitions for nursing concepts, such as with the NANDA-I nursing diagnoses. The definition can be within reference text with the diagnostic name. The nurse can "hover" over the nursing diagnosis to see the definition, or "right click" or select a link to open a message box to view the definition. The EHR functions may differ, so nurses should try both options to access the definitions and read the underlying information provided within the EHR. This definition can also include the list of defining characteristics and related or risk factors that are evidence for the nursing diagnoses, as seen in the example in Box 4.2. Unfortunately, not all EHRs provide this level of CDS for students and new nursing staff. When these electronic evidence-based resources are not available, the *NANDA-I Definitions & Classifications* text or personal digital assistants that include this information can be useful to confirm the choice for a nursing diagnosis.

Box 4.2 *Impaired Swallowing*

Definition: Abnormal functioning of the swallowing mechanism associated with deficits in oral, pharyngeal, or esophageal structure or function
Defining characteristics include: epigastric pain, food refusal, acidic-smelling breath, abnormality in esophageal phase by swallow study, heartburn, repetitive swallowing, vomiting (signs and symptoms within the patient assessments)
Related factors include: upper airway abnormalities, esophageal defect, mechanical obstruction

---

This type of added knowledge allows students, nurses, and others to better understand what one would like to describe about the patient. The ability to open or look up the definitions in the EHR and see a list of the defining characteristics, risks, or related factors is a level of evidence to help decision-makers. The ability to reference additional information helps the student and new nurse to fully understand what is already documented and to use evidence-based definitions to help select and document the appropriate nursing diagnosis within the EHR. Lunney (2006) describes a few tools available to guide student learning and skills for practices. These tools are sometimes placed within the EHRs to support those who are still learning. Students and practicing nurses are encouraged to use the CDS resources often to look up definitions and other reference information to help with decision-making, until they are comfortable with their level of expertise on these diagnoses.

In summary, when documenting the nursing diagnosis, a student should specify the risk factors or related factors and defining characteristics, or indicate another nursing diagnosis that supports the documented decision in the EHR. More often, the nursing student is encouraged to document the nursing diagnosis with supporting defining characteristics and related or risk factors to justify the decision.

Relationship of Nursing Diagnoses to Assessments

A nurse collects and assimilates information about the patient; ultimately, these data are used to make a decision. An admission assessment with the patient should provide nurses with data for critical thinking and reasoning to make decisions about nursing diagnosis and additionally help physicians and nurse practitioners with medical diagnoses. These assessments and diagnoses become historical information within the longitudinal EHR. A nurse needs to verify and update the patient information with each subsequent assessment, but, for the most part, the history contributes to a nurse's judgment and decisions about care. Those risk factors and related factors for nursing diagnoses are sometimes found within the history of the patient's record, and a nurse could use this information in combination with the current assessment findings. A nurse does not want to make a mistake or to miss something important that guides nursing care.

It is important for a student or new nurse to know how to organize the assessment findings and the past information from the longitudinal EHR to support current clinical decision-making. Questions for the student or practicing nurse include: What nursing diagnoses may be occurring in this patient based on my assessment data and his or her history? What other data may I need to collect or review? What nursing diagnosis or medical diagnoses relate to another potential nursing diagnosis? For example, using clinical reasoning, you may find that one human response (such as *Acute Pain*) potentiates another human response (including *Impaired Physical Mobility* and *Sleep Deprivation*).

Linking Nursing Diagnoses to Other Documentation

The EHR helps nurses collect information and communicate information. Yet EHRs are different. If you see one EHR, you have seen *one* EHR. EHR design components that support nursing decisions and provide linkages include the following.

An Organizing Framework for Nursing Assessments

Gordon's Functional Health Patterns (Gordon, 2010), the domains and classes of the NANDA-I nursing taxonomy (Von Krogh, 2008), and the critical care Synergy Model (Curley, 2007; Hardin and Kaplow, 2005; Pacini, 2005) have been used as infrastructures for nursing documentation in EHRs.

Each framework is a useful evidence-based guide to find where to document the observations and interview findings so that others can view the same findings within an organized structure (see Part 1, *The NANDA International Taxonomy*). A common framework that is used globally is Gordon's Functional Health Patterns (Gordon, 2010). More often, the nursing assessments are interspersed into a medical assessment framework (a review of body systems, or a head-to-toe assessment), and no nursing assessment framework is viewed. When this exists, nurses report instances where assessments cannot be easily captured into the EHR because there is no guidance on where to document findings such as assessments on relationships and family problems, or feelings related to fear, loneliness, hopelessness, or powerlessness. These findings that are identified through Functional Health Pattern assessments do not fit within the body systems. When this happens, each nurse may document within a different location of the EHR, or document within a free-text comment field. Always ask nurse faculty and nurse managers where information should be documented when there is no organizing framework.

Link Between Assessment and a Short List of Nursing Diagnoses

Some EHRs have provided a short "pick-list" of nursing diagnoses based on a domain and class subset of assessments. Often the domain (e.g., physiological, safety, or family) and subset class (these include elimination, protection, and role relationship) guide where assessments can be documented, and the short list increases the selection of an appropriate nursing diagnosis.

Link Between Nursing Diagnosis and Patient Outcome, Current State, and Mutual Goal for an Outcome

This information is not always available in an EHR. The nursing-sensitive patient outcomes have been directly linked to the nursing diagnosis in the plan of care, and the steps to measure the patient's current state with the outcome have been documented, but often the step to set the patient's outcome goal is lacking in EHR systems. One exception is with pain assessment and management, where the patient states a pain level as an expected outcome. When the patient sets his or her outcome, the progress towards that patient's outcome is a measurable indicator using an assessment.

This linkage of interventions with the patient's risks and problems or health enhancements (nursing diagnoses) is where evidence-based interventions are used to support nursing practice. In this relationship, nursing interventions are selected as options for the nursing diagnoses and packaged as care sets. The care sets help nurses decide on the plan of care with a level of efficiency.

The EHRs have provided linkages between nursing diagnoses, nursing outcomes, and nursing interventions within the plan of care. These linkages between nursing diagnosis, outcomes, and interventions allow nurses to quickly select the patient's plan of care. This plan is accessible to adjust or modify with input from the patient. In some hospital and ambulatory EHRs, the nurse's care plan is a separate application, while other EHRs integrate the nursing care plan within interdisciplinary orders. These EHR features have linked orders to the nurses' documentation. A feature of direct linkages to the electronic documentation forms (screens) reminds nurses to document according to the plan of care. This ensures that nurses follow through with the plan and also evaluate the patient's progress towards the outcome goal, enabling them to revise the plan as needed.

Nursing Informatics Specialist/Graduate Student – Guiding Clinical Decision Support (CDS) within the EHR

The purpose of this section is to describe how the role of an informatics nurse specialist works to support practicing nurses, nurse administrators, and nurse researchers. The nursing informatics specialist facilitates the translation of conceptual models, empirical knowledge, and evidence into all practice settings. Builders of successful EHRs need first to identify the theories and conceptual models that guide the information infrastructure for the health-related data, and second to understand the needs of nurses and other clinicians who use and reuse the information within their context of knowledge (Razzaque & Jala-Karim, 2010). This information needs to be uniform and fully understood when exchanged with others to benefit the patient.

The informatics nurse specialist and graduate student will find a variety of tools to help with decision-making, planning care, and follow-through reminders to help nurses and others care for the patient. Osheroff (2009) describes the CDS interventions as intelligently filtering the information for a clinician (including nursing students, nurses, and other professionals) to guide their actions and decisions. CDS interventions are provided to help new nurse clinicians and students learn nursing practice.

One of the more common and simple types of CDS intervention is to find the definitions for the nursing diagnosis by hovering or right-clicking to open reference text, which may include more knowledge about the defining characteristics and related factors (e.g. InfoButtons; evidence-based reference content). This type of CDS facilitates the selection of the most accurate diagnosis, the patient outcome to measure, and the nursing interventions.

A second type of CDS intervention is the translation of nursing knowledge into screen designs to facilitate collection of information and organizing information to support decisions. This is a way of having knowledge designed directly into the

EHR. The display screens can present or showcase a nursing framework to organize patient assessments and guide the collection of the information. The display screens more often include interview questions with the nursing taxonomy domains and classes. The taxonomy provides an approach to organizing nursing assessments. Additionally, these screens may present instructions for collecting the information or scoring measurements (age-appropriate pain scales, Glasgow Coma Scale, Morse Fall Scale, Braden Scale, Beck II Depression Inventory, etc.). The assessment scores, interview questions, and physiological measures often require instructions for use to guide students and new nurses in the use of nursing diagnoses.

A third type of CDS includes logical use of the information that is present within the EHR. This type of CDS application automates searches of patient information, identifies patterns of information, and sends a message to the nurse with recommendations for care. One example of this is when a nurse documents the patient's regurgitation and problem of difficulty swallowing in a nutrition screen; this automates the selection of the nursing diagnosis for *Risk for Aspiration* and the aspiration precautions, as well as a referral to the rehabilitation therapists and dietitian. The logic alerts, by way of a message to the physician, automate a referral order to the therapist, and suggest adding the nursing diagnoses to the problem list. This type of complex CDS can be called a best practice alert or CDS or expert rule, which supports the nurse by automatically contacting members of the interdisciplinary team (Brokel, Shaw & Nicholson, 2006).

Other types of CDS intervention use the nursing diagnosis to guide nurse decisions. These interventions support nurses in administering medications safely, communicating referrals to other disciplines, ordering care sets using best practice guidelines, and guiding clinical documentation using standardized nursing languages and other medical and laboratory terms.

Role of Nursing Informatics

The nurse informatics role facilitates EHR and CDS development and the analysis of care effectiveness using data warehouses. Another major role is to evaluate an EHR and to improve the EHR applications for nurses. Evaluation of health information technology is based upon standards and criteria to support nursing practice, education, research, and administration of nursing services. Informatics specialists learn about the professional, international, and national standards that impact the development and design of technology and information infrastructures. Types of standards that impact the use of EHRs include standardized terminologies, linkages, and associations of elements for the nursing dataset, Health Level Seven International (HL7) reference information models, nursing evidence and protocols, security procedures, and use cases for workflow (for example, nursing process for acute, ambulatory, emergency and long term services).

In this chapter, we focus on the nursing diagnosis concepts for the EHR. One example of evaluation is using the NANDA-I Taxonomy for nursing practice to evaluate the framework for the assessment and nursing diagnoses. The nurse informatics specialist works with clinical nurse specialists, nurse practitioners, nurse administrators, researchers, and practicing nurses to understand what nursing theories and conceptual models guide practice and therefore guide the design of the EHR to support nursing practice. The nursing taxonomy provides such a framework to guide the design and improvements for documentation. The nursing informatics role is involved in the education of nurses for improving nursing workflow and purchasing the nursing knowledge, drug databases, or medicine and health science resources for nurses. These resources are often linked into the EHR for bedside use.

During the past decade, many institutions have adopted EHRs within hospitals and home-care agencies, and now more long-term care facilities and other ambulatory and community settings are also adopting these systems. The goal is to achieve interoperability for health information and patient care technologies using standards, and to use evidence-based terminologies, linkages, and protocols with EHRs (Halley, Sensmeier & Brokel, 2009).

Faculty Guide for Students in the Use of Nursing Diagnoses in the EHR

Teacher
Resources

The educator of students uses a variety of EHRs in different settings. The EHRs have different designs for nursing information infrastructures. The differences in the nursing information infrastructures will create some initial confusion for students in knowing where clinical documentation should be placed within the EHR. The placement of clinical documentation is important when the information is used and reused for clinical summary displays, for CDS alerts, messages or reminders, and for exchange of essential information when a patient moves to the next level of care. This chapter has been written first to guide the student or practicing nurse in use of the EHR, second to guide the graduate student of nursing informatics or the nursing informatics specialist, and finally to guide the educator who is directing the students' self-learning and clinical practice experiences.

This section provides additional content to explain the background that guides the student's learning of skills to document nursing diagnoses in the most appropriate location in the EHR. The placement of documentation with the longitudinal EHR impacts the continuation of care for nursing diagnoses that cannot be resolved while within a one-encounter setting. For example, the risk nursing diagnoses that are unresolved can be reused within the EHR when the patient returns to the setting. This reuse of longitudinal data such as nursing diagnoses provides nurses with new efficiencies to save time in work effort, and eliminate wastes in recreating a plan for nursing interventions that is proven to be working for a patient, family, group, or community. Students need to first look for pre-existing nursing diagnoses and the plan of care, and then validate that these fit with their own clinical assessments.

Nursing practice has been and continues to be redesigned or re-engineered with the new health information technologies including the longitudinal EHR, CDS applications, knowledge databases within the EHR, HIE, and personal health record (PHR). All of these technologies provide opportunities to document on the patient's long-term health needs, to find efficiencies through the reuse of historical information, and to select proven interventions that work for individual patients. The future is exciting but also requires some cautious optimism. Not all EHRs are created equally, so students will need to understand the capabilities and limitations of the EHRs and the type of information available within the HIEs. When there are limitations, students and nurses need to know how to overcome the gaps within current technologies and foster improvements within the health information technologies to ensure safe patient care (Keenan, Yake, Tschanen & Mandeville, 2008). There is great potential with the use of CDS interventions available in EHRs to facilitate a nurse's decision-making to select the diagnoses. There are opportunities to prioritize nursing diagnoses, to measure patient outcomes beyond one setting, and to maintain a plan of care that has proven beneficial for the patient's mental and family needs. Often EHRs have paid ample attention to the physiological parameters and less to the other domains of nursing practice. Educators need to help students bridge this evolution of technologies and foster better development.

Documentation

The capacity to assess patients begins with the nurse and how she or he identifies what to collect and what to document from interviews, physical examination, and ongoing observations, as well as what to compile from historical documents. These assessment findings and history contain the defining characteristics, risk factors, and related factors to build evidence for a decision about actual patient problems, health-promotion opportunities, or risks. The historical factors may help students identify patient risks or actual problems. Encourage the student to use the chapters in this book to guide decision-making and to use the EHR tools discussed earlier to document the nursing diagnosis, with the rationale for this decision.

Using the EHR

Students should describe what assessment framework was used within the EHR. Ask the student to describe where data are located, how data are collected, where information should be, and when information is important to use and reuse. Students may not remember where assessment data are found in the EHR, so ask students where they can find information. Do not be surprised if students report they could not document an assessment because they did not know where to enter data. When the assessment framework for nursing is disguised within the medical body systems framework, graduate and undergraduate students have reported instances of no location to document. The longitudinal EHR can be organized to assist nurses in their daily work, but this is not always the case. Not all EHRs have been designed with a nurse's conceptual nursing practice model and nursing languages. It is for this reason that this chapter has been written to help students and novice nurses and faculty to handle the variation in EHRs.

Guiding Student Learning

To guide student learning, nursing faculty need to showcase the NANDA-I Taxonomy for nursing practice. Students need to locate within the EHR how all aspects of the nursing framework have been assessed. When using the NANDA-I Taxonomy, faculty can ask students to explain how each of the domains of nursing was used to assess the patient. The student can outline what assessments were part of the domains of Health Promotion, Nutrition, Elimination and Exchange, Activity/Rest, Perception/Cognition, Self-Perception, Role Relationships, Sexuality, Coping/Stress Tolerance, Life Principles, Safety/Protection, Comfort, and Growth/

Development. Having the student purposefully learn and speak to all the domains of the NANDA-I Taxonomy increases the student's holistic approach to assess the patient's human responses. Refer to Chapter 1 on the NANDA-I Taxonomy II to review the scope of what should and could be assessed with patients, families, groups, and communities.

Learning the EHR, CDS and Health Information Exchange (HIE)

The information infrastructure for health information technologies such as the EHR should have common features within different vendor systems. All EHRs have a clinical documentation feature to capture the assessments, measure the outcomes, and record the interventions performed. The infrastructure of the information is very different. Some EHRs are technically designed using the medical model, whereas others use an interdisciplinary approach. The EHRs have common structures that include a problem list, an allergy profile, a drug database for patient education and drug alerts, a medication profile for home lists, and electronic medication administration record for drugs given. Other application features have different designs for the plan of care, often called computerized provider order entry or care planning process, and a discharge navigator feature to prepare instructions. Not all EHRs are the same; consequently students may find that they need to document in different locations. Students have reported their challenges in finding where to document patient assessments and outcomes when the framework is limited to a medical model. Educators need to help students discern the nursing frameworks for clinical documentation and find the established internal workflows (i.e., paper and textbooks) that can be used to bridge the gaps until upgrades in EHRs occur.

Assessment Framework

In the initial use of an EHR, the student should learn what assessment framework is used to identify patient risks, problems, needs, and health-promotion opportunities. The student's electronic documentation should be used to match assessments to the defining characteristics, related factors or risk factors that justify the selection of a nursing diagnosis. This exercise helps students learn how to link clinical findings to the nursing diagnoses of the patient's risks, actual problems, and/or health-promotion needs.

Knowledge Resources (Library)

In the EHR, the student can use the knowledge about definitions, defining characteristics, related factors, and risk factors as evidence to support clinical decisions about the patient. When the EHR integrates the nursing evidence to support decision-making at the bedside or within the clinic setting, the student can look up definitions and associated defining characteristics, risk factors, and related factors to help with decision-making. When not in the EHR, the students will need the NANDA-I textbook or a personal digital assistant version of NANDA-I.

Problem List

The longstanding problems and risks are profiled for the patient on the problem lists. This problem list exists as a data set for all visits, and is accessible with the HIE record locator service for others to obtain. This problem list is useful for nursing homes, home-care services, and pharmacies, as well as the patient's primary care providers. The problem list is a standard feature.

Interdisciplinary Care Planning

This feature is not the same among EHRs. Some vendor systems integrate the orders placed by all clinical disciplines, while other vendor systems separate the nursing orders from the patient orders entered by the physicians. This is where much of the uniqueness of clinical EHRs is challenging for students. When the EHR is integrated, the physician and all others see the plan for nursing care within the same EHR ordering function. When separate, the nurse and student must take steps to keep the physician and others informed of the nursing care because they may not see the nurse's plan for care.

Clinical Decision Support

This feature is the most complex because it involves the use of many of the above features and an expert application. Some advanced students in nursing informatics learn how to design, build, and evaluate the validity, reliability, and effectiveness of CDS interventions. The use of standardized nursing languages such as NANDA-I nursing diagnoses is necessary to develop such a CDS support application.

Health Information Exchange

This feature is part of the statewide HIEs and national health information network within the United States to move standard formatted information from one location to another. The problem list, allergies, medication list, immunizations, and care plan are data sets that are standardized using health information vocabularies. The problem list and care plan are two items in the continuity of care document (HL7v3). The standard nursing diagnoses are documented by nurses and therefore can be exchanged between and among settings for the patient and family. Nurses access the web portal to sign on to the record locator service to search for the patient, and to find the problem list and care plan. The nursing diagnoses that often are long-lasting risks, problem or health-promotion needs are retained on the longitudinal health record to continue care across locations. Examples are provided in Table 4.1.

Personal Health Records

One type of health information technology that is on the horizon is the use of PHRs. The PHR is driven by the patient's use of his or her information for work-related, family, and/or school needs. Patients are involved in receiving and sending

Table 4.1 *Nursing diagnoses to add to the problem list in the electronic health record*

Nursing diagnosis	Assessment domains	Location documented
Risk for unstable blood glucose	Nutrition	Care plan if temporary, or problem list if longitudinal risk
Risk for bleeding	Activity/Rest	Care plan
Risk for caregiver role strain	Role Relationships	Problem list
Constipation	Elimination and Exchange	Problem list
Social isolation	Comfort	Problem list
Impaired memory	Perception/Cognition	Problem list
Delayed growth and development	Growth/Development	Problem list
Risk of self-directed violence	Safety/Protection	Care plan

messages from their healthcare providers when PHRs are linked with the EHR. The nurse will need to involve and teach patients how to monitor and document signs, symptoms, and changes in their conditions for their PHR. Nurses will have opportunities to use the health-promotion nursing diagnoses to engage patients in identifying health needs and finding interventions to address those needs and to monitor progress over time. The PHR is central to patient-centered care, and will contain information that nurses should access to find patient assessments for diagnosing human responses and planning care in the home setting.

References

Barrett, M.J. (2000). The evolving computerized medical record. *Healthcare Informatics, 17*(5), 85–92.

Brokel, J.M., Shaw, M.G., & Nicholson, C. (2006). Expert clinical rules automate steps in delivering evidence-based care in the electronic health record. *Computers, Informatics, and Nursing, 24*(4), 197–205.

Curley, M.A.Q. (2007). *Synergy: The unique relationships between nurses and patients.* Indianapolis: Sigma Theta Tau.

Englebardt, S.P., & Nelson, R. (2002). *Health care informatics: An interdisciplinary approach.* St. Louis, MO: Mosby.

Figoski, M.R., & Downey, J. (2006). Perspectives in continuity of care. Facility charging and Nursing Intervention Classification (NIC): The new dynamic duo. *Nursing Economics, 24*(2), 102–111, 115.

Gordon, M. (2010). *Manual of nursing diagnoses* (12th ed.). St. Louis, MO: Mosby.

Halley, E.C., Sensmeier, J., & Brokel., J.M. (2009). Nurses exchanging information: Understanding electronic health record standards and interoperability. *Urologic Nursing, 29*(5), 305–313.

Hardin, S.R., & Kaplow, R. (2005). *Synergy for clinical excellence: The AACN synergy model for patient care.* Sudbury, MA: Jones & Bartlett.

Keenan, G.M., Yake, E., Tschanen, D., & Mandeville, M. (2008). Documentation and the nurse care planning process. In R.G. Hughes (ed.), *Patient safety and quality: An EVIDENCE-based handbook for nurses.* Rockville, MD: AHRQ, pp. 1317–1349.

Lunney, M. (2006). Staff development helping nurses use NANDA, NOC, and NIC. *Journal of Nursing Administration, 36*(3), 118–125.

Murphy, G.F., Waters, K.A., & Amatayakul, M. (1999). EHR vision, definition, and characteristics. In G.F. Murphy, M.A. Hanken, & K.A. Waters (eds), *Electronic health records: Changing the vision*. Philadelphia: W.B. Saunders.

Osheroff, J.A. (2009). *Improving medication use and outcomes with clinical decision support: a step by step guide*. Chicago, IL: Healthcare Information and Management Systems Society. Available at: www.himss.org/cdsguide.

Pacini, C.M. (2005). Synergy: A framework for leadership development and transformation. *Critical Care Nursing Clinics of North America, 17*, 113–119.

Razzaque, A., Jalal-Karim, A. (2010). Conceptual healthcare knowledge management model for adaptability and interoperability of EHR. Proceedings form the European, Mediterranean, and Middle Eastern Conference on Information Systems, April 12–13.Abu Dhabi, UAR.

Von Krogh, G. (2008). An examination of the NANDA International taxonomy for domain completeness, ontological, homogeneity, and clinical functionality. *International Journal of Nursing Terminologies and Classifications, 19*(2), 65–75.

Chapter 5

Nursing Diagnosis and Research

Margaret Lunney, Maria Müller-Staub

Since 1973, the diagnoses approved for the NANDA-I Taxonomy of nursing diagnoses have been developed and submitted by nurses using a variety of research methods. Each diagnosis is research-based, with some diagnoses having stronger research evidence than others (Berger, 2008; Herdman, 2009). Over the last four decades, the research methods have become more sophisticated, and the Diagnosis Development Committee has required more stringent evidence as the basis for approving new diagnoses (Herdman, 2009).

To remain evidence-based, however, the NANDA-I Taxonomy needs ongoing research support. Some of the types of studies needed are concept analyses, content validation, construct-related, criterion-related, and consensus validation. Additionally, studies that establish the sensitivity, specificity, and predictive value of clinical indicators in specific populations, studies of accuracy of nurses' diagnoses, and implementation studies are necessary. The references cited in each of the following descriptions can be used as resources for these research methods.

Concept Analyses

Concept analyses have been and continue to be an important aspect of the development and approval of new diagnoses (Avant, 1990). Concept identification and formulation are the first steps in developing new diagnoses and refining previously accepted diagnoses. Each nursing diagnosis is a concept that needs to be developed using systematic methods (Walker and Avant, 2005). A classic study, for example, was Whitley's (1992) concept analysis of *fear*.

At the 2006 NANDA-I–NIC–NOC (NNN) Alliance conference, a concept analysis was reported to develop a new wellness health-promotion diagnosis: *Supportive Family Role Performance* (Lamont, 2006). Melo Ade, Carvalho & Pelà (2007) used concept analyses to recommend changes in the diagnoses of *Sexual Dysfunction* and *Ineffective Sexuality Pattern*.

Content Validation

Content validation studies are often foundational for refining approved diagnoses and developing new diagnoses. In these studies, there are two possible groups of

NANDA International Nursing Diagnoses: Definitions & Classification 2012–2014, First Edition.
Edited by T. Heather Herdman.
© 2012 NANDA International. Published 2012 by Blackwell Publishing Ltd.

subjects – nurses who work with patients who experience the specific diagnoses, and patients who currently are experiencing the diagnosis (Fehring, 1986). A problem with nurses as subjects, however, especially if it is a new diagnosis, is that they are being asked to state from memory the relevance of defining characteristics. Clinical validation studies, in which patients are assessed for defining characteristics at the time that they experience the specific human response, provide better data for content validation studies.

Chaves, Barros & Marini (2010) conducted a content validation study using nurse experts of the diagnosis *Impaired Memory*. The definition, defining characteristics, related factors, and proposed related factor "aging" were evaluated using the Fehring method (1986). In another nurse expert study, a descriptive correlational design was used (Guirao-Goris & Duarte-Climents, 2007) with a population of Spanish nurses to evaluate the diagnosis of *Sedentary Lifestyle*. The authors used Fehring's Diagnostic Content Validity (DCV) index to determine the DCV for each of the defining characteristics, analyze the factorial and convergent validity of the label, and determine how the characteristics of expert profiles affected the DCV of the diagnosis. The DCV index for experts was 0.70, and the factorial validity showed two different factors: (1) the expression of laziness, and (2) the performance of activities of daily living. With factor analysis of nurse expert demographics, the two factors of experience and education were identified.

For decades, the data from clinical validation studies have served as support for nursing diagnoses (e.g., Bartek, Lindeman & Hawks, 1999; Carlson-Catalano et al., 1998; Kim, et al., 1984; Zeitoun, Barros, Michel & Bettencourt, 2007). The challenges of conducting clinical studies are significant but worthwhile because data are from actual patients who are currently experiencing the human response of interest to the researcher. Methodological considerations for such studies were described by Carlson-Catalano and Lunney (1995), Grant, Kinney & Guzzetta (1990), and Maas, Hardy & Craft (1990). Sparks and Lien-Gieschen (1994) provided revised guidelines for scoring and interpreting defining characteristics as highly or moderately relevant for making a diagnosis. These scoring guidelines are important to avoid the development of long lists of defining characteristics. Some of the currently approved diagnoses have long lists of defining characteristics that could be reduced if clinical studies were done using the aforementioned guidelines.

A three-phase clinical study was performed to validate 18 defining characteristics of *Ineffective Peripheral Tissue Perfusion* (Silva, Cruz, Bortolotto, Irigoyen, Krieger, Palomo, & Consolim-Colombo, 2006). Prior to the study, defining characteristics were identified by a literature review. The first phase of the study consisted of the construction and validation of a data collection instrument. During the second phase, patients underwent a clinical nursing evaluation that consisted of an interview, a physical examination, and tests to evaluate peripheral perfusion. The third phase was the clinical validation of the defining characteristics of *Ineffective Peripheral Tissue Perfusion*, and involved evaluation of vasomotor function by three methods: analysis of vasodilation in response to reactive hyperemia, intra-arterial infusion of acetylcholine, and pulse wave velocity measurements. A vasomotor function assessment was completed in 24 patients with hypertensive cardiomyopathy. Statistical analysis was conducted using the Student's *t*-test and Kruskal–Wallis test to determine the significance of the relationships between the defining characteristics and vasomotor function data. The defining characteristics of the diagnosis were highly associated with the data found in clinical vasomotor function assessments and tests that functioned as "gold standards" for *Ineffective Peripheral Tissue Perfusion*.

Construct- and Criterion-Related Validity

"Knowledge development of diagnoses in the NANDA-I Taxonomy means that a series of studies needs to be done for each individual diagnosis as well as groups of diagnoses" (Parker & Lunney, 1998, p. 146). The various types of study needed to establish construct- and criterion-related validity are reliability, epidemiological, outcome, causal analysis, and generalizability studies (Parker & Lunney, 1998). Reliability studies can establish the stability and coherence of diagnoses.

Epidemiological studies of the incidence and prevalence of specific diagnoses in settings and populations can show the importance and co-occurrence of diagnoses. For example, in retrospective analyses of 123,241 sequential admissions to a university hospital, Welton and Halloran (2005) demonstrated that nursing diagnoses were good predictors of hospital outcomes, adding 30–146% of explanatory power to diagnosis-related groups and all payer-refined diagnosis-related groups. Epidemiological studies can also be done to show the relationships among diagnoses, interventions, and outcomes.

Outcome, or effectiveness, studies can illustrate the prognoses of diagnoses and the best interventions to help people who are experiencing specific diagnoses. Effectiveness studies are being conducted by a research team in Iowa (Shever Titler, Dochterman, Fei & Picone, 2007). Studies of teaching nurses to use nursing diagnoses and interventions showed improved patient outcomes (Müller-Staub, Needham, Odenbreit, Lavin & van Achterberg, 2007, 2008).

A symposium of three examples of effectiveness studies was presented at the 2006 NNN Alliance conference (Dochterman, 2006). Causal analysis studies, using experimental designs, can show the relation of diagnoses to theories and the importance of using standardized diagnoses to achieve high-quality nursing care.

Generalizability studies can show the importance of nursing diagnoses across institutions and medical diagnoses (International Classification of Diseases, 1987). A good resource for conducting validity and reliability studies is a book on measurement (e.g., Waltz, Strickland & Lenz, 2005).

Consensus Validation

Consensus validation techniques are being used to establish the connections of NANDA-I, the Nursing Interventions Classification (NIC), and the Nursing Outcomes Classification (NOC) with specific populations for the purposes of developing standards of practice and identifying the specific terms to be included in electronic health records (Carlson, 2006a, 2006b; Westmoreland, Wesorick, Hanson & Wyngarden, 2000). The study by Westmoreland et al. validated that their clinical practice guidelines delineated the right services and knowledge related to these services (2000, p. 19). Carlson (2006a, 2006b) recommended participatory action research methods for practicing nurses to identify the specific NANDA-I, NIC, and NOC terms that apply to patients served by their agency or unit. This process is being used in a variety of settings, and can be adopted by nurses in any setting and locality (Lunney, McGuire, Endoza & Waddy-McIntosh, 2010; Lunney, Caffrey & Umbro, 2010; Minthorn, 2006; Minthorn & Lunney, 2010).

Sensitivity, Specificity, and Predictive Value of Clinical Indicators

The sensitivity, specificity, and predictive value of clinical indicators are needed for populations that are expected to experience a specific response to a health problem or life process. For example, hospitalized children with congenital heart disease are expected to experience *Ineffective Airway Clearance* (IAC). In a study of 45 children aged 1 year or under with congenital heart disease (Silva, Lopes, Araujo, Ciol, & Carvalho, 2009). only 31% of children with IAC were identified with the first assessment, whereas 71% were identified with the last assessment. Measuring the sensitivity, specificity, and predictive value of clinical indicators made a significant difference in the number of children identified with IAC. Presumably identifying the diagnosis improved nursing interventions and the health outcomes of these children.

The sensitivity, specificity, and predictive value of the defining characteristics of the nursing diagnosis *Impaired Spirituality* were calculated in 120 adults with chronic renal disease receiving hemodialysis treatment (Chaves, Carvalho, Goyata & Souza, 2010). *Impaired Spirituality* was identified in 27.5% of the patients. The highest sensitivity, specificity, and predictive values were found with the defining characteristics of: anger, feels abandoned, questions suffering, and expresses alienation.

Studies of Accuracy of Nurses' Diagnoses

Studies of the accuracy of nurses' diagnoses and factors that influence accuracy are needed because previous studies have established that accuracy varies widely (Lunney, 2008). The accuracy of nurses' diagnoses is important because this is the foundation for choices of interventions and outcomes. Examples of accuracy studies are a clinical study by Lunney, Karlick, Kiss, and Murphy (1997), a mail survey by Hasegawa, Ogasawara & Katz (2007), a study of teaching critical thinking to experienced nurses (Cruz, Pimenta & Lunney, 2009), and a study of teaching critical thinking to nursing students (Collins, 2010).

The prevalence of accurate nursing documentation was assessed in patient records ($n = 341$) from 35 wards in 10 randomized hospitals in The Netherlands (Paans, Sermeus, Nieweg & van der Schans, 2010a). The D-Catch instrument was used to quantify the accuracy of the: (1) record structure, (2) admission data, (3) nursing diagnosis, (4) nursing interventions, (5) progress and outcome evaluations, and (6) legibility of nursing reports. The quantity and quality criteria of diagnostic accuracy scored as "incomplete" and "ambiguous" led to an accuracy average sum score of 4 (range 2–8 points) for records that listed diagnostic labels but no related factors or diagnostic labels, and no signs or symptoms.

Implementation Studies

The importance of using nursing diagnoses in clinical practice is that the quality of nursing care is expected to improve (Lunney, 2008). Yet there are insufficient data at the present time to convince others that this is so. Two recent studies demonstrated the positive effects of implementing standardized nursing languages (Müller-Staub et al., 2007; Thoroddsen & Ehnfors, 2007), but many more such studies are needed.

Guided Clinical Reasoning (GCR) as an implementation method was evaluated in a cluster randomized trial by Müller-Staub et al. (2008). The quality of 225 randomly selected nursing records, containing 444 documented nursing diagnoses, corresponding interventions, and patient outcomes, was evaluated by applying the instrument Quality of Nursing Diagnoses, Interventions and Outcomes (Q-DIO). The effect of GCR was tested against classic case discussions using Student t-tests and mixed effects model analyses. Implementing nursing diagnoses by GCR showed significantly higher accuracy in diagnoses, in related factors, and in defining characteristics ($P < 0.0001$). Nurses also performed significantly more effective nursing interventions ($P < 0.0001$), which led to better nursing-sensitive patient outcomes ($P < 0.0001$). In the control group, the accuracy of diagnoses, the effectiveness of interventions, and the nursing outcomes did not change (Müller-Staub et al., 2008).

Two instruments were developed to measure the accuracy and effects of nursing diagnoses implementation: the Q-DIO and the D-Catch (Müller-Staub, Lunney, Odenbreit, Needham, Lavin, & van Achterberg, 2009; Müller-Staub, Lunney, Lavin, Needham, Odenbreit, & van Achterberg, 2010; Paans, Sermeus, Niewig, & van der Schans, 2010a, 2010b). The Q-DIO measures the quality and accuracy of nursing diagnoses, related factors and defining characteristics, the effectiveness of nursing interventions, and the quality of nursing outcomes in nursing documentation (Müller-Staub et al., 2009). The D-Catch measures accuracy of nursing diagnoses and of nursing documentation (Paans et al., 2010a, 2010b). Methodological studies of the psychometric properties of both instruments demonstrated satisfactory validity and reliability.

Prevalence Studies

Studies addressing the prevalence of nursing diagnoses were performed in specialty settings, and more studies are needed. In a cross-sectional study, the prevalence of *Sedentary Lifestyle* and the common defining characteristics were identified (Guedes, Lopes, Moreira, Calvalcante & Araujo, 2010). The prevalence of nursing diagnoses was assessed in a geriatric rehabilitation setting. The highest prevalence diagnoses were *Chronic Confusion*, *Imbalanced Nutrition: Less Than Body Requirements*, *Risk for Falls*, *Self-Care Deficits*, *Impaired Physical Mobility (Transfer Ability, Bed Mobility, Walking)*, and *Urinary Incontinence (Urge, Functional, Stress, Reflex, Total)* (Heering, 2010). The diagnoses of *Risk for Falls, Disturbed Thought Process*, and *Disturbed Sleep Pattern* were found to be prevalent in psychiatric nursing units (Shiraishi et al., 2009).

In a systematic literature review, *Pain* was the most frequently stated nursing diagnosis (Müller-Staub, Lavin, Needham, & van Achterberg, 2006). This systematic literature review included data from nursing studies of 4051 patients from 12 different sites.

Summary

Nursing diagnosis studies are needed to maintain and enhance the evidence base of the NANDA-I Taxonomy. The NANDA-I Education and Research Committee is available to provide assistance to anyone considering undertaking a study. For support, please contact the chair of the Education & Research Committee via the NANDA-I website.

References

Avant, K.C. (1990). The art and science in nursing diagnosis development. *Nursing Diagnosis, 1*(2), 51–56.

Bartek, J.K., Lindeman, M., & Hawks, J.H. (1999). Clinical validation of characteristics of the alcoholic family. *Nursing Diagnosis: Journal of Nursing Language and Classification, 10*, 158–168.

Berger, S. (2008). *Validation studies on NANDA-I diagnoses: Methodological demands, overview of studies, and critical evaluation.* Paper presented at the NNN conference, Miami, FL, November.

Carlson, J.M. (2006a). Consensus validation process: A standardized research method to identify and link their relevant NANDA, NIC and NOC terms for local populations. *International Journal of Nursing Terminologies and Classifications, 17*, 23–24 [Abstract].

Carlson, J.M. (2006b). Professional nursing latent tuberculosis infection standards of practice development using NANDA, NIC and NOC [Abstract]. *International Journal of Nursing Terminologies and Classifications, 17*, 62.

Carlson-Catalano, J. & Lunney, M. (1995). Quantitative methods for clinical validation of nursing diagnoses. *Clinical Nurse Specialist: Journal of Advanced Nursing Practice, 9*, 306–311.

Carlson-Catalano, J., Lunney, M., Paradiso, C., Bruno, J., Luise, B., Martin, T., Massoni, M. & Pachter, S. (1998). Clinical validation of ineffective breathing pattern, ineffective airway clearance, and impaired gas exchange. *Image: Journal of Nursing Scholarship, 30*, 243–248.

Chaves, E.C.L., Carvalho, E.C., Goyata, S.L.T., & Souza, L. (2010a). Sensitivity, specificity and predictive value of the defining characteristics of the nursing diagnosis Impaired Spirituality. Paper presented at the AENTDE-NANDA International Conference, Madrid, Spain, May.

Chaves, E.H.B., de Barros, A.L.B., & Marini, M. (2010a). Aging as a related factor of the nursing diagnosis Impaired Memory: A content validation. *International Journal of Nursing Terminologies and Classifications, 21*, 14–20.

Collins, A. (2010). *Nursing students: Improving accuracy of and attitude to nursing diagnosis.* Paper presented at the AENTDE-NANDA International conference, Madrid, Spain, May.

Cruz, D.A.L.M., Lopes, N.V., Araujo, T.L., Ciol, M.A., & Carvalho, E.C. (2009). Improving critical thinking and clinical reasoning with a continuing education course. *Journal for Continuing Education in Nursing, 40*, 121–127.

Dochterman, J. (2006). Effectiveness research: Three examples. *International Journal of Nursing Terminologies and Classifications, 17*, 85–87 [Abstracts].

Fehring, R.J. (1986). Validating diagnostic labels: Standardized methodology. In Hurley, M. (ed.), *Classification of nursing diagnoses: Proceedings of the sixth conference.* St. Louis, MO: NANDA, pp. 183–90.

Grant, J.S., Kinney, M., & Guzzetta, C.E. (1990). Using magnitude estimation scaling to examine the validity of nursing diagnoses. *Nursing Diagnosis, 1*(2), 64–69.

Guedes, N.G., Lopes, M.V.O., Moreira, R.P., Cavalcante, T.F., & Araujo, T.L. (2010). Prevalence of sedentary lifestyle in individuals with high blood pressure. *International Journal of Nursing Terminologies and Classifications, 21*, 50–56.

Guirao-Goris, J.A., & Duarte-Climents, G. (2007). The expert nurse profile and diagnostic content validity of sedentary lifestyle: The Spanish validation. *International Journal of Nursing Terminologies and Classifications, 18*, 84–92.

Hasegawa, T., Ogasawara, C., & Katz, E.C. (2007). Measuring diagnostic competency and the analysis of factors influencing competency using written case studies. *International Journal of Nursing Terminologies and Classifications, 18*, 93–102.

Heering, C. (2010). *Prevalence of nursing diagnoses in an acute geriatric rehabilitation clinic.* Paper presented at the AENTDE-NANDA International Conference, Madrid, Spain, May.

Herdman, T.H. (ed.) (2009). *NANDA International nursing diagnoses: Definitions and classifications, 2009–2011.* Chichester, UK: Wiley-Blackwell.

International Classification of Diseases. (n.d.). Retrieved from ftp://ftp.cdc.gov/pub/Health_Statistics/NCHS/Publications/ICD-9/ucod.txt.

International Statistical Classification of Diseases and Related Health Problems. (2007). Retrieved from http://apps.who.int/classifications/apps/icd/icd10online/.

Kim, M.J., Amoroso-Seritella, R., Gulanick, M., et al. (1984). Clinical validation of cardiovascular nursing diagnoses. In: Kim, M.J., McFarland, G.K., & McLane, A.M. (eds), *Classification of nursing diagnoses: Proceedings of the fifth national conference*. St. Louis, MO: Mosby, pp. 128–138.

Lamont, S.C. (2006). Supportive role performance: Development of a new wellness diagnosis. *International Journal of Nursing Terminologies and Classifications*, 17, 40–41 [Abstract].

Lunney, M. (2008). Critical need to address accuracy of nurses' diagnoses. *OJIN: Online Journal of Issues in Nursing*. Retrieved from http://www.nursingworld.org/MainMenuCategories/ANAMarketplace/ANAPeriodicals/OJIN/TableofContents/vol132008/No1Jan08/ArticlePreviousTopic/AccuracyofNursesDiagnoses.aspx .

Lunney, M., Karlik, B.A., Kiss, M., & Murphy, P. (1997). Accuracy of nurses' diagnoses of psychosocial responses. *Nursing Diagnosis*, 8, 157–166.

Lunney, M., McGuire, M., Endozo, N., & Waddy-McIntosh, D. (2010a). Consensus-validation study identifies relevant nursing diagnoses, nursing interventions, and health outcomes for people with traumatic brain injuries. *Rehabilitation Nursing*, 35, 161–166.

Lunney, M., Caffrey, P., & Umbro, S. (2010b). *Action research to identify nursing diagnoses, patient outcomes, and nursing interventions for end of life care*. Paper presented at the AENTDE-NANDA International Conference, Madrid, Spain, May.

Maas, M.L., Hardy, M.A., & Craft, M. (1990). Methodologic considerations in nursing diagnosis research. *Nursing Diagnosis*, 1(1), 24–30.

Melo Ade, S., Carvalho, E.C., & Rotter Pelà, N.T. (2007). Proposed revisions for the nursing diagnoses sexual dysfunction and ineffective sexuality patterns. *International Journal of Nursing Terminologies and Classifications*, 18, 150–155.

Minthorn, C. (2006). Meeting Magnet criteria with studies of NANDA, NIC and NOC. *International Journal of Nursing Terminologies and Classifications*, 17, 46 [Abstract].

Minthorn, C., & Lunney, M. (2010). Participant action research with bedside nurses to identify NANDA, Nursing Interventions Classification, and Nursing Outcomes Classification categories for hospitalized persons with diabetes. *Applied Nursing Research*. Epub ahead of print.

Müller-Staub, M., Lavin, M.A., Needham, I., & van Achterberg, T. (2006). Nursing diagnoses, interventions and outcomes – application and impact on nursing practice: A systematic literature review. *Journal of Advanced Nursing*, 56, 514–531.

Müller-Staub, M., Needham, I., Odenbreit, M., Lavin, M.A., & van Achterberg, T. (2007). Improved quality of nursing documentation: Results of a nursing diagnoses, interventions and outcomes implementation study. *International Journal of Nursing Terminologies and Classifications*, 18, 5–17.

Müller-Staub, M., Needham, I., Odenbreit, M., Lavin, M. A., & van Achterberg, T. (2008). Implementing nursing diagnostics effectively: Cluster randomized trial. *Journal of Advanced Nursing*, 63, 291–301.

Müller-Staub, M., Lunney, M., Odenbreit, M., Needham, I., Lavin, M. A., & van Achterberg, T. (2009). Development of an instrument to measure the quality of documented nursing diagnoses, interventions and outcomes: The Q-DIO. *Journal of Clinical Nursing*, 18, 1027–1037.

Müller-Staub, M., Lunney, M., Lavin, M.A., Needham, I., Odenbreit, M., & van Achterberg, T. (2010). Testtheoretische Gütekriterien des Q-DIO, eines Instruments zur Messung der Qualität der Dokumentation von Pflegediagnosen, -interventionen und -ergebnissen. *Pflege: Die wissenschaftliche Zeitschrift für Pflegeberufe*, 23, 119–128.

Paans, W., Sermeus, W., Nieweg, R.M.B., & van der Schans, C.P. (2010a). D-Catch instrument: Development and psychometric testing of a measurement instrument for nursing documentation in hospitals. *Journal of Advanced Nursing*, 66, 1388–1400.

Paans, W., Sermeus, W., Nieweg, R.M.B., & van der Schans, C.P. (2010b). Prevalence of accurate nursing documentation in patient records. *Journal of Advanced Nursing*, 66(11), 2481–2489.

Parker, L., & Lunney, M. (1998). Moving beyond content validation of nursing diagnoses. *International Journal of Nursing Terminologies and Classifications*, 9(Suppl. 2), 144–150.

Shever, L.L., Titler, M., Dochterman, J., Fei, Q., & Picone, D.M. (2007). Patterns of nursing intervention use across 6 days of acute care hospitalization for three older patient populations. *International Journal of Nursing Terminologies and Classifications*, 18, 18–29.

Shiraishi, S., Sano, Y., Yatabe, K., Takemasa, N., Motegi, Y., Yamakatsu, Y., Shikazawa, K., Sakai, K., Nomura, C., Shinohara, Y., & Fujiki, M. (2009). Current state and problems of introducing nursing diagnoses in psychiatric nursing units. *Journal of Japan Society of Nursing Diagnosis*, 14(1), 27–33.

Silva, V.M., Lopes, M.V., de Araujo, T.L., Ciol, M.A., & de Carvalho, E.C. (2009). Clinical indicators of ineffective airway clearance in children with congenital heart disease. *Journal of Clinical Nursing, 18*(5), 729–736.

Silva, R.C.G., Cruz, D.A.L.M., Bortolotto, L.A., Irigoyen, M.C.C., Krieger, E.M., Palomo, J.S.H., & Consolim-Colombo, F.M. (2006). Ineffective peripheral tissue perfusion: Clinical validation in patients with hypertensive cardiomyopathy. *International Journal of Nursing Terminologies and Classifications, 17*, 97–107.

Sparks, S.M., & Lien-Gieschen, T. (1994). Modification of the diagnostic content validity model. *Nursing Diagnoses, 5*(1), 31–35.

Thoroddsen, A., & Ehnfors, M. (2007). Putting policy into practice: Pre-and posttests of implementing standardized languages for nursing documentation. *Journal of Clinical Nursing, 16*, 1826–1838.

Walker, L.O. & Avant, K.C. (2005). *Strategies for theory construction in nursing* (4th ed.). Norwalk, CT: Appleton & Lange.

Waltz, C.F., Strickland, O.L., & Lenz, E.R. (2005). *Measurement in nursing and health sciences research* (3rd ed.). New York: Springer.

Welton, J.M. & Halloran, E.J. (2005). Nursing diagnoses, diagnosis-related groups, and hospital outcomes. *Journal of Nursing Administration, 35*, 541–549.

Westmoreland, D., Wesorick, B., Hanson, D., & Wyngarden, K. (2000). Consensus validation of clinical practice model practice guidelines. *Journal of Nursing Care Quality, 14*(4), 16–27.

Whitley, G.G. (1992). Concept analysis of fear. *Nursing Diagnoses, 3*(4), 155–161.

Zeitoun, S.S., Barros, A.L.B.L., & Bettencourt, A.R., (2007). Clinical validation of the signs and symptoms and the nature of the respiratory nursing diagnoses in patients under invasive mechanical ventilation. *Journal of Clinical Nursing, 16*, 1417–1426.

Chapter 6

Clinical Judgment and Nursing Diagnoses in Nursing Administration

T. Heather Herdman, Marcelo Chanes

Nurses in administrative roles have a variety of requirements, regulations, and strategies for which they are responsible. During the past two decades, the major shifts in demographics – with the increased number of elderly and the concurrent increase in comorbidities – has begun to force a shift from episodic-based care to health-promotion/disease prevention strategies across the continuum of healthcare services. This change comes at the same time as one of the most devastating economic crises the world has faced, which places additional burdens on already taxed healthcare systems. In the midst of all of this change, growth, and economic challenge has come a nursing shortage, and the increasing age of nurses worldwide suggests that this shortage will worsen over the next decades (Allen, 2008; Fox & Abrahamson, 2009; Yun, Jie & Anli, 2010). All of these realities create an environment in which nurses must work more efficiently, while being able to demonstrate the efficacy of our impact on patients, or risk being replaced by uneducated, unskilled workers who demand lower salaries.

The increasing complexity of human responses, coupled with the nursing shortage and economic realities at hand, demand professional nurses with excellent assessment, clinical judgment, and diagnostic reasoning abilities. Nurses need to understand how to differentiate between nursing diagnoses, how to identify patient outcomes that are appropriate given the length of stay and number of nursing visits each patient will have, and how to determine the most effective and efficient interventions based on evidence, whenever possible (Bolton, Donaldson, Rutledge, Bennett & Brown, 2007; Halm, 2010; Preston & Flynn, 2010). Evidence-based practice is a major topic of discussion, and it is being discussed as one of the most critical issues for nursing in this decade (Ahrens, 2005; Krainovich-Miller, Haber, Yost & Jacobs, 2009; Prior, Wilkinson & Neville, 2010; Scott & McSherry, 2009). Yet there are many questions still to be answered: What practice changes will have the best return on investment? How can nurses efficiently implement research-based practice? Is it really possible to have evidence for *all* decisions made by nurses or for all things that nurses do – or for any other discipline?

Nursing Research Priorities of Importance to Nurse Administrators

It has been suggested that nursing research should focus on the study of principles for effective and efficient nursing practice, and factors affecting perceptions of health and well-being among individuals, families, communities, and healthcare services, in order to expand nursing's scientific knowledge base (Evers, 2003; Hinshaw, 2000). These same aims are important for nurse administrators, who must justify the need for professional nurses at all levels of healthcare, to promote patient safety, health promotion, disease prevention, and positive patient outcomes.

In order to identify critical issues in nursing with which nurse administrators need to be concerned, it is helpful to look at international nursing research priorities. Studies across Europe, the United Kingdom, Asia, and the Americas have several consistent themes. The results of these studies have some variation, but they also demonstrate consistencies, including: outcomes of care delivery, staffing issues in practice, communication in clinical practice, nursing input into health policy and decision-making, implementing nursing knowledge in clinical practice and evaluating the beneficence to the patient, determining means to evaluate the relationship between the supervision of nurses and quality improvement, the effect of decision-making, and the nurse:patient ratio and its effect on patient outcomes. The National Institute of Nursing Research in the United States has identified research priorities in areas including: health outcomes measurement in health-promotion and prevention intervention studies, studies of patients at risk for disease states, investigations of adherence to treatment regimes, and evaluations of technology-based interventions (Reeve, Burke, Chiang, Clauser, Colpe, Elias, 2007). Other studies consider the effectiveness of interventions on patient outcomes, factors influencing decision-making in nurses, and the implementation of evidence-based practice (Back-Pettersson, Hermansson, Sernert & Bjorkelund, 2008; Drennan, Meehan, Kemple, Johnson, Treacy & Butler, 2007; Lopez, 2003; Wiener, Chacko, Brown, Cron & Cohen, 2009).

Nursing's Role in Patient Safety

Seven subcultures of patient safety culture were identified through a comprehensive review of the culture of safety literature within the US hospital setting using meta-analysis: (1) leadership, (2) teamwork, (3) evidence-based, (4) communication, (5) learning, (6) just, and (7) patient-centered (Sammer, Lykens, Singh, Mains & Lackan, 2010). In looking at the results of this review, the subcultures with a direct relationship to the implementation of clinical judgment/critical thinking/diagnostic reasoning are: leadership, evidence-based, communication, learning, and patient-centered.

According to these authors, *leaders* must acknowledge that the healthcare environment is high risk, and move to align vision/mission, competency of staff, and fiscal and human resources across the organization. *Evidence-based practice* encourages standardization to reduce variation whenever possible, with processes implemented to improve reliability. *Communication* includes hand-off communication in a structured communication method between healthcare providers so that information is transferred cohesively across shifts, departments, and units. *Learning* begins with the leaders who show a willingness to learn from internal and external models of high-performing safety cultures. Education and training incorporates performance improvement processes and understanding of the science of safety. The organization becomes transparent in the collection and reporting of nurse-sensitive patient safety indicators, and those results are shared routinely with all nursing staff. Finally, *patient-centered* organizations ensure that all care is centered around the recipient of care (individual, family, group, or community).

The role of clinical judgment/critical thinking/diagnostic reasoning on patient safety has been discussed in many articles (Clarke & Aiken, 2003; del Bueno, 2005; Eisenhauer, Hurley & Dolan, 2007; Lunney, 2010; Myers, Reidy, French, McHale, Chisholm & Griffin, 2010; Page, 2004). Van Gelder (2005) argued that critical thinking must be studied and practiced in its own right; it must be an explicit part of nursing education curricula. Four central themes have been identified as defining the specific impact of the nursing professional on patient safety. It is the nurse's responsibility to: (1) place the patient in safety; (2) generate a broader knowledge base on safety across the continuum of care; (3) create a safe culture and healthy work environment to mitigate current threats to patient safety; and (4) advance the translation of evidence to practice at the organizational and clinical levels (Jeffs, Macmillan, McKey & Ferris, 2009).

An emerging body of research shows that nurses are more likely than any other healthcare professional to recognize, interrupt, and correct errors that are often life-threatening (Rothschild, Hurley, Landrigan & Cronin, 2006). Because nurses assess, plan, implement, and evaluate patient care, their education on and involvement in patient safety and quality care initiatives are vital (Smith, 2006). When considering the seven subcultures of patient safety culture identified by Sammer et al. (2010), it is difficult not to see applications for the use of NANDA-I nursing diagnoses, the Nursing Outcomes Classification (NOC), and the Nursing Interventions Classifications (NIC). The use of clinical judgment in nursing – as with other healthcare professions – logically results in the identification of areas of concern to the discipline: human responses to actual or potential health problems/life processes, as well as health-promotion opportunities. It also logically follows that the use of standardized terminology that is clearly defined, and has objective and subjective clinical defining characteristics (signs/symptoms), related (etiologic) factors, and/or risk factors that are derived from nursing assessments, will enable clarity in communication and hand-off of patient care. Likewise, the use of clearly defined, nurse-sensitive outcomes and nursing interventions is critical for trending efficient and effective nursing care.

Without conceptual and operational definitions that are contained within the component parts of standardized terminologies such as NANDA-I, NOC, and NIC, this is simply not possible. Creating nursing terms at the bedside defeats the purpose of standardization, and prohibits any long-term or multisite research on diagnoses, interventions, or outcomes because there is no way to identify accuracy in diagnosis, or that the same concepts are being discussed in regard to diagnosis, outcome, or intervention. Indeed, it should be argued that this is a patient safety concern because inaccuracy in communication – thinking that a term represents one concept when it is actually being used to represent something different – can lead to inappropriate outcome setting and intervention choices.

Nurse administrators have a role to play in improving clinical judgment skills by expecting nurses to use these skills and rewarding them for doing so. Strategies for improving the clinical judgment/diagnostic reasoning abilities of nursing in clinical practice need to be assured by nurse administrators; they cannot assume that this critical function has been mastered in nursing educational preparation and that all professional nurses are experts. Clinical judgment evolves and improves over time, with experience and practice. Administrators should ensure that their organizations provide a variety of opportunities to improve these skills. It is important that students and nurses consider clinical judgment and diagnostic reasoning as *separate from* the documentation tool of nursing care plans. Documentation is critically important, but if the nurses do not understand how to apply clinical judgment and diagnostic reasoning and how to use the nursing process to improve patient outcomes – if they see it simply as a documentation tool – it will never become engrained as part of their identity as a nurse, but instead will be seen as "yet another task to be completed." This prevents nurses from seeing the nursing process as a way to frame, consider, and drive care, so it instead becomes a documentation task that many see as irrelevant and separate from the "real work" of nursing. Nurse administrators are responsible for creating, developing, and maintaining an organizational culture in which expertise in these critical areas is valued and considered in every decision related to nursing care.

Teacher
Resources

Triple Model for Nursing Administrators

Nurse administrators need to assume a very strategic role to implement a working process for their areas of accountability. Strategy for clinical practice should be based on concepts of nursing process, nursing autonomy, nursing quality, and evidence-based practice, all of which can be used in conjunction with the nursing taxonomies of NANDA-I, NOC, and NIC. Administrators can support the appropriate use of the nursing process as a method of integrating clinical judgment through educational programs in their organizations. Research has shown that guided clinical reasoning/diagnostic ability supports clinicians' abilities to derive accurate diagnoses, and to reach favorable patient outcomes through the selection of effective interventions (Beullens, Struyf & Van Damme, 2006; Müller-Staub, Needham, Odenbreit, Lavin & van Achterberg, 2007, 2008; Durak, Caliskan, Bor & Van Der Vleuten, 2007).

Transformational nurse leaders must be capable of influencing staff to align with organizational goals, by translating organizational vision, objectives, and strategy to staff at the unit level. Critical thinking skills and the inclination to engage in critical thinking are as essential for the nurse manager to function as a transformational leader as they are for the clinical nurse to function as a safe practitioner (Kjervik & Leonard, 2001; Robbins & Davidhizar, 2007). The use of a model can be a helpful mechanism for understanding the requirements to motivate staff to adopt and implement practice changes. The Triple Model of Nursing Manager Behavior (Chanes, 2010) is offered as a method that can support nursing staff in adopting nursing diagnosis, improving clinical judgment and patient safety (Figure 6.1). The model has three components: developing the desire to work with nursing diagnoses, adopting a viable implementation and utilization of nursing diagnoses, and articulating the importance of clinical judgment and nursing diagnosis across the layers of power within the healthcare organization.

The first part of the Triple Model is to create a desire for nursing staff to work with nursing diagnoses. This kind of model is based on holographic leadership in which the beliefs of the whole organization are built upon every single organizational cell, beyond the leader's demonstration of beliefs (Morgan, 2006). Considering that the use of clinical judgment and nursing diagnoses impact the time nurses spend with their patients, there may be staff who complain that these changes are not a good idea, or cannot be effectively implemented. Therefore, it is normal to expect that resistance forces will arise inside the nursing staff.

Figure 6.1 *Triple Model of Nursing Manager's behavior. Adapted from Chanes (2010)*

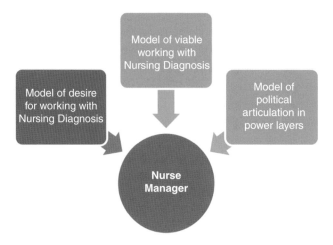

Resistance generally comes from those that are against change: in this instance, they may oppose a change from a medical or disease-focused model to a human response-focused nursing. It is therefore important that the nurse administrator helps nurses understand what nursing really is, the phenomena of concern to the discipline, and their accountability for identifying those concepts of concern to nursing practice. In other words, the nurse administrator must create new beliefs. Beliefs are created through observation of demonstration; someone or something showing us that a belief is real helps to create new beliefs for other individuals (March & Olsen, 1975). A process of belief creation is based on creating a response/reaction that serves as a demonstration that beliefs are correct. The nurse administrator must be aware of those forces and weaken them by showing that nursing diagnoses are desirable because the additional time spent with patients reduces errors and miscommunication, while supporting nurses in understanding what is really happening with patients.

The clear identification of nursing accountability that occurs with the use of defined, clearly described standardized nursing terminologies impacts positively on the nursing image inside the healthcare organization, across disciplines, and with patients and their families. The nurse administrator needs to meet with staff, and identify nurse-sensitive outcome indicators that will be collected and evaluated before and after the implementation of nursing diagnoses. It is important that in those meetings, and at every suitable opportunity, the nurse administrator speaks enthusiastically about nursing diagnoses, the reason nurses are required for safe patient care, and the ability for nursing diagnoses to support the justification of nurses in the organization. The nurse administrator needs to speak consistently about the scientific basis for nursing practice and clinical judgment, how it can be made obvious through the use of nursing diagnoses, and how the linkage of nursing diagnoses to nursing-sensitive patient outcome measures and nursing interventions supports the importance of nursing practice.

Finally, it is important to ensure that the nurses understand that nursing diagnoses are developed internationally, and therefore provide culturally sensitive terms to describe nursing practice worldwide. This means that there may be nursing diagnoses within the NANDA-I Taxonomy that would not be considered appropriate for use within a particular specialty or in some geographical regions. Therefore, all nurses must know their own standards of practice and the regional laws and regulations regarding nursing practice, and should not utilize nursing diagnoses that would be considered inappropriate within their scope of nursing practice, or their own competency.

Another strategy that leaders can use to improve the adoption of nursing diagnoses is the development of clinical mentors. Those individuals who are early adopters of change, and/or who demonstrate a strong understanding of and who believe in the use of nursing diagnoses, must be identified and developed to serve as mentors for implementation of the new practice model. It is not necessary to begin to implement nursing diagnoses in all units at same time. Pilot units can be identified that have strong clinical nurses who are in favor of and have a clear vision of what is and what is not a nursing diagnosis. Information about nursing-sensitive indicators linked to nursing diagnoses, and performance on quality-of-care indicators before and after implementation should be collected on these pilot units to serve as a basis of comparison between units working with nursing diagnoses and those that are not. Facts based on indicators will speak for themselves, and nurses will have the possibility to see their performance and judge their own beliefs in an evidence-based manner. It is helpful to remind staff that researchers worldwide have shown that indicators improve with the implementation and correct use of nursing diagnoses (Müller-Staub, Lavin, Needham & van Achterberg, 2006).

Simultaneously, it is critical to help those nurses who are not working in the pilot units to begin to understand the real importance of clinical judgment and nursing diagnoses during the time that the pilot units are collecting data. They need to understand that nursing diagnoses are not "one more task" or another documentation tool, but that they represent the actual knowledge of nursing, are critical to the nursing process, and are the basis for obtaining positive patient health outcomes within their healthcare organizations. Only after these processes have been used to sensitize resistant nurses will it be possible to implement nursing diagnoses across all units.

The second part of the Triple Model has the nurse administrator serving as a champion for the adoption, implementation, and viable utilization of nursing diagnoses in clinical practice. One of the roles of a leader is to facilitate the work of the nursing staff. Nurse administrators must provide nurses with a workable structure and framework of knowledge about nursing diagnoses to ensure their successful implementation. Training must be provided for all staff, ongoing work with case studies should be utilized, and a system of grand rounds based on nursing diagnoses can be an effective learning tool. A continuous program of training and competency evaluation must be offered yearly for all staff. It is important that nursing diagnoses and their requisite competencies – interpersonal, intellectual, and technical (Lunney, 2010) – be included in the training and evaluation on an annual basis.

Mentors must be empowered to resolve nurses' concerns and to answer their questions as they arise. One nurse can be assigned as the reference person on each shift to respond to doubts and questions from the nurses as they begin to use nursing diagnoses. A resource page located within the organization's internal website can include a "frequently asked questions" section. A monitored e-mail for questions can be identified and made available for all staff, with responses given within a preset period of time (e.g., within 24 hours). The important thing is that the nurse administrator must create a variety of communication channels for all nurses to express any difficulties or doubts that they may have, and a way to have questions addressed. Nurses should feel safe asking for help, and responses should be tailored in a way that not only provides information, but also gives encouragement and support.

Various recommendations have been made with regard to improving critical thinking/clinical judgment skills in nurses working in patient care areas. Preceptors for new nurses can be a key strategy for developing critical thinking skills and diagnostic reasoning (del Bueno, 2005; Forneris & Peden-McAlpine, 2009). The use of clinical preceptors who coach by asking specific questions based on patient assessment findings, to encourage nurses to consider the patient's human responses (nursing diagnosis), appropriate nurse-sensitive patient outcomes, and effective interventions can be critical to success. Encouraging nurses to consider what additional data they need to collect to rule out a diagnosis, or differentiate between two similar diagnoses, should be incorporated into daily clinical experiences.

Training needs to not only offer learning strategies to conceptualize nursing diagnoses, but to do so using interactive methodologies. The Living Learning Cycle is used to help nurses to think about the concepts they encounter during their education (including their formal nursing education, and the training being provided specific to the implementation of nursing diagnoses in their organization). It is important to have a framework of training for nurses to develop critical thinking, and not simply a class where concepts are taught, and nurses are expected to memorize them. Nurse administrators must emphasize to those doing the education that it is important that the nurses practice clinical judgment skills on their own – learning to think in a critical manner, without reliance on "the teacher" to give the answer, or a protocol to make decisions for them. According to the Living Learning Cycle, after a learning experience with a video, a game, an exercise, or even a lecture where new concepts are introduced, it is important to follow with these steps of report, processing, and generalization:

- *Report* is achieved when the facilitator asks the nurses to discuss their feelings about the experience or the new concepts, or to verbalize their perceptions of what has been discussed in the training sessions. In this phase, the nurses can report their point of view about the concepts or experiences and can help the facilitator to identify the stage of group development regarding these new concepts.
- *Processing* is the phase in which the teacher asks students *why* they think that their feelings and perceptions occur. The answers to this question will help the nurses to analyze their own thoughts and points of view, giving them the possibility to think about their thoughts; this "thinking about thinking" is known as metacognition (Lunney, 2008).
- Finally, *generalization* is the bridge between learning and applying the concepts, and the nurses are asked to discuss how they can use the new concepts in their own clinical practice environment. This enables the nurses to consider and discuss the structure they may need, or behavioral changes that will be required, in order to implement the concepts covered in the training.

Ongoing strategies for reinforcement of clinical judgment/diagnostic reasoning skills and accuracy in nursing diagnoses should be organized. Clinical nurses must be invited to present cases that were challenging, or cases that provide rich learning experiences. This strategy helps nurses to be recognized, while also supporting their development and maturity in clinical and critical thinking and reasoning skills. This strategy gives nursing diagnoses a formal importance in nursing staff agenda, and gives all the opportunity to understand the taxonomy structure. It can also provide a moment for staff to understand the process of diagnostic reasoning and how it serves as a basis for outcomes and interventions planning and implementation.

Having the nurse administrator not only support these methods, but also actually participate in and lead some of them, provides a strong statement that the administration of the organization understands and supports the importance of this work. The presence and participation of the nurse administrator demonstrates to staff that training and case studies are considered strategic to the success of the organization, and focuses attention on the importance of the nursing department's mission and role inside the health institution. Nurses recognize that activities which are truly considered to be important by the nurse administrator will receive more of that individual's attention; if the administrator reserves time to participate in these activities, it will create a culture in which clinical judgment and nursing diagnoses are understood to be important.

The third component of the Triple Model is embodied by the nurse administrator articulating the importance of clinical judgment and nursing diagnoses across the layers of power within the healthcare organization. Other healthcare professionals may not initially understand why nursing is focusing on clinical judgment or nursing diagnoses. This may be especially true if those professionals do not truly understand the scope of nursing practice. It is therefore possible that some of these professionals, including other administrators and perhaps physicians, might not support the emphasis or resources being placed on clinical judgment and nursing diagnoses. They may see this activity as a "task to be done that is taking too much time of nurses," or one that is potentially threatening to their own disciplines. The nurse administrator should anticipate such concerns, and provide education to all healthcare administrators and key leaders across other disciplines to introduce them to the importance of clinical judgment and nursing diagnoses. Data from research studies should be used to show the impact of clinical judgment and nursing diagnoses on critical indicators, such as overall length of stay, length of stay in intensive care units, number of rehospitalizations, and the percent of patients experiencing pressure ulcers, falls, deep vein thrombosis, effective risk management, and others.

In every situation in which a resistant healthcare professional tries to challenge a nurse applying clinical judgment or working with nursing diagnoses, the nurse administrator must be the voice of nursing and stand firm on the importance of these concepts to improved patient safety. Administrators must be willing to explain to other professions the role of nursing, why clinical judgment is as important to nursing practice as to other healthcare disciplines, and how the use of standardized terminology can improve patient safety, inter- and intradisciplinary communication, and continuity of care. The level of confidence with which the nurse administrator approaches these conversations will set the tone for the entire organization; she or he is the role model for all nurses across the organization, and this is a crucial component of establishing clinical judgment and nursing diagnoses as being of critical importance for patient care.

Ultimately, the nurse administrator as a professional leader must speak to the current evidence base that supports the need for clinical judgment, evidence-based practice, and the improvement in patient safety and nurse-sensitive patient outcomes that can be achieved with standardized nursing terminologies that provide definitions, defining characteristics, related factors, risk factors, clinical outcome indicators, and nursing activities. NANDA-I, NOC, and NIC provide the level of necessary information to support clinical judgment and use of the nursing process at the bedside. A comparison to the similar use of defined, standardized terminologies within other healthcare disciplines helps to provide a common basis of understanding, while demonstrating that NANDA-I, NOC, and NIC are necessary not just for the nursing profession, but for improved patient safety and quality of care as well.

Conclusion

Nurses have a unique perspective and critical role in assuring patient safety across all areas of healthcare service delivery. Clinical judgment skills are more important than ever due to the increasing number of comorbidities patients are experiencing, extremes of patient age (from care of very early neonates to care of the very old), decreased lengths of stay, and shortage of professional nurses. The focus on patient safety and evidence-based care is of primary importance to nurses, as they are on the front line of patient care, and are best positioned to identify and prevent patient complications. The use of nursing diagnoses that have standardized definitions, defining characteristics, and related and risk factors, provides a consistent terminology for inter- and intradisciplinary communication, hand-off of patient care, and identification of those phenomena of concern to nurses in clinical practice.

Nurse administrators must champion the need for nurses with expertise in clinical judgment and diagnostic reasoning, and the appropriate utilization of the entire nursing process. They must also understand the importance of using nursing classifications that are truly standardized, well researched, and peer reviewed to ensure patient safety and the appropriate selection of outcomes and nursing indicators. NANDA-I, NOC, and NIC provide the requisite components of a standardized classification: they are not terms that are developed "as needed" at the bedside, and that therefore lack consistency of meaning. Rather, they provide linkages to assessment data (defining characteristics, and related and risk factors) to assure diagnostic accuracy, and provide indicators for outcome measurement, and nursing activities to further explain nursing interventions. Without these components, it is impossible not only to assure standardization in use, but also to accurately educate nurses on the use of the classifications. Without clearly identified assessment criteria, it is impossible to know whether a diagnosis that is made is accurate, because there is no way to review assessment data to see if the required objective and subjective data were present in the patient. These component parts provide nurse administrators with the justification they need to support the use of these classifications in supporting an organizational cuture of patient safety, with regard for nursing clinical judgment.

References

Ahrens, T. (2005). Evidence-based practice: priorities and implementation strategies. *AACN Clinical Issues: Advanced Practice in Acute and Critical Care*, 16(1), 36–42.

Allen, L. (2008). The nursing shortage continues as faculty shortage grows. *Nursing Economic$*, 26(1), 35–40.

Back-Pettersson, S., Hermansson, E., Sernert, N., & Bjorkelund, C. (2008). Research priorities in nursing – a Delphi study among Swedish nurses. *Journal of Clinical Nursing*, 17(16), 2221–2231.

Beullens, J., Struyf, E., & Van Damme, B. (2006). Diagnostic ability in relation to clinical seminars and extended-matching questions examinations. *Medical Education*, 40(12), 1173–1179.

Bolton, L.B., Donaldson, N.E., Rutledge, D.N., Bennett, C., & Brown, D.S. (2007). The impact of nursing interventions: Overview of effective interventions, outcomes, measures, and priorities for future research. *Medical Care Research and Review*, 64(2 Suppl.), 123S–143S.

Chanes, M. (2010). Managing nursing process using and integrating NANDA-I, NOC and NIC taxonomies. In: W. Malagutti, & S.M.R.C. de Miranda. *Nursing paths – from Florence to globalization*. São Paulo: Phorte, pp. 179–192.

Chanes, M., & Leite, M.M.J. (2008). Measuring knowledge acquired though leadership educational game. *Nursing, São Paulo*, 10(17), 70–74.

Clarke, S. P., & Aiken, L.H. (2003). Failure to rescue. *American Journal of Nursing*, 103(1), 42–47.

del Bueno, D. (2005). A crisis in critical thinking. *Nursing Education Perspectives*, 26(5), 278–282.

Drennan, J., Meehan, T., Kemple, M., Johnson, M., Treacy, M., & Butler, M. (2007). Nursing research priorities for Ireland. *Journal of Nursing Scholarship*, 39(4), 298–305.

Durak, H.I., Caliskan, S.A., Bor, S., & Van Der Vleuten, C. (2007). Use of case-based exams as an instructional teaching tool to teach clinical reasoning. *Medical Teacher*, 29, e170–e174.

Eisenhauer, L.A., Hurley, A.C., & Dolan, N. (2007). Nurses' reported thinking during medication administration. *Journal of Nursing Scholarship*, 39(1), 82–87.

Evers, G. (2003) Developing nursing science in Europe. *Journal of Nursing Scholarship*, 35(1), 9–13.

Forneris, S.G., & Peden-McAlpine, C. (2009). Creating context for critical thinking in practice: The role of the preceptor. *Journal of Advanced Nursing*, 65(8), 1715–1724.

Fox, R.L., & Abrahamson, K. (2009). A critical examination of the U.S. nursing shortage: Contributing factors, public policy implications. *Nursing Forum*, 44(4), 235–244.

Halm, M. (2010). "Inside looking in" or "Inside looking out"? How leaders shape cultures equipped for evidence-based practice. *American Journal of Critical Care*, 19(4), 375–378.

Hinshaw, A.S. (2000) Nursing knowledge for the 21st century: Opportunities and challenges. *Journal of Nursing Scholarship*, 32(2), 117–123.

Jeffs, L., Macmillan, K., McKey, C., & Ferris, E. (2009). Nursing leaders' accountability to narrow the safety chasm: Insights and implications from the collective evidence base on healthcare safety. *Nursing Leadership*, 22(1), 86–98.

Kjervik, D.K., & Leonard, D.J. (2001). Nurse responses to re-tooling practice, education, and management roles. *Journal of Continuing Education in Nursing*, 32(6), 254–259, 284–285.

Krainovich-Miller, B., Haber, J., Yost, J., & Jacobs, S.K. (2009). Evidence-based practice challenge: Teaching critical appraisal of systematic reviews and clinical practice guidelines to graduate students. *Journal of Nursing Education*, 48(4), 186–195.

Lopez, V. (2003). Critical care nursing research priorities in Hong Kong. *Journal of Advanced Nursing*, 43(6), 578–587.

Lunney, M. (2008). Current knowledge related to intelligence and thinking with implications for the development and use of case studies. *International Journal of Nursing Terminologies and Classifications*, 19(4), 158–162.

Lunney, M. (2010). Use of critical thinking in the diagnostic process. *International Journal of Nursing Terminologies and Classifications*, 21(2), 82–88.

March, J.G., & Olsen, J.P. (1975). The uncertainty of the past: Organizational learning under ambiguity. *European Journal of Political Research*, 3(2), 147–171.

Morgan, G. (2006). *Images of organization*. São Paulo, Brazil: ATLAS.

Müller-Staub, M., Lavin, M.A., Needham, I., & van Achterberg, T. (2006). Nursing diagnoses, interventions and outcomes – application and impact on nursing practice: A systematic literature review. *Journal of Nursing Administration*, 56(5), 514–531.

Müller-Staub, M., Needham, I., Odenbreit, M., Lavin, M.A., & van Achterberg, T. (2007). Improved quality of nursing documentation: Results of a nursing diagnoses, interventions, and outcomes implementation study. *International Journal of Nursing Terminologies and Classifications*, *18*(1), 5–17.

Müller-Staub, M., Needham, I., Odenbreit, M., Lavin, M.A., & van Achterberg, T. (2008). Implementing nursing diagnostics effectively: Cluster randomized trial. *Journal of Advanced Nursing*, *63*(3), 291–301.

Myers, S., Reidy, P., French, B., McHale, J., Chisholm, M., & Griffin, M. (2010). Safety concerns of hospital-based new-to-practice registered nurses and their preceptors. *Journal of Continuing Education in Nursing*, *41*(4), 163–171.

Page, A. (ed.). (2004). Keeping patients safe: Transforming the work environment of nurses. Retrieved from www.nap.edu/catalog/10851.html .

Preston, R., & Flynn, D. (2010). Observations in acute care: Evidence-based approach to patient safety. *British Journal of Nursing*, *19*(7), 442–447.

Prior, P., Wilkinson, J., & Neville, S. (2010). Practice nurse use of evidence in clinical practice: A descriptive study. *Nursing Praxis in New Zealand*, *26*(2), 14–25.

Reeve, B.B., Burke, L.B., Chiang, Y., Clauser, S.B., Colpe, L.J., Elias, J.W. et al. (2007). Enhancing measurement in health outcomes research supported by Agencies within the US Department of Health and Human Services. *Quality of Life Research*, *16*(2), 175–186.

Robbins, B., & Davidhizar, R. (2007). Transformational leadership in health care today. *Health Care Manager*, *26*(3), 234–239.

Rothschild, J.M., Hurley, A.C., Landrigan, C.P., & Cronin, J.W. (2006). Recovering from medical errors: The critical care safety net. *Joint Commission on Quality and Patient Safety*, *32*(2), 63–72.

Sammer, C.E., Lykens, K., Singh, K.P., Mains, D.A., & Lackan, N.A. (2010). What is patient safety culture? A review of the literature. *Journal of Nursing Scholarship*, *42*(2), 156–165.

Scott, K., & McSherry, R. (2009). Evidence-based nursing: Clarifying the concepts for nurses in practice. *Journal of Clinical Nursing*, *18*(8), 1085–1095.

Smith, E.L. (2006). NNSDO update: National nursing staff development organization. *Journal for Nurses in Staff Development*, *22*(3), 160–161.

Van Gelder, T. (2005). Teaching critical thinking: Some lessons from cognitive science. *College Teaching*, *53*(1), 41–46.

Wiener, B., Chacko, S., Brown, T. R., Cron, S.G., & Cohen, M.Z. (2009) Delphi survey of research priorities. *Journal of Nursing Management*, *17*(5), 532–538.

Yun, H., Jie, S., & Anli, J. (2010). Nursing shortage in China: State, causes, and strategy. *Nursing Outlook*, *58*(3), 122–128.

Chapter 7

Nursing Classifications: Criteria and Evaluation

Matthias Odenbreit, Maria Müller-Staub, Jane M. Brokel, Kay C. Avant, Gail Keenan

Nursing diagnosis classifications categorize patients' responses to health problems/ life processes for which nurses provide nursing interventions designed to positively impact patient outcomes. Nursing diagnoses are internationally accepted as a part of systematic and individualized nursing care (American Nurses Association, 2009; Departement des Innern, 2003; Venturini, Matsuda & Waidman, 2009). The increasing use of biomedical technology, reducing length of hospital stay, and escalating healthcare costs place nurses under increasing performance pressure even as the demands increase for nurses to describe their contribution (Keenan, Tschannen & Wesley, 2008; Kurashima, Kobayashi, Toyabe & Akazawa, 2008). Often, only the most urgent needs in direct patient contact are met, and adequate documentation of nursing care is neglected. Nursing documentation is frequently incomplete, the relationship between nursing diagnoses and nursing interventions is not logically indicated, and progress toward meeting patient-focused outcomes is deficient (Müller-Staub, Needham, Odenbreit, Lavin & van Achterberg, 2007a). The use of nursing diagnoses facilitates comprehensive nursing documentation by providing defined concepts in a common language to represent and easily track the priority patient issues of concern to nurses, while simultaneously increasing the efficiency of data management (Kurashima, Kobayashi, Toyabe & Akazawa, 2008; Lundberg, Warren, Brokel, Bulecheck, Butcher, Dochterman, Johnson, et al., 2008). Thus, standardized, computer-compatible professional classifications are becoming a requirement, especially by institutions and healthcare systems that bear the costs of healthcare (Keenan, Tschannen & Wesley, 2008; Lunney, Delaney, Duffy, Moorhead & Welton, 2005).

Nursing diagnoses have been introduced in many hospitals to make data collection electronically retrievable from electronic health records (EHRs) (Burri, Odenbreit & Schärer, 2010). However, administrators and clinical nurses may be unfamiliar with the criteria that a nursing classification should include, and to what degree existing classification systems meet these criteria. These deficiencies render the selection of nursing classification systems difficult. This chapter is intended to serve as a decision-making aid in choosing nursing classifications for implementation in practice and in EHRs. The aim is to describe literature-based classification criteria and to assess classifications according to these criteria.

NANDA International Nursing Diagnoses: Definitions & Classification 2012–2014, First Edition.
Edited by T. Heather Herdman.
© 2012 NANDA International. Published 2012 by Blackwell Publishing Ltd.

Characteristics of Classifications

Seven classifications are addressed in this chapter: the Clinical Care Classification (CCC), the International Classification of Nursing Practice (ICNP), the International Classification of Functioning, Disability and Health (ICF), the Omaha System, the NANDA International Nursing Diagnosis Classification (NANDA-I), the Nursing Interventions Classification (NIC), and the Nursing Outcomes Classification (NOC).

The *CCC* (formerly called Home Health Care Classification, developed by Dr. Virginia Saba) was first developed for home healthcare and adapted to the CCC by adding NANDA-I terms (Saba, 2007).

The *ICNP* is a multiaxial system intended to describe and serve nursing practice. The ICNP Beta Version lists nursing diagnoses (formerly named phenomena) and intervention labels. The gathering and organization of terms is not conceptually driven but hierarchical in nature (Bartolomeyczik, 2003; Hinz, Dörre, König & Tackenberg, 2003; International Council of Nurses, 2010). In the ICNP, the assignment and linkages are not prescribed by the classification, but are to be determined individually for each patient by each individual nurse. Although diagnostic terms are described in the ICNP, defining characteristics, etiologies, and related factors or risk factors are not provided for the diagnoses. ICNP does not relate to nursing theory (Bartolomeyczik, 2003), nor does it provide a theoretical background for teaching or improving clinical reasoning, or for introduction into clinical practice.

The *ICF* was chosen for evaluation despite the fact that it is not a nursing classification (World Health Organization, 2005, 2010). Because the ICF is promoted as a complementary system to be used with the International Classification of Diseases, 10th edition (ICD-10) for interdisciplinary use, it is sometimes perceived as aiming to represent nursing or the nursing process. As a general healthcare classification, it was not designed by nurses or specifically for nursing care. This can explain some difficulties when nurses attempt to use this terminology, as well as the rather low levels of agreement that were found in a study that explored the relevance of ICF for nursing diagnoses (Van Achterberg, Holleman, Heijnen-Kaales, Van der Brug, Roodbol, Stallinga, et al., 2005). When prompted to choose a nursing classification, nurse administrators often require information about the meaning of the ICF for nursing, and therefore it was included in this analysis. The Omaha System includes three components – assessment (Problem Classification Scheme), intervention (Intervention Scheme), and outcomes (Problem Rating Scale for Outcomes) – but not nursing diagnoses with defined etiologies (Martin, 2005).

NANDA-I diagnoses are defined as "A clinical judgment about individual, family, group or community experiences/responses to actual or potential health problems or life processes. Nursing diagnoses provide the basis for the selection of nursing interventions to achieve outcomes for which the nurse has accountability" (NANDA International, 2009). The *NIC* includes the full range of nursing interventions from general practice to specialty areas (Bulechek, Butcher & Dochterman, 2008). The *NOC* is a comprehensive classification of patient outcomes developed to evaluate the effects of nursing interventions (Moorhead, Johnson, Maas & Swanson, 2008). The three classifications NANDA-I, NIC, and NOC are systematically connected in the NNN Taxonomy (Herdman, 2012; NANDA International, 2004). The NIC, CCC, Omaha, and NNN are embedded in a nursing framework, with linkages between diagnoses, interventions, and outcomes described in these systems (Johnson, Bulechek, Butcher, McCloskey Dochtermann, Maas, Moorhead, et al., 2006).

Classification Criteria

General criteria were based on four sources that were identified: the works of Gordon (1994), Van der Bruggen (2002), Olsen (2001), and Müller-Staub et al. (2007a). These authors indicate that the goal of a classification is twofold: to divide a domain of knowledge or information into classes or categories, and to facilitate communication among those who rely upon it for professional or scientific purposes. In addition, these authors point out that a classification system organizes groups of classes or categories in such a way that the relationship of the classes to each other and their respective characteristics are apparent. They also point out that a class consists of several concepts all possessing the same class characteristics. Their analyses led to the development of the following general criteria for evaluating classifications:

- The classification describes the domain and subject matter for which the domain is accountable.
- The purpose, objectives, and development procedures of the classification should be transparent, and the parameters clearly established.
- The classification system should demonstrate coherence. That means that every class is part of a central, superordinate concept. In other words, the classification is conceptually driven. Each concept must also be clearly defined.
- The conceptual focus and the classes of phenomena should be identified and have an exact conceptual definition.

With regard to nursing classifications, this requires the following:

- A nursing classification must comprehensively describe the knowledge base and the subject matter for which the nursing profession is responsible and accountable.
- As the purpose of nursing diagnosis classifications is to classify diagnoses, classification procedures should be transparent, and parameters should be clearly established: each class fits within a central concept of nursing or, in other words, is conceptually driven.
- Each within-class diagnosis possesses an exact definition including valid diagnostic criteria, key diagnostic features (or defining characteristics), and etiologies, with an exactness that allows for differentiation among diagnoses (Delaney, Mehmert, Prophet, Bellinger, Gardner-Huber & Ellerbe, 1992; Gordon, 1994; Gordon & Bartolomeyczik, 2001; Müller-Staub, 2004; Olsen, 2001; Van der Bruggen, 2002).
- Interventions and outcome classifications classify nursing interventions and nursing-sensitive patient outcomes. The purpose of the classification and the development procedures should be transparent, and parameters should be clearly established: each class fits within a central concept of nursing or, in other words, is conceptually driven.
- Each within-class intervention or outcome possesses an exact concept definition including valid criteria, intervention key features (actions/activities), or outcome indicators, with an exactness that allows for differentiation among concepts (Delaney et al., 1992; Gordon, 1994; Gordon & Bartolomeyczik, 2001; Müller-Staub, 2004; Olsen, 2001; Van der Bruggen, 2002).

Figure 7.1 *Illustration of coherent structure*

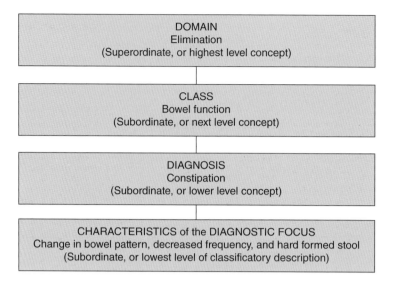

Specific criteria for nursing classifications have been described in the literature (Gordon & Bartolomeyczik, 2001; Müller-Staub et al., 2007a; Olsen, 2001; Van der Bruggen, 2002). The validity and reliability criteria used in the Classification Criteria Matrix (Table 7.1) were developed by an expansion and modification of Olsen's criteria (Just, 2005; Olsen, 2001; Müller-Staub, Lavin, Needham & van Achterberg, 2007b). Each system was assessed on its fulfilment of the criteria based on literature reviews and former evaluations (Just, 2005; Müller-Staub et al., 2007a; Olsen, 2001; Van der Bruggen, 2002). The validity of a nursing classification refers to the degree to which the classification succeeds at categorizing the domain of nursing knowledge and its phenomena of concern. A classification must organize all levels coherently. Any subordinate concept must have at least one characteristic that distinguishes it from its superordinate concept (e.g., domains, classes, diagnosis or diagnostic structure). An example to illustrate a coherent structure is shown in Figure 7.1.

The reliability of a classification reflects the degree of consistency and exactness of the classification when used or applied by different persons. "Internal consistency" describes exactly how nursing diagnoses and their characteristics are presented within class and domain categories, and how well the classes represent the domains of nursing (Müller-Staub et al., 2007a; Van der Bruggen, 2002). The elucidation of these principles of nursing diagnosis classifications lays the foundation for a continual improvement of classification systems, the utility of which extends beyond that of the simpler nursing terminology (nomenclature or lexicon) (Van der Bruggen, 2002). Table 7.1 presents the criteria and literature-based evaluation of the seven classifications reviewed.

Discussion

Based on the literature and as outlined in the Classification Criteria Matrix, the NANDA-I, NIC, and NOC fulfil the most criteria; NNN is also the most

Table 7.1 *Classification Criteria Matrix and Evaluation*

Nursing classification criteria	CCC[1]	ICF	ICNP	NANDA-I	NIC	NOC	Omaha
Established as clinical/nursing interface classification for point of care use	Y	N	N	Y	Y	Y	Y
Applicable as reference terminology	P	Y	Y	P	P	P	P
Transparent classification procedures with clearly established validation parameters: each class fits within a central concept of nursing and is conceptually driven	N	P	N	Y	Y	Y	P
Elements of the classification are coded concepts, with possibly multiple synonymous text representations including definitions, and hierarchical or definitional linkages to other coded concepts	Y	Y	–	Y	Y	Y	P
Each within-class nursing diagnostic concept possesses an exact description including valid diagnostic criteria, key diagnostic features, and etiologies, with an exactness that allows for differentiation among the diagnoses concepts within the classification	N	–	N	Y	–	–	N
Nursing diagnoses described by label and definition	Y	–	N	Y	–	–	Y
Nursing diagnoses contain related factors	N	N	N	Y	–	–	N
Nursing diagnoses contain defining characteristics (signs/symptoms)	N	N	N	Y	–	–	Y
Nursing diagnoses degree/severity is described	N	Y	Y	P	–	–	P
Actual/problem and risk diagnoses are included	Y	N	Y	Y	–	–	Y

Continued

Table 7.1 *Continued*

Nursing classification criteria	CCC[1]	ICF	ICNP	NANDA-I	NIC	NOC	Omaha
Health-promotion diagnoses are included in the classification	Y	N	N	Y	–	–	Y
Nursing interventions are described by label and definition	Y	–	N	–	Y	Y	Y
Nursing intervention concept is specified by activities	N	–	N	–	Y	–	N
Allotted time weight (dose) for nursing interventions is described	N	–	N	–	Y	–	N
Required job qualification or educational level to practice the nursing interventions of the classification are described	N	N	N	Y	Y	Y	N
Nursing outcomes are described by label and definition	N	–	N	–	–	Y	P
Outcomes are operationalized by indicators and outcome measurement scales	P	–	P	–	–	Y	P
Classification represents and defines physiological, psychosocial, spiritual, functional, and environmental domains	P	–	–	Y	Y	Y	P
Classification organizes all levels coherently; any subordinate concept has at least one characteristic that distinguishes it from its superordinate concept (domains, classes, and diagnostic structure)	P	–	N	Y	Y	Y	P
Classification represents the scope of nurses' accountability	Y	–	Y	Y	Y	Y	Y

Table 7.1 *Continued*

Nursing classification criteria	CCC[1]	ICF	ICNP	NANDA-I	NIC	NOC	Omaha
Classification defines nursing care needed by individuals, families, groups, and populations	Y	–	P	Y	Y	Y	Y
Number of published validity studies (PubMed-Search; search term: classification name AND validity)	1	116	6	938	38	35	2
Number of studies (PubMed-Search; search term: classification name)	12[2]	850	131	2535	730	685	60
Classification developed by nurses to represent nursing practice	Y	N	P	Y	Y	Y	Y
Classification based on a nursing framework/ nursing models/ theories; connections between classification and nursing theories are described (studies, textbooks)	N	–	N	Y	Y	Y	P
Guidelines published for use of the classification	Y	Y	Y	Y	Y	Y	Y
Multiple nursing textbooks published for meaningful and safe use of the classification, and are an integral part of international nursing curricula	P	–	N	Y	Y	Y	P
Textbooks published address clinical decision-making and critical thinking, including studies on application of the classification	N	–	N	Y	Y	Y	N
Theory-based linkages connecting nursing diagnoses, interventions, and outcomes are tested and published	P	–	N	Y	Y	Y	P

Continued

Table 7.1 *Continued*

Nursing classification criteria	CCC[1]	ICF	ICNP	NANDA-I	NIC	NOC	Omaha
Nursing diagnoses, interventions, and outcomes are coded for computer usage	Y	–	Y	Y	Y	Y	Y
According to systematic literature reviews, is the most widely implemented classification	N	N	N	Y	Y	Y	N
Classification is recognized by the American Nurses Association as being specific to nursing, and is included in the 2003 AA edition of the UMLS Metathesaurus	Y	N	N	Y	Y	Y	Y

N, no, criterion not fulfilled; P, partially, criterion partially fulfilled; Y, yes, criterion fulfilled; –, not applicable/not in the scope of the classification.
[1]Formerly named the Home Health Care Classification.
[2]Including articles addressing the Home Health Care Classification.

internationally disseminated classification (Anderson, Keenan & Jones, 2009; Lavin, 2004; Müller-Staub et al., 2007a). Scientific research on the NANDA-I classification is extensive, whereas research related to the majority of other classifications that include nursing diagnoses is limited (Anderson et al., 2009; Bernhard-Just Hillewerth, Holzer-Pruss, Paprotny & Zimmermann Heinrich, 2009). Based on these results presented in the Classification Criteria Matrix (Table 7.1), NANDA-I and other languages such as NOC and NIC have been recommended for implementation into EHRs because of their dispersion in textbooks and journals and the number of studies and validation research conducted on these classifications (Anderson, Keenan & Jones, 2009; Bernhard-Just Hillewerth, Holzer-Pruss, Paprotny & Zimmermann Heinrich, 2009; Cordova, Lucero, Hyun, Quinlan, Price & Stone, 2010; Müller-Staub, Lunney, Odenbreit, Needham, Lavin & van Achterberg, 2009). NOC and NIC have shown similar granularity to NANDA-I because of their provision of background knowledge to assist the practicing nurse at the bedside and within the clinic setting.

State-of-the-art EHRs contain all concepts (diagnoses, interventions, and outcomes labels including definitions), related or risk factors, and defining characteristics that are linked with theory-based interventions and outcomes, including outcome indicators (Odenbreit, 2008, 2010a, 2010b; von Krogh & Naden, 2008a, 2008b). An intelligent expert EHR system that guides nurses through the whole nursing process – including linkages among assessment, diagnoses, interventions, and outcomes planning and documentation, as well as outcomes evaluation – was developed and implemented (Burri et al., 2010; Odenbreit, 2008, 2010a). Such intelligent expert systems function as decision-making support tools and guide nurses in daily practice (Brokel, Schwichtenberg, Wakefield, Ward, Shaw & Kramer, 2011; Dougherty, 2007; Hendrix, 2009; Lunney, 2008; Lunney et al., 2005; Odenbreit, 2008, 2010a; Reyes, 2010; Van Horn & Kautz, 2010). Over 2000 peer-reviewed manuscripts have been published about decision-making with one or more of the NNN classifications (Anderson et al., 2009). This level of dissemination and evaluation within the nursing profession on a global scale within the past 30 years provides criteria to guide the meaningful use of nursing knowledge with health information technologies (Boyd, Funk, Schwartz, Kaplan & Keenan, 2010; Van Horn & Kautz, 2010).

Although the scope of this chapter is not to discuss education or implementation, it is important to acknowledge and emphasize that, in order for classifications to be safely used in clinical practice, nurses must be familiar with the content of the NNN classifications and with professional language. For this reason, theory-based nursing diagnoses, interventions, and outcomes must be carefully implemented into clinical practice by those knowledgeable in the classifications. These theory-based languages provide nurses with resources for assessment and accurate diagnosing, because the defining characteristics, risk factors, and/or related factors present knowledge that is required for safe decision-making.

Conclusion

Choosing nursing classifications for implementation into practice and EHRs has been shown to be a difficult task for clinical nurses and nurse administrators. The Classification Criteria Matrix and Evaluation presented in this chapter can serve as a guide for selecting a nursing classification. Based on study results, the NNN is recommended for implementation into practice and EHRs. Educating nurses about nursing classifications and how to apply theory-based diagnoses, interventions, and outcomes is key for the success of safe and meaningful use of nursing classifications.

References

American Nurses Association. (2009). *Nursing: A social policy statement*. Kansas: American Nurses Publishing.

Anderson, C.A., Keenan, G., & Jones, J. (2009). Using bibliometrics to support your selection of a nursing terminology set. *CIN: Computers, Informatics, Nursing*, 27(2), 82–90.

Bartolomeyczik, S. (2003). Zur Formalisierung der Sprache in der Pflege. In M. Hinz, F. Dörre, P. König, & P. Tackenberg (eds), *ICNP: Internationale Klassifikation für die Pflegepraxis*. Bern: Huber, pp. 77–87.

Bernhard-Just, A., Hillewerth, K., Holzer-Pruss, C., Paprotny, M., & Zimmermann Heinrich, H. (2009). Die elektronische Anwendung der NANDA-, NOC- und NIC-Klassifikationen und Folgerungen für die Pflegepraxis. *Pflege*, 22(6), 443–454.

Boyd, A.D., Funk, E.A., Schwartz, S.M., Kaplan, B., & Keenan, G.M. (2010). Top EHR challenges in light of the stimulus. Enabling effective interdisciplinary, intradisciplinary and cross-setting communication. *Journal of Healthcare Information Management: JHIM*, 24(1), 18–24.

Brokel, J.M., Schwichtenberg, T.J., Wakefield, D.S., Ward, M.M., Shaw, M.G., & Kramer, J.M. (2011). Evaluating clinical decision support rules as an intervention in clinician workflows with technology. *Computers, Informatics, Nursing*, 29(1), 36–42.

Bulechek, G., Butcher, H., & Dochterman, J. (2008). *Nursing Interventions Classification (NIC)* (5th ed.). St. Louis, MO: Mosby/Elsevier.

Burri, B., Odenbreit, M., & Schärer, S. (2010). Elekronische Pflegedokumentation: Zum Papier zurük-kehren möchte niemand. *Krankenpflege*, *103*(4), 16–18.

Cordova, P.B., Lucero, R.J., Hyun, S., Quinlan, P.K., Price, K., & Stone, P.W. (2010). Using the Nursing Interventions Classification as a potential measure of nurse workload. *Journal of Nursing Care Management*, *25*(1), 39–45.

Delaney, C., Mehmert, P.A., Prophet, C., Bellinger, S.L.R., Gardner-Huber, D., & Ellerbe, S. (1992). Standardized nursing language for healthcare information systems. *Journal of Medical Systems*, *16*(4), 145–159.

Departement des Innern. (2003). *Richtlinien des Departements des Innern: Pflege und Betreuungsdokumentation*: Solothurn: Departement des Innern Kt.

Dougherty, L. (2007). Using nursing diagnoses in prevention and management of chemotherapy-induced alopecia in the cancer patient. *International Journal of Nursing Terminologies and Classifications*, *18*(4), 142–149.

Gordon, M. (1994). *Nursing diagnosis: Process and application* (3rd ed.). St. Louis, MO: Mosby.

Gordon, M., & Bartolomeyczik, S. (2001). *Pflegediagnosen: Theoretische Grundlagen*. München: Urban & Fischer.

Hendrix, S.E. (2009). An experience with implementation of NIC and NOC in a clinical information system. *Computer, informatics, nursing*, *27*(1), 7–11.

Herdman, T.H. (ed.). (2012). *NANDA International nursing diagnoses: Definitions and classification, 2012–2014*. Singapore: Wiley-Blackwell.

Hinz, M., Dörre, F., König, P., & Tackenberg, P. (eds). (2003). *ICNP: Internationale Klassifikation für die Pflegepraxis*. Bern: Huber.

International Council of Nurses. (2010). ICNP® Definition. Retrieved from http://www.icn.ch/pill-arsprograms/definition-a-elements-of-icnpr/ .

Johnson, M., Bulechek, G., Butcher, H., McCloskey Dochtermann, J., Maas, M., Moorhead, S., et al. (2006). *NANDA, NOC and NIC linkages: Nursing diagnoses, outcomes, & interventions* (2nd ed.). St. Louis, MO: Mosby.

Just, A. (2005). *Ordnungssysteme zur Abbildung des Pflegeprozesses im elektronischen Patientendossier: Eine Empfehlung zuhanden der Pflegedienst-Kommission der Gesundheitsdirektion des Kantons Zürich*. Zurich.

Keenan, G., Tschannen, D., & Wesley, M.L. (2008). Standardized nursing teminologies can transform practice. *Jona*, *38*(3), 103–106.

Kurashima, S., Kobayashi, K., Toyabe, S., & Akazawa, K. (2008). Accuracy and efficiency of computer-aided nursing diagnosis. *International Journal of Nursing Terminologies and Classifications*, *19*(3), 95–101.

Lavin, M.A. (2004). *Stages of diffusion of an innovation: Nursing diagnosis classification*. Paper presented at the NANDA, NIC & NOC Conference, Chicago.

Lundberg, C., Warren, J., Brokel, J., Bulecheck, G., Butcher, H., Dochterman, J., Johnson, M., Maas, M., Martin, K., Moorhead, S., Spisla, C., Swanson, E., & Giarrizzo-Wilson, S. (2008). Selecting a standard-ized terminology for the electronic health record that reveals the impact of nursing on patient care. *Online Journal of Nursing Informatics*, *12*(2). Retrieved from http://ojni.org/12_2/lundberg.pdf.

Lunney, M. (2008). Critical need to address accuracy of nurses' diagnoses. *Online Journal of Issues in Nursing*, *13*(1).

Lunney, M., Delaney, C., Duffy, M., Moorhead, S., & Welton, J. (2005). Advocating for standardized nursing languages in electronic health records. *Journal of Nursing Administration*, *35*(1), 1–3.

Martin, K. S. (2005). *The Omaha system: A key to practice, documentation, and information management*. Omaha: Health Connections Press.

Moorhead, S., Johnson, M., Maas, M., & Swanson, E. (2008). *Nursing outcomes classification (NOC)* (4th ed.). St. Louis, MO: Mosby.

Müller-Staub, M. (2004). Pflegeklassifikationen im Vergleich. *PRINTERNET: Die wissenschaftliche Fachzeitschrift für die Pflege*, *6/04*, 359–377.

Müller-Staub, M., Needham, I., Odenbreit, M., Lavin, M.A., & van Achterberg, T. (2007a). Improved quality of nursing documentation: Results of a nursing diagnoses, interventions and outcomes imple-mentation study. *International Journal of Nursing Terminologies and Classifications*, *18*(1), 5–17.

Müller-Staub, M., Lavin, M.A., Needham, I., & van Achterberg, T. (2007b). Meeting the criteria of a nursing diagnosis classification: Evaluation of ICNP®, ICF, NANDA and ZEFP. *International Journal of Nursing Studies*, *44*(5), 702–713.

Müller-Staub, M., Lunney, M., Odenbreit, M., Needham, I., Lavin, M.A., & van Achterberg, T. (2009). Development of an instrument to measure the quality of documented nursing diagnoses, interventions and outcomes: The Q-DIO. *Journal of Clinical Nursing*, *18*(7), 1027–1037.

NANDA International. (2004). *Working together for quality nursing care: Striving toward harmonization*. Paper presented at the NANDA, NIC, NOC Conference, Chicago.

NANDA International (2009). Minutes of the International Think Tank. Retrieved from: www.nanda.org/Resources.aspx .

Odenbreit, M. (2008). *Electronically supported nursing documentation*. Paper presented at the NANDA International 2008 Conference: Capturing the expert knowledge of nursing, Miami.

Odenbreit, M. (2010a). Entwicklung und Implementierung der elektronischen Pflegedokumentation der Solothurner Spitäler AG: Eine Erfolgsstory. *Swiss Medical Informatics, 69*(2), 23–27.

Odenbreit, M. (2010b). *Pflegeleistung und DRG: Sichtbar durch Pflegediagnosen?* Paper presented at the DRG und elektronische Pflegedokumentation: Risiken und Chancen. Retrieved from http://www.pflege-pbs.ch/kongresse/100125/kongress100125.html .

Olsen, P.S. (2001). *Classificatory review of ICNP prepared for the Danish Nurses' Organization*. Brussels: PSO Sundhedsinformatiko.

Reyes, D. (2010). My first patient as a nurse practitioner: A man with low literacy. *International Journal of Nursing Terminologies and Classifications, 21*(4), 177–181.

Saba, V. (2007). *Clinical Care Classification (CCC) system manual*. New York: Springer.

Van Achterberg, T., Holleman, G., Heijnen-Kaales, Y., Van der Brug, Y., Roodbol, G., Stallinga, H.A., et al. (2005). Using a multidisciplinary classification in nursing: The International Classification of Functioning, Disability and Health. *Journal of Advanced Nursing, 49*(4), 432–441.

Van der Bruggen, H. (2002). *Pflegeklassifikationen*. Bern: Huber.

Van Horn, E.R., & Kautz, D.D. (2010). NNN language and evidence-based practice guidelines for acute cardiac care: retaining the essence of nursing. *Dimensions of Critical Care Nursing, 29*(2), 69–72.

Venturini, D., Matsuda, L., & Waidman, A. (2009). Produçâo científica Brasileira sobre sistematizaçao da assistência de enfermagem. *Ciência Cuidado e Saúde, 8*(4):707–715.

von Krogh, G., & Naden, D. (2008a). A nursing-specific model of EPR documentation: Organizational and professional requirements. *Journal of Nursing Scholarship, 40*(1), 68–75.

von Krogh, G., & Naden, D. (2008b). Implementation of a documentation model comprising nursing terminologies – theoretical and methodological issues. *Journal of Nursing Management, 16*(3), 275–283.

World Health Organization. (2005). International Classification of Functioning, Disability and Health: Introduction. Retrieved from http://www3.who.int/icf/icftemplate.cfm?myurl=introduction.html%20&mytitle=Introduction.

World Health Organization. (2010). *International Classification of Functioning, Disability and Health (ICF)*. Retrieved from http://www.who.int/classifications/icf/en/.

Part 3
NANDA-I Nursing Diagnoses 2012–2014

NANDA International Nursing Diagnoses: Definitions & Classification 2012–2014, First Edition.
Edited by T. Heather Herdman.
© 2012 NANDA International. Published 2012 by Blackwell Publishing Ltd.

International Considerations on the Use of the *NANDA-I Taxonomy of Nursing Diagnoses*

T. Heather Herdman

As noted in earlier chapters, NANDA International initially began as a North American organization, and therefore the earliest nursing diagnoses were primarily developed by nurses from the United States and Canada. However, over the past 20 years, there has been an increasing involvement of nurses from around the world, and membership in NANDA-I includes nurses from nearly 40 countries. Work is occurring across all continents using NANDA-I nursing diagnoses in curricula, clinical practice, research, and informatics applications. Development and refinement of diagnoses is ongoing across multiple countries. As a reflection of this increased international activity, contribution, and utilization, the North American Nursing Diagnosis Association changed its scope to an international organization in 2002, changing its name to **NANDA International** (it is therefore no longer accurate to refer to the organization as the *North American Nursing Diagnosis Association*).

As NANDA-I experiences increased worldwide adoption, issues related to differences in the scope of nursing practice, diversity of nurse practice models, divergent laws and regulations, nurse competency, and educational differences must be addressed. At the 2009 Think Tank Meeting, which included 86 individuals representing 16 countries, significant discussions occurred on how best to handle these and other issues. Nurses in some countries are not able to utilize nursing diagnoses of a more physiological nature because they are in conflict with their current scope of nursing practice. Nurses in other nations are facing regulations to ensure that everything done within nursing practice can be demonstrated to be evidence based, and therefore face difficulties with some of the older nursing diagnoses and/or linked interventions that are not supported by a strong level of research literature. Discussions were therefore held with international leaders in nursing diagnosis use and research, looking for the direction that would meet the needs of the worldwide community.

These discussions resulted in a unanimous decision to maintain the taxonomy as an intact body of knowledge in all languages, in order to enable nurses around the world to view, discuss, and consider diagnostic concepts being used by nurses within and outside of their countries, and to engage in discussions, research, and debate regarding the appropriateness of all of the diagnoses. The full minutes of the Think Tank Summit can be found in Part 4 of this text. However, a critical point is noted here prior to introducing the nursing diagnoses themselves.

Not every nursing diagnosis within the NANDA-I taxonomy is appropriate for every nurse in practice – nor has it ever been. Some of the diagnoses are specialty-specific, and would not necessarily be used by all nurses in clinical practice. In addition, there are diagnoses within the taxonomy that may be outside the scope or standards of nursing practice governing a particular geographical area in which a nurse practices.

Those diagnoses would, in these instances, not be appropriate for practice, and should not be used if they lie outside the scope or standards of nursing practice for a particular geographical region. However, it is appropriate for these diagnoses to

NANDA International Nursing Diagnoses: Definitions & Classification 2012–2014, First Edition.
Edited by T. Heather Herdman.
© 2012 NANDA International. Published 2012 by Blackwell Publishing Ltd.

remain visible in the taxonomy because the taxonomy represents clinical judgments made by nurses around the world, and not just those made in a particular region or country. Every nurse should be aware of, and work within, the standards and scope of practice and any laws or regulations within which he or she is licensed to practice. However, it is also important for all nurses to be aware of the areas of nursing practice that exist globally, as this informs discussion and may over time support the broadening of nursing practice across other countries. Conversely, these individuals may be able to provide evidence that would support the removal of diagnoses from the current taxonomy, which, if they were not shown in their translations, would be unlikely to occur.

Ultimately, nurses must identify those diagnoses that are appropriate for their area of practice, that fit within their scope of practice or legal regulations, and for which they have competency. Nurse educators, clinical experts, and nurse administrators are critical to ensuring that nurses are aware of diagnoses that are truly outside the scope of nursing practice in a particular geographical region. Multiple textbooks in many languages are available that include the entire NANDA-I taxonomy, so for the NANDA-I text to remove diagnoses from country to country would no doubt lead to a great level of confusion worldwide. Publication of the taxonomy in no way requires that a nurse utilize every diagnosis within it, nor does it justify practicing outside the scope of an individual's nursing license or regulations to practice.

Domain 1
Health Promotion

NANDA International Nursing Diagnoses: Definitions & Classification 2012–2014, First Edition.
Edited by T. Heather Herdman.
© 2012 NANDA International. Published 2012 by Blackwell Publishing Ltd.

Deficient Diversional Activity (00097)

(1980)

Domain 1: Health Promotion
Class 1: Health Awareness

Definition Decreased stimulation from (or interest or engagement in) recreational or leisure activities

Defining Characteristics

- Reports feeling bored (e.g., wishes there was something to do, to read)
- Usual hobbies cannot be undertaken in the current setting

Related Factors

- Environmental lack of diversional activity

Sedentary Lifestyle (00168)

(2004, LOE 2.1)

Domain 1: Health Promotion
Class 1: Health Awareness

Definition Reports a habit of life that is characterized by a low physical activity level

Defining Characteristics

- Chooses a daily routine lacking physical exercise
- Demonstrates physical deconditioning
- Reports preference for activities low in physical activity

Related Factors

- Deficient knowledge of the health benefits of physical exercise
- Lack of interest
- Lack of motivation
- Lack of resources (e.g., time, money, companionship, facilities)
- Lack of training for accomplishment of physical exercise

References

Blair, S., & Panffenbarguer R.(1989). Physical fitness and all-cause mortality. *Journal of the American Medical Association*, 262, 2395–2401.

Campbell, K., Waters, E., O'Meara, S., Kelly, S., & Summerbell, C. (2003). Interventions for preventing obesity in children. *Cochrane Database of Systematic Reviews*, (2).

Del Pino Casado, R., & Ugalde Apalategui, M. (1999) Líneas de investigación en diagnóstico enfermero. *Enfermería Clínica*, 9(3), 115–120.

Guirao-Goris, J.A., Moreno, P., & Martínez-Del, P. (2000). Validación del contenido diagnóstico de la etiqueta diagnóstica enfermera "sedentarismo". *Enfermería Clínica*, 4(11), 135–140.

Lizán Tudela, L., & Reig Ferrer, A. (1999) Adaptación transcultural de una medida de la calidad de vida relacionada con la salud: La versión española de las viñetas COOP/WONCA. *Atención Primaria*, 23(2), 75–83.

Montgomery, P., & Dennis, J. (2003). Physical exercise for sleep problems in adults aged 60+. *Cochrane Database of Systematic Reviews*, (2).

U.S. Department of Health and Human Services. (1996). *Physical activity and health: A report of the Surgeon General*. Atlanta, GA: US Department of Health and Human Services, Centers for Disease Control and Prevention, National Center for Chronic Disease Prevention and Health Promotion.

Vázquez Altuna, J. (1994). Evaluación de la efectividad de un programa de ejercicio físico en la disminución del peso graso. *Atención Primaria*, 14(4), 711–716.

Deficient Community Health (00215)
(2010, LOE 2.1)

Domain 1: Health Promotion
Class 2: Health Management

Definition Presence of one or more health problems or factors that deter wellness or increase the risk of health problems experienced by an aggregate

Defining Characteristics

- Incidence of risks relating to hospitalization experienced by aggregates or populations
- Incidence of risks relating to physiological states experienced by aggregates or populations
- Incidence of risks relating to psychological states experienced by aggregates or populations
- Incidence of health problems experienced by aggregates or populations
- No program available to enhance wellness for an aggregate or population
- No program available to prevent one or more health problems for an aggregate or population
- No program available to reduce one or more health problems for an aggregate or population
- No program available to eliminate one or more health problems for an aggregate or population

Related Factors

- Lack of access to public healthcare providers
- Lack of community experts
- Limited resources
- Program has inadequate budget
- Program has inadequate community support
- Program has inadequate consumer satisfaction
- Program has inadequate evaluation plan
- Program has inadequate outcome data
- Program partly addresses health problem

References

Edmundson, S., Stuenkel, D.L., & Connolly, P. M. (2005). Upsetting the apple cart: A community antico-agulation clinic survey of life event factors that undermine safe therapy. *Journal of Vascular Nursing*, 23(3), 105–111.

Francis, E., Hughes, P., & Schinka, J. (1999). Improving cost-effectiveness in a substance abuse treatment program. *Psychiatric Services*, 50(5), 633–635.

Goetzel, R.Z., Ozminkowski, R. J., Bruno, J.A., Rutter, K. R., Isaac, F., & Wang, S. (2002). The long-term impact of Johnson & Johnson's Health & Wellness Program on employee health risks. *Journal of Occupational and Environmental Medicine*, 44(5), 417–424.

Hawkins, J.D., Catalano, R.F., & Arthur, M.W. (2002). Promoting science-based prevention in communi-ties. *Addictive Behaviors*, 27(6), 951–976.

Keller, L.O., Schaffer, M.A., Lia-Hoagberg, B., & Strohschein, S. (2002). Assessment, program planning, and evaluation in population-based public health practice. *Journal of Public Health Management and Practice, 8*(5), 30–43.

McGinnis, J.M., Williams-Russo, P., & Knickman, J.R. (2002). The Case for More Active Policy Attention to Health Promotion. *Health Affairs, 21*(2), 78–93.

Pegus, C., Bazzarre, T.L., Brown, J.S., & Menzin, J. (2002). Effect of the Heart at Work program on awareness of risk factors, self-efficacy, and health behaviors. *Journal of Occupational and Environmental Medicine, 44*(3), 228–236.

Porter, H.B., Avery, S., Edmond, L., Straw, R., & Young, J. (2002). Program evaluation in pediatric education. *Journal for Nurses in Staff Development, 18*(5), 258–266.

Rome, S. (2002). Developing a fall-prevention program for patients. *American Journal of Nursing, 102*(6), 24A, 24C–D.

Swallow, A.D., & Dykes, P.C. (2004). Tobacco cessation at Greenwich Hospital. *American Journal of Nursing, 104*(12), 61–62.

Woodward, D. (2005). Developing a pain management program through continuous improvement strategies. *Journal of Nursing Care Quality, 20*(3), 261–267.

Risk-Prone Health Behavior (00188)
(1986, 1998, 2006, 2008, LOE 2.1)

Domain 1: Health Promotion
Class 2: Health Management

Definition Impaired ability to modify lifestyle/behaviors in a manner that improves health status

Defining Characteristics

- Demonstrates nonacceptance of health status change
- Failure to achieve optimal sense of control
- Failure to take action that prevents health problems
- Minimizes health status change

Related Factors

- Excessive alcohol
- Inadequate comprehension
- Inadequate social support
- Low self-efficacy
- Low socioeconomic status
- Multiple stressors
- Negative attitude toward healthcare
- Smoking

References

Alder, J., & Bitzer, J. (2003). Retrospective evaluation of the treatment for breast cancer: How does the patient's personal experience of the treatment affect later adjustment to the illness? *Archives of Women's Mental Health, 6*(2), 91–97.

American Medical Association. (2001). Executive summary of the third report of the National Cholesterol Education Program (NCEP) expert panel on detection, evaluation, and treatment of high blood cholesterol in adults (Adult Treatment Panel III). *Journal of the American Medical Association, 285*(19), 2486–2497.

Bandura, A. (1982). Self efficacy mechanism in human agency. *American Psychologist, 37*(2), 122–147.

Bornstein, J., & Bahat-Sterensus, H. (2004). Predictive factors for noncompliance with follow-up among women treated for cervical intraepithelial neoplasia. *Gynecologic and Obstetric Investigation, 58*(4), 202–206.

DiMatteo, R.M., Lepper, H.S., & Croghan, T.W. (2000). Depression is a risk factor for non-compliance with medical treatment. *Archives of Internal Medicine, 160*(14), 2101–2107.

Jager, B., Liedtke, R., Lamprecht, F., & Freyberger, H. (2004). Social and health adjustment of bulimic women 7–9 years following therapy. *Acta Psychiatrica Scandinavia, 110*(2), 138–145.

Kiefe, C.L., Heudebert, G., Box, J.B., Farmer, R.M., Micahel, M., & Clancy, C.M. (1999). Compliance with post-hospitalization follow-up visits: Rationing by inconvenience? *Ethnicity and Disease, 9*(3), 387–395.

Koenigsberg, M., Barlett, D., & Carmer, J.S. (2004). Facilitating treatment adherence with lifestyle changes in diabetes. *American Family Physician, 69*(2), 309–316, 319–320, 323–334.

Lifshitz, H., & Glaubman, R. (2004). Caring for the people with disabilities in the Haredi community: Adjustment mechanism in action. *Disability and Society, 19*(5), 469–486.

Medline. *Medline plus medical encyclopedia.* Retrieved from http://www/nlm.nih.gov/medlineplus/ency/article/000932.htm .

Merriam-Webster (1993). *Webster's third new international dictionary, unabridged.* Springfield, MA: Merriam-Webster.

National Heart, Lung, and Blood Institute. *How you can lower your cholesterol level?* Retrieved from www. nhlbi.nih.gov/chd/lifestyles.htm.

National Heart, Lung, and Blood Institute. (2003). *Seventh report of the Joint National Committee of the Prevention, Detection, Evaluation, and Treatment of High Blood Pressure (JNC 7).* Retrieved from http://www.nhlbi.nih.gov/guidelines/hypertension/jnc7full.htm .

National Kidney Foundation/Kidney Disease Outcomes Institute Guidelines. (2002). *K/DOQI Clinical practice guidelines for chronic kidney disease: Evaluation, classification, and stratification.* Retrieved from http://www.kidney.org/professionals/kdoqi/p4_class_g2.htm .

Newsom, J.T., Kaplan, M.S., Huguet, N., & Mcfarland, B.H. (2004). Health behaviors in a representative sample of older Canadians: Prevalences, reported change, motivation to change, and perceived barriers. *Gerontologist, 44*(2), 193–205.

Nosè, M., & Barbui, C. (2003). Efficacia delle strategie per migliorare l'aderenza ai trattamenti nelle psicosi: Revisione sistematica [Systematic review of clinical interventions for reducing treatment nonadherence in psychosis]. *Epidemiologia e Psichiatria Sociale, 12*(4), 272–286.

Pinto, M.B., Maruyama, N.C., Clark, M.M., Cruess, D.G., Park, E., & Roberts, M. (2002). Motivation to modify lifestyle risk behaviors in women treated for breast cancer. *Mayo Foundation for Medical Education and Research, 77*(2), 122–129.

Prelow, H.M., Danoff-Burg, S., Swenson, R.R., & Pulgiano, D. (2004). The impact of ecological risk and perceived discrimination on the psychological adjustment of African American and European youth. *Journal of Community Psychology, 32*(4), 375–389.

Psyweb. *Adjustment disorders.* Retrieved from http://www.psyweb.com/Mdisord/adjd.html .

Shemesh, E. (2004). Non-adherence to medications following pediatric liver transplantation. *Pediatric Transplantation, 8*(6), 600–605.

Uphold C.R., & Graham, M.R. (2003) *Clinical guidelines in family practice* (4th ed.). Gainesville, FL: Barmarrae Books.

Ineffective Health Maintenance (00099)

(1982)

Domain 1: Health Promotion
Class 2: Health Management

Definition Inability to identify, manage, and/or seek out help to maintain health

Defining Characteristics

- Demonstrated lack of adaptive behaviors to environmental changes
- Demonstrated lack of knowledge about basic health practices
- History of lack of health-seeking behavior
- Inability to take responsibility for meeting basic health practices
- Impairment of personal support systems
- Lack of expressed interest in improving health behaviors

Related Factors

- Cognitive impairment
- Complicated grieving
- Deficient communication skills
- Diminished fine motor skills
- Diminished gross motor skills
- Inability to make appropriate judgments
- Ineffective family coping
- Ineffective individual coping
- Insufficient resources (e.g., equipment, finances)
- Lack of fine motor skills
- Lack of gross motor skills
- Perceptual impairment
- Spiritual distress
- Unachieved developmental tasks

Readiness for Enhanced Immunization Status (00186)*
(2006, LOE 2.1)

Domain 1: Health Promotion
Class 2: Health Management

Definition A pattern of conforming to local, national, and/or international standards of immunization to prevent infectious disease(s) that is sufficient to protect a person, family, or community and can be strengthened

Defining Characteristics

- Expresses desire to enhance behavior to prevent infectious disease
- Expresses desire to enhance identification of possible problems associated with immunizations
- Expresses desire to enhance identification of providers of immunizations

- Expresses desire to enhance immunization status
- Expresses desire to enhance knowledge of immunization standards
- Expresses desire to enhance record-keeping of immunizations

References

Bundt, T.S., & Hu, H.M. (2004). National examination of compliance predictors and the immunization status of children: Precursor to a developmental model for health systems. *Military Medicine, 169,* 740–745.

Centers for Disease Control. (1997). Recommended childhood immunization schedule. United States 1997. *Mortality and Morbidity Weekly Report, 46*(2), 35–40.

Centers for Disease Control. (2002). Recommended adult immunization schedule: United States, 2002–2003. *Mortality and Morbidity Weekly Report, 51*(18), 904–908.

Das, J., & Das, S. (2003). Trust, learning and vaccination: A case study of a North Indian village. *Social Science & Medicine, 57*(1), 97–112.

Davis, T.C., Frederickson, D.D., Kennen, E.M., Arnold, C., Shoup, E., Sugar, M., Humiston, S.G., & Bocchini, J.A. (2004). Childhood vaccine risk/benefit communication among public health clinics: A time motion study. *Public Health Nursing, 21*(2), 228–236.

Hull, S., Hagdrup, N., Hart, B., Griffiths, C., & Hennessy, E. (2002). Boosting uptake of influenza immunization: A randomised controlled trial of telephone appointing in general practice. *British Journal of General Practice, 52*(482), 712–716.

Lambert, J. (1995). Every child by two. A program of the American Nurses Foundation. *American Nurse, 27*(8), 12.

Lopreiato, J.O., & Ottolini, M.C. (1996). Assessment of immunization compliance among children in the Department of Defense health care system. *Pediatrics, 97*(3), 308–311.

McMurray, R., Cheater, F.M., Weighall, A., Nelson, C., Schweiger, M., & Mukherjee, S. (2004). Managing controversy through consultation: A qualitative study of communication and trust around MMR vaccination decisions. *British Journal of General Practice, 54*(504), 520–525.

Mell, L.K., Ogren, D.S., Davis, R.L., Mullooly, J.P., Black, S.B., Shinefield, et al.; Centers for Disease Control and Prevention Vaccine Safety Datalink Project. (2005). Compliance with national immunization guidelines for children younger than 2 years, 1996–1999. *Pediatrics, 115*(2), 461–467.

*This diagnosis is to be retired in the next edition.

Scarborough, M.L., & Landis, S.E. (1997). A pilot study for the development of a hospital-based immunization program. *Clinical Nurse Specialist, 11*(2), 70–5.

Shui, I., Kennedy, A., Wooten, K., Schwartz, B., & Gust, D. (2005). Factors influencing African–American mothers' concerns about immunization safety: A summary of focus group findings. *Journal of the National Medical Association, 97*(5), 657–66.

Taylor, J.A., Darden, P.M., Slora, E., Hasemeier, C.M., Asmussen, L., & Wasserman, R. (1997). The influence of provider behavior, parental characteristics, and a public policy initiative on the immunization status of children followed by private pediatricians: A study from Pediatric Research in Office Settings. *Pediatrics, 99*(2), 209–215.

Wood, D., Donald-Shelbourne, C., Halfon, N., Tucker, M.B., Ortiz, V., Hamlin, J.S. et al. (1995). Factors related to immunization status among inner-city Latino and African–American preschoolers. *Pediatrics, 96*(2 Pt 1), 295–301.

Ineffective Protection (00043)
(1990)

Domain 1: Health Promotion
Class 2: Health Management

Definition Decrease in the ability to guard self from internal or external threats such as illness or injury

Defining Characteristics

- Altered clotting
- Anorexia
- Chilling
- Cough
- Deficient immunity
- Disorientation
- Dyspnea
- Fatigue
- Immobility
- Impaired healing
- Insomnia
- Itching
- Maladaptive stress response
- Neurosensory alteration
- Perspiring
- Pressure ulcers
- Restlessness
- Weakness

Related Factors

- Abnormal blood profiles (e.g., leukopenia, thrombocytopenia, anemia, coagulation)
- Cancer
- Extremes of age
- Immune disorders
- Inadequate nutrition
- Pharmaceutical agents (e.g., antineoplastic, corticosteroid, immune, anticoagulant, thrombolytic)
- Substance abuse
- Treatment-related side effects (e.g., surgery, radiation)

Ineffective Self-Health Management (00078)
(1994, 2008, LOE 2.1)

Domain 1: Health Promotion
Class 2: Health Management

Definition Pattern of regulating and integrating into daily living a therapeutic regimen for the treatment of illness and its sequelae that is unsatisfactory for meeting specific health goals

Defining Characteristics

- Failure to include treatment regimens in daily living
- Failure to take action to reduce risk factors
- Ineffective choices in daily living for meeting health goals
- Reports desire to manage the illness
- Reports difficulty with prescribed regimens

Related Factors

- Complexity of healthcare system
- Complexity of therapeutic regimen
- Decisional conflicts
- Deficient knowledge
- Economic difficulties
- Excessive demands made (e.g., individual, family)
- Family conflict
- Family patterns of healthcare
- Inadequate number of cues to action
- Perceived barriers
- Perceived benefits
- Perceived seriousness
- Perceived susceptibility
- Powerlessness
- Regimen
- Social support deficit

References

Banister, N.A., Jastrow, S.T., Hodges, V., Loop, R., & Gillham, M.B. (2004). Diabetes self-management training program in a community clinic improves patient outcomes at modest cost. *Journal of the American Dietetic Association, 104*(5), 807–810.

Benavides-Vaello, S, Garcia, A.A., Brown, S.A., & Winchell, M. (2004). Using focus groups to plan and evaluate diabetes self-management interventions for Mexican Americans. *Diabetes Educator, 30*(2), 238, 242–244, 247–250.

Bodenheimer, T., Lorig, K., Holman, H., & Grumbach, K. (2002). Patient self-management of chronic disease in primary care. *Journal of the American Medical Association, 288*(19), 2469–2475.

Blyth, F.M., March, L.M., Nicholas, M.K., & Cousins, M.J. (2005). Self-management of chronic pain: a population-based study. *Pain, 113*(3), 285–292.

Brown, C.M., & Segal, R. (1996). Ethnic differences in temporal orientation and its implications for hypertension management. *Journal of Health & Social Behavior, 37*(4), 350–361.

Chinn, M.H., Polonsky, T.S., Thomas, V.D., & Nerney, M.P. (2000). Developing a conceptual framework for understanding illness and attitudes in older, urban African Americans with diabetes. *Diabetes Educator, 26*(3), 439–449.

Cousins, S.O. (2000). My heart can't take it: Older women's beliefs about exercise benefits and risks. *Journals of Gerontology Series B: Psychological Sciences and Social Sciences, 55B*(5), 283–294.

Curtin, R.B., Sitter, D.C.B., Schatell, D., & Chewning, B.A. (2004). Self-management, knowledge, and functioning and well-being of patients on hemodialysis. *Nephrology Nursing Journal, 31*(4), 378–396.

Deakin, T., McShane, C.E., Cade, J.E., & Willams, R.D. (2005). Group based training for self-management strategies in people with type 2 diabetes mellitus. *Cochrane Database of Systematic Reviews, 18*(2), CD003417.

DeWalt, D.A., Pignone, M., Malone, R., Rawls, C., Kosnar, M.C., George, G., Bryant, B., Rothman, R.L., & Angel, B. (2004). Development and pilot testing of a disease management program for low literacy patients with heart failure. *Patient Education and Counseling, 55*(1), 78–86.

DiLorio, C., Shafer, P.O., Letz, R., Henry, T.R., Schomer, D.L., Yeager, K., & Project EASE study group. (2004). Project EASE: A study to test a psychosocial model of epilepsy medication management. *Epilepsy and Behavior, 5*(6), 926–936.

Funnell, M.M., & Anderson, R.M. (2004). Empowerment and self-management of diabetes. *Clinical Diabetes, 22*(3), 123–127.

Gallant, M.H., Beaulieu, M.C., & Carnevale, F.A. (2002). Partnership: An analysis of the concept within the nurse–client relationship. *Journal of Advanced Nursing, 40*(2), 149–157.

Georges, C.A., Bolton, L.B., & Bennett, C. (2004). Functional health literacy: An issue in African–American and other ethnic and racial communities, *Journal of the National Black Nurses Association, 15*(1), 1–4.

Goldberg, H.I., Lessier, D.S., Mertens, K., Eytan, T.A., & Cheadle, A.D. (2004). Self management support in a web-based medical record: A pilot randomized controlled trial. *Joint Commission Journal of Quality and Safety, 30*, 629–635, 589.

Goodwin, J.S., Black, S.A., & Satish, S. (1999). Aging versus disease: The opinions of older black, Hispanic, and non-Hispanic white Americans about the causes and treatment of common medical conditions. *Journal of the American Geriatric Society, 47*(8), 973–979.

Gray, J.A. (2004). Self-management in chronic illness. *Lancet, 364*(9444), 1523–1527.

Grey, M., Knafl, K., & McCorkle R. (2006). A framework for the study of self- and family management of chronic conditions. *Nursing Outlook, 54*(5), 278–286.

Griffiths, R., Johnson, M., Piper, M., & Langdon, R. (2004), A nursing intervention for the quality use of medicines by elderly community clients. *International Journal of Nursing Practice, 10*(4), 166–176.

Haidet, P., Kroll, T., & Sharf, B. (2006). The complexity of patient participation: Lessons learned from patients' illness narratives. *Patient Education and Counseling, 62*(3), 323–329.

Harmon, M., Castro, F., & Coe, K. (1996). Acculturation and cervical cancer: Knowledge, beliefs, and behaviors of Hispanic women. *Women's Health, 24*(3), 37–57.

Harvey, I.S. (2006). Self management of a chronic illness: An exploratory study on the role of spirituality among older African American women. *Journal of Women and Aging, 18*(3), 75–88.

Hibbard, J.H. (2004). Perspective: Moving toward a more patient-centered health care delivery system. *Health Affairs*, 2004. Retrieved from http://content.healthaffairs.org/content/early/2004/10/07/hlthaff.var.133.citation .

Huang, C.L., Wu, S.C., Jeng, C.Y., & Lin, L.C. (2004). The efficacy of a home-based nursing program in diabetic control of elderly people with diabetes mellitus living alone. *Public Health Nurse, 21*(1), 49–56.

Kastermans, M.C., & Bakker, R.H. (1999). Managing the impact of health problems on daily living. In M.J. Ranz, & P. Lemone (eds), *Classification of nursing diagnoses: Proceedings of the thirteenth conference*. Glendale, CA: CINAHL Information Systems.

Kennedy, A.P., Nelson, E., Reeves, D., Richardson, G., Roberts, C., Robinson, J.A., Rogerts, A.E., Sculpher, M., & Thomson, D.G. (2004). A randomised controlled trial to assess the effectiveness and cost of a patient oriented self management approach to chronic inflammatory bowel disease. *Gut, 53*(11), 1639–1645.

Kennedy, M.S. (2005). Education benefits women with IBS: Nurses teach self management techniques. *American Journal of Nursing, 105*(1), 22.

Koch, T., Jenkin, P., & Kralik, D. (2004). Chronic illness self-management: Locating the "self". *Journal of Advanced Nursing, 48*(5), 484–492.

Krein, S., Heisler, M., Piette, J., Makki, F., & Kerr, E. (2005). The effect of chronic pain on diabetes patients' self-management. *Diabetes Care, 28*(1), 65–70.

McMurray, S.D., Johnson, G., Davis, S., & McDougall, K. (2002). Diabetes education and care management significantly improve patient outcomes in a dialysis unit. *American Journal of Kidney Disease, 40*, 566–575.

Marabini, A., Brugnami, G., Curradi, F., Casciola, G., Stopponi, R., Pettinari, L., & Siracusa, A. (2002). Short term effectiveness of an asthma educational program: Results of a randomized controlled trial. *Respiratory Medicine, 96*, 933–938.

Midwest Bioethics Center (2001). Healthcare narratives from diverse communities – a self-assessment tool for health-care providers. *Bio-ethics Forum*, *17*(3–4), SS1.

Millard, L., Hallett, C., & Luker, K. (2006). Nurse–patient interaction and decision making in care: Patient involvement in community nursing. *Journal of Advanced Nursing*, *55*(2), 142–150.

Mohammadi, E., Abedi, H.A., Gofranipour, F., & Jalali, F. (2002). Partnership caring: A theory of high blood pressure control in Iranian hypertensives. *International Journal of Nursing Practice*, *8*(6), 324–329.

Munir, F., Leka, S., & Griffiths, A. (2005). Dealing with self-management of chronic illness at work: Predictors for self-disclosure. *Social Science Medicine*, *60*(6), 1397–1407.

Neafsey, P.J., Strickler, Z., Shellman, J., et al. (2002). An interactive technology approach to educate older adults about drug interactions arising from over-the-counter self medication practices. *Public Health Nursing*, *19*(4), 255–262.

Newman, S., Steed, L., & Mulligan, K. (2004). Self management interventions for chronic illness. *Lancet*, *364*(9444), 1523–1537.

Nguyen, H.Q., Carrieri-Kohlman, V., Rankin, S.H., Slaughter, R., & Stulberg, M. (2005). Is Internet-based support for dyspnea self-management in patients with chronic obstructive pulmonary disease possible? Results of a pilot study. *Heart and Lung*, *34*(1), 51–62.

Ogedegbe, G., Mancuso, C.A., & Allegrante, J.P. (2004). Expectations of blood pressure management in hypertensive African–American patients: a qualitative study. *Journal of the National Medical Association*, *96*(4), 442–449.

Opler, L.A., Ramirez, P.M., Dominguez, L.M., Fox, M.S., & Johnson, P.B. (2004). Rethinking medication prescribing practices in an inner-city Hispanic mental health clinic. *Journal of Psychiatric Practice*, *10*(2), 134–140.

Patterson, B.L., Russell, C., & Thorne, S. (2003). Critical analysis of everyday self care decision making in chronic illness. *Journal of Advanced Nursing*, *35*(3), 335–341.

Pearson, J., Mensing, C., & Anderson, R. (2004). Medicare reimbursement and diabetes self-management training: national survey results. *Diabetes Educator*, *30*(6), 914, 916, 918.

Robbins, B., Rausch, K.J., Garcia, R.I., & Prestwood, K.M. (2004). Multicultural medication adherence: A comparative study. *Journal of Gerontological Nursing*, *30*(7), 25–32.

Rogers, A., Kennedy, A., Nelson, E., & Robinson, A. (2005). Uncovering the limits of patient centeredness: Implementing a self management trail for chronic illness. *Qualitative Health Research*, *15*(2), 224–239.

Stevens, S., & Sin, J. (2005). Implementing a self-management model of relapse prevention for psychosis into routine clinical practice. *Journal of Psychiatric Mental Health Nursing*, *12*(4), 495–501.

Thackeray, R., Merrill, R.M., & Neiger, B.L. (2004). Disparities in diabetes management practice between racial and ethnic groups in the United States. *Diabetes Educator*, *30*(4), 665–675.

Thorne, S.E., & Paterson, B.L. (2000). Two decades of insider research: What we know and don't know about chronic illness experience. *Annual Review of Nursing Research*, *18*, 3–25.

Warsi, A., Wang, P.S., LaValley, M.P., Avorn, J., & Solomon, D. (2004). Self management education programs in chronic disease. *Archives of Internal Medicine*, *164*(15),1641–1649.

Watts, T., Merrell, J., Murphy, F., & Williams, A. (2004). Breast health information needs of women from minority ethnic groups. *Journal of Advanced Nursing*, *47*(5), 526–535.

Wen, L.K., Shepard, M.D., & Parchman, M.L. (2004). Family support, diet, and exercise among older Mexican Americans with type 2 diabetes. *Diabetes Educator*, *30*(6), 980–993.

Whittemore, R., Melkus, G.D., & Grey, M. (2005). Metabolic control, self management and psychosocial adjustment in women with type 2 diabetes. *Journal of Clinical Nursing*, *14*(2), 195–203.

Readiness for Enhanced Self-Health Management (00162)

(2002, 2008 LOE 2.1)

Domain 1: Health Promotion
Class 2: Health Management

Definition A pattern of regulating and integrating into daily living a therapeutic regimen for the treatment of illness and its sequelae that is sufficient for meeting health-related goals and can be strengthened

Defining Characteristics

- Choices of daily living are appropriate for meeting goals (e.g., treatment, prevention)
- Describes reduction of risk factors
- Expresses desire to manage the illness (e.g., treatment, prevention of sequelae)
- Expresses little difficulty with prescribed regimens
- No unexpected acceleration of illness symptoms

References

Banister, N.A., Jastrow, S.T., Hodges, V., Loop, R., & Gillham, M.B. (2004). Diabetes self-management training program in a community clinic improves patient outcomes at modest cost. *Journal of the American Dietetic Association, 104*(5), 807–810.

Benavides-Vaello, S, Garcia, A.A., Brown, S.A., & Winchell, M. (2004). Using focus groups to plan and evaluate diabetes self-management interventions for Mexican Americans. *Diabetes Educator, 30*(2), *238*, 242–244, 247–250.

Bodenheimer, T., Lorig, K., Holman, H., & Grumbach, K. (2002). Patient self-management of chronic disease in primary care. *Journal of the American Medical Association, 288*(19), 2469–2475.

Blyth, F.M., March, L.M., Nicholas, M.K., & Cousins, M.J. (2005). Self-management of chronic pain: a population-based study. *Pain, 113*(3), 285–292.

Brown, C.M., & Segal, R. (1996). Ethnic differences in temporal orientation and its implications for hypertension management. *Journal of Health & Social Behavior, 37*(4), 350–361.

Chinn, M.H., Polonsky, T.S., Thomas, V.D., & Nerney, M.P. (2000). Developing a conceptual framework for understanding illness and attitudes in older, urban African Americans with diabetes. *Diabetes Educator, 26*(3), 439–449.

Cousins, S.O. (2000). My heart can't take it: Older women's beliefs about exercise benefits and risks. *Journals of Gerontology Series B: Psychological Sciences and Social Sciences, 55B*(5), 283–294.

Curtin, R.B., Sitter, D.C.B., Schatell, D., & Chewning, B.A. (2004). Self-management, knowledge, and functioning and well-being of patients on hemodialysis. *Nephrology Nursing Journal, 31*(4), 378–396.

Deakin, T., McShane, C.E., Cade, J.E., & Willams, R.D. (2005). Group based training for self-management strategies in people with type 2 diabetes mellitus. *Cochrane Database of Systematic Reviews, 18*(2), CD003417.

DeWalt, D.A., Pignone, M., Malone, R., Rawls, C., Kosnar, M.C., George, G., Bryant, B., Rothman, R.L., & Angel, B. (2004). Development and pilot testing of a disease management program for low literacy patients with heart failure. *Patient Education and Counseling, 55*(1), 78–86.

DiIorio, C., Shafer, P.O., Letz, R., Henry, T.R., Schomer, D.L., Yeager, K., & Project EASE study group. (2004). Project EASE: A study to test a psychosocial model of epilepsy medication management. *Epilepsy and Behavior, 5*(6), 926–936.

Funnell, M.M., & Anderson, R.M. (2004). Empowerment and self-management of diabetes. *Clinical Diabetes*, 22(3), 123–127.

Gallant, M.H., Beaulieu, M.C., & Carnevale, F.A. (2002). Partnership: An analysis of the concept within the nurse–client relationship. *Journal of Advanced Nursing*, 40(2), 149–157.

Georges, C.A., Bolton, L.B., & Bennett, C. (2004). Functional health literacy: An issue in African–American and other ethnic and racial communities, *Journal of the National Black Nurses Association*, 15(1), 1–4.

Goldberg, H.I., Lessier, D.S., Mertens, K., Eytan, T.A., & Cheadle, A.D. (2004). Self management support in a web-based medical record: A pilot randomized controlled trial. *Joint Commission Journal of Quality and Safety*, 30, 629–635, 589.

Goodwin, J.S., Black, S.A., & Satish, S. (1999). Aging versus disease: The opinions of older black, Hispanic, and non-Hispanic white Americans about the causes and treatment of common medical conditions. *Journal of the American Geriatric Society*, 47(8), 973–979.

Gray, J.A. (2004). Self-management in chronic illness. *Lancet*, 364(9444), 1523–1527.

Grey, M., Knafl, K., & McCorkle R. (2006). A framework for the study of self- and family management of chronic conditions. *Nursing Outlook*, 54(5), 278–286.

Griffiths, R., Johnson, M., Piper, M., & Langdon, R. (2004), A nursing intervention for the quality use of medicines by elderly community clients. *International Journal of Nursing Practice*, 10(4), 166–176.

Haidet, P., Kroll, T., & Sharf, B. (2006). The complexity of patient participation: Lessons learned from patients' illness narratives. *Patient Education and Counseling*, 62(3), 323–329.

Harmon, M., Castro, F., & Coe, K. (1996). Acculturation and cervical cancer: Knowledge, beliefs, and behaviors of Hispanic women. *Women's Health*, 24(3), 37–57.

Harvey, I.S. (2006). Self management of a chronic illness: An exploratory study on the role of spirituality among older African American women. *Journal of Women and Aging*, 18(3), 75–88.

Hibbard, J.H. (2004). Perspective: Moving toward a more patient-centered health care delivery system. *Health Affairs*, 2004. Retrieved from http://content.healthaffairs.org/content/early/2004/10/07/hlthaff.var.133.citation .

Huang, C.L., Wu, S.C., Jeng, C.Y., & Lin, L.C. (2004). The efficacy of a home-based nursing program in diabetic control of elderly people with diabetes mellitus living alone. *Public Health Nurse*, 21(1), 49–56.

Kastermans, M.C., & Bakker, R.H. (1999). Managing the impact of health problems on daily living. In M.J. Ranz, & P. Lemone (eds), *Classification of nursing diagnoses: Proceedings of the thirteenth conference*. Glendale, CA: CINAHL Information Systems.

Kennedy, A.P., Nelson, E., Reeves, D., Richardson, G., Roberts, C., Robinson, J.A., Rogerts, A.E., Sculpher, M., & Thomson, D.G. (2004). A randomised controlled trial to assess the effectiveness and cost of a patient oriented self management approach to chronic inflammatory bowel disease. *Gut*, 53(11), 1639–1645.

Kennedy, M.S. (2005). Education benefits women with IBS: Nurses teach self management techniques. *American Journal of Nursing*, 105(1), 22.

Koch, T., Jenkin, P., & Kralik, D. (2004). Chronic illness self-management: Locating the "self". *Journal of Advanced Nursing*, 48(5), 484–492.

Krein, S., Heisler, M., Piette, J., Makki, F., & Kerr, E. (2005). The effect of chronic pain on diabetes patients' self-management. *Diabetes Care*, 28(1), 65–70.

McMurray, S.D., Johnson, G., Davis, S., & McDougall, K. (2002). Diabetes education and care management significantly improve patient outcomes in a dialysis unit. *American Journal of Kidney Disease*, 40, 566–575.

Marabini, A., Brugnami, G., Curradi, F., Casciola, G., Stopponi, R., Pettinari, L., & Siracusa, A. (2002). Short term effectiveness of an asthma educational program: Results of a randomized controlled trial. *Respiratory Medicine*, 96, 933–938.

Midwest Bioethics Center (2001). Healthcare narratives from diverse communities – a self-assessment tool for health-care providers. *Bio-ethics Forum*, 17(3–4), SS1.

Millard, L., Hallett, C., & Luker, K. (2006). Nurse–patient interaction and decision making in care: Patient involvement in community nursing. *Journal of Advanced Nursing*, 55(2), 142–150.

Mohammadi, E., Abedi, H.A., Gofranipour, F., & Jalali, F. (2002). Partnership caring: A theory of high blood pressure control in Iranian hypertensives. *International Journal of Nursing Practice*, 8(6), 324–329.

Munir, F., Leka, S., & Griffiths, A. (2005). Dealing with self-management of chronic illness at work: Predictors for self-disclosure. *Social Science Medicine*, 60(6), 1397–1407.

Neafsey, P.J., Strickler, Z., Shellman, J., et al. (2002). An interactive technology approach to educate older adults about drug interactions arising from over-the-counter self medication practices. *Public Health Nursing, 19*(4), 255–262.

Newman, S., Steed, L., & Mulligan, K. (2004). Self management interventions for chronic illness. *Lancet, 364*(9444), 1523–1537.

Nguyen, H.Q., Carrieri-Kohlman, V., Rankin, S.H., Slaughter, R., & Stulberg, M. (2005). Is Internet-based support for dyspnea self-management in patients with chronic obstructive pulmonary disease possible? Results of a pilot study. *Heart and Lung, 34*(1), 51–62.

Ogedegbe, G., Mancuso, C.A., & Allegrante, J.P. (2004). Expectations of blood pressure management in hypertensive African–American patients: a qualitative study. *Journal of the National Medical Association, 96*(4), 442–449.

Opler, L.A., Ramirez, P.M., Dominguez, L.M., Fox, M.S., & Johnson, P.B. (2004). Rethinking medication prescribing practices in an inner-city Hispanic mental health clinic. *Journal of Psychiatric Practice, 10*(2), 134–140.

Patterson, B.L., Russell, C., & Thorne, S. (2003). Critical analysis of everyday self care decision making in chronic illness. *Journal of Advanced Nursing, 35*(3), 335–341.

Pearson, J., Mensing, C., & Anderson, R. (2004). Medicare reimbursement and diabetes self-management training: national survey results. *Diabetes Educator, 30*(6), 914, 916, 918.

Robbins, B., Rausch, K.J., Garcia, R.I., & Prestwood, K.M. (2004). Multicultural medication adherence: A comparative study. *Journal of Gerontological Nursing, 30*(7), 25–32.

Rogers, A., Kennedy, A., Nelson, E., & Robinson, A. (2005). Uncovering the limits of patient centeredness: Implementing a self management trail for chronic illness. *Qualitative Health Research, 15*(2), 224–239.

Stevens, S., & Sin, J. (2005). Implementing a self-management model of relapse prevention for psychosis into routine clinical practice. *Journal of Psychiatric Mental Health Nursing, 12*(4), 495–501.

Thackeray, R., Merrill, R.M., & Neiger, B.L. (2004). Disparities in diabetes management practice between racial and ethnic groups in the United States. *Diabetes Educator, 30*(4), 665–675.

Thorne, S.E., & Paterson, B.L. (2000). Two decades of insider research: What we know and don't know about chronic illness experience. *Annual Review of Nursing Research, 18*, 3–25.

Warsi, A., Wang, P.S., LaValley, M.P., Avorn, J., & Solomon, D. (2004). Self management education programs in chronic disease. *Archives of Internal Medicine, 164*(15),1641–1649.

Watts, T., Merrell, J., Murphy, F., & Williams, A. (2004). Breast health information needs of women from minority ethnic groups. *Journal of Advanced Nursing, 47*(5), 526–535.

Wen, L.K., Shepard, M.D., & Parchman, M.L. (2004). Family support, diet, and exercise among older Mexican Americans with type 2 diabetes. *Diabetes Educator, 30*(6), 980–993.

Whittemore, R., Melkus, G.D., & Grey, M. (2005). Metabolic control, self management and psychosocial adjustment in women with type 2 diabetes. *Journal of Clinical Nursing, 14*(2), 195–203.

Ineffective Family Therapeutic Regimen Management (00080)
(1992)

Domain 1: Health Promotion
Class 2: Health Management

Definition A pattern of regulating and integrating into family processes a program for the treatment of illness and its sequelae that is unsatisfactory for meeting specific health goals

Defining Characteristics

- Acceleration of illness symptoms of a family member
- Failure to take action to reduce risk factors
- Inappropriate family activities for meeting health goals
- Lack of attention to illness
- Reports desire to manage the illness
- Reports difficulty with prescribed regimen

Related Factors

- Complexity of healthcare system
- Complexity of therapeutic regimen
- Decisional conflicts
- Economic difficulties
- Excessive demands
- Family conflict

Domain 2
Nutrition

NANDA International Nursing Diagnoses: Definitions & Classification 2012–2014, First Edition.
Edited by T. Heather Herdman.
© 2012 NANDA International. Published 2012 by Blackwell Publishing Ltd.

Insufficient Breast Milk (00216)

(2010, LOE 2.1)

Domain 2: Nutrition
Class 1: Ingestion

Definition Low production of maternal breast milk

Defining Characteristics

Infant

- Constipation
- Does not seem satisfied after sucking time
- Frequent crying
- Long breastfeeding time
- Refuses to suck
- Voids small amounts of concentrated urine (less than four to six times a day)
- Wants to suck very frequently
- Weight gain is lower than 500 g in a month (comparing two measures)

Mother

- Milk production does not progress
- No milk appears when mother's nipple is pressed
- Volume of expressed breast milk is less than prescribed volume

Related Factors

Infant

- Ineffective latching on
- Ineffective sucking
- Insufficient opportunity to suckle
- Rejection of breast
- Short sucking time

Mother

- Alcohol intake
- Fluid volume depletion (e.g., dehydration, hemorrhage)
- Malnutrition
- Medication side effects (e.g., contraceptives, diuretics)
- Pregnancy
- Tobacco smoking

References

Aragaki, I.M.M., Silva, I.A., & Santos, J.L.F. (2006). Traço e estado de ansiedade de nutrizes com indica-dores de hipogalactia e nutrizes com galactia normal [Trait and state anxiety of nursing mothers with indicators of nursing mothers with insufficient and normal lactation]. *Revista Da Escola De Enfermagem Da U S P*, 40(3), 396–403.

Daly, S.E.J., & Hartmann, P.E. (1995). Infant demand and milk supply. Part 1: Infant demand and milk production in lactating women. *Journal of Human Lactation, 11*(1), 21–26.

Dewey, K.G. (2001). Maternal and fetal stress are associated with impaired lactogenesis in humans. *Journal of Nutrition, 131*(11), 3012S–3015S.

Dewey, K.G., Nommsen-Rivers, L.A., Heinig, M.J., & Cohen, R.J. (2002). Lactogenesis and infant weight change in the first weeks of life. *Advances in Experimental Medicine and Biology, 503,*159–166.

Dykes, F., & Williams, C. (1999). Falling by the wayside: A phenomenological exploration of perceived breast-milk inadequacy in lactating women. *Midwifery, 15*(4), 232–246.

Hill, P.D., Aldag, J.C., Chatterton, R.T., & Zinaman, M. (2005). Psychological distress and milk volume in lactating mothers. *Western Journal of Nursing Research, 27*(6), 676–693; discussion 694–700.

Milsom, S.R., Rabone, D.L., Gunn, A.J., & Gluckman, P.D. (1998). Potential role for growth hormone in human lactation insufficiency. *Hormone Research, 50*(3), 147–150.

Page-Goertz, S. (2005). Weight gain concerns in the breastfed infant. Maternal factors. *Advance for Nurse Practitioners, 13*(2), 45–48, 72.

Powers, N.G. (1999). Slow weight gain and low milk supply in the breastfeeding dyad. *Clinical Perinatology, 26*(2), 399–430.

Sievers, E., Haase, S., Oldigs, H.D., & Schaub, J. (2003). The impact of peripartum factors on the onset and duration of lactation. *Biology of the Neonate, 83*(4), 246–252.

Silva, I.A. (2000). Enfermagem e aleitamento materno: combinando práticas seculares [Nursing and breastfeeding: combining secular practices]. *Revista Da Escola De Enfermagem Da U S P, 34*(4), 362–369.

Winberg, J. (2002). Breastfeeding – an evolutionary and neuroendocrine perspective. *Advances in Experimental Medicine and Biology, 503*, 149–157.

World Health Organization, Division of Diarrhoeal and Acute Respiratory Disease Control. (1996). *Not enough milk*. Update 1996: 21.

Zeitlyn, S., & Rowshan, R. (1997). Privileged knowledge and mothers, perceptions: The case of breast-feeding and insufficient milk in Bangladesh. *Medical Anthropology Quarterly, 11*(1), 56–68.

Ineffective Infant Feeding Pattern (00107)

(1992, 2006, LOE 2.1)

Domain 2: Nutrition
Class 1: Ingestion

Definition Impaired ability of an infant to suck or coordinate the suck/swallow response resulting in inadequate oral nutrition for metabolic needs

Defining Characteristics

- Inability to coordinate sucking, swallowing, and breathing
- Inability to initiate an effective suck
- Inability to sustain an effective suck

Related Factors

- Anatomical abnormality
- Neurological delay
- Neurological impairment
- Oral hypersensitivity
- Prematurity
- Prolonged nil by mouth (NPO) status

References

Hazinski, M.F. (1992). *Nursing care of the critically ill child*. St. Louis, MO: Mosby.

Shaker, C.S. (1991). Nipple feeding premature infants: A different perspective. *Neonatal Network: Journal of Neonatal Nursing, 8*(5), 9–17.

VandenBerg, K. (1990). Nippling management of the sick neonate in the NICU: The disorganized feeder. *Neonatal Network: Journal of Neonatal Nursing, 9*(1), 9–16.

Imbalanced Nutrition: Less Than Body Requirements (00002)

(1975, 2000)

Domain 2: Nutrition
Class 1: Ingestion

Definition Intake of nutrients insufficient to meet metabolic needs

Defining Characteristics

- Abdominal cramping
- Abdominal pain
- Aversion to eating
- Body weight 20% or more below ideal weight range
- Capillary fragility
- Diarrhea
- Excessive hair loss
- Hyperactive bowel sounds
- Lack of food
- Lack of information
- Lack of interest in food
- Loss of weight with adequate food intake
- Misconceptions
- Misinformation
- Pale mucous membranes
- Perceived inability to ingest food
- Poor muscle tone
- Reports altered taste sensation
- Reports food intake less than recommended daily allowance (RDA)
- Satiety immediately after ingesting food
- Sore buccal cavity
- Steatorrhea
- Weakness of muscles required for mastication
- Weakness of muscles required for swallowing

Related Factors

- Biological factors
- Inability to absorb nutrients
- Inability to digest food
- Inability to ingest food
- Insufficient finances
- Psychological factors

Imbalanced Nutrition: More Than Body Requirements (00001)

(1975, 2000)

Domain 2: Nutrition
Class 1: Ingestion

Definition Intake of nutrients that exceeds metabolic needs

Defining Characteristics

- Concentrating food intake at the end of the day
- Dysfunctional eating pattern (e.g., pairing food with other activities)
- Eating in response to external cues (e.g., time of day, social situation)
- Eating in response to internal cues other than hunger (e.g., anxiety)
- Sedentary lifestyle
- Triceps skin fold >15 mm in men
- Triceps skin fold >25 mm in women
- Weight 20% over ideal for height and frame

Related Factors

- Excessive intake in relation to metabolic need
- Excessive intake in relation to physical activity (caloric expenditure)

Readiness for Enhanced Nutrition (00163)
(2002, LOE 2.1)

Domain 2: Nutrition
Class 1: Ingestion

Definition   A pattern of nutrient intake that is sufficient for meeting metabolic needs and can be strengthened

Defining Characteristics

- Attitude toward drinking is congruent with health goals
- Attitude toward eating is congruent with health goals
- Consumes adequate fluid
- Consumes adequate food
- Eats regularly
- Expresses knowledge of healthy fluid choices
- Expresses knowledge of healthy food choices
- Expresses willingness to enhance nutrition
- Follows an appropriate standard for intake (e.g., the food pyramid or American Diabetic Association guidelines)
- Safe preparation of fluids
- Safe preparation of food
- Safe storage of fluids
- Safe storage of food

Risk for Imbalanced Nutrition: More Than Body Requirements (00003)

(1980, 2000)

Domain 2: Nutrition
Class 1: Ingestion

Definition At risk for an intake of nutrients that exceeds metabolic needs

Risk Factors

- Concentrating food intake at the end of the day
- Dysfunctional eating patterns
- Eating in response to external cues (e.g., time of day, social situation)
- Eating in response to internal cues other than hunger (e.g., anxiety)
- Higher baseline weight at beginning of each pregnancy
- Observed use of food as a comfort measure
- Observed use of food as a reward
- Pairing food with other activities
- Parental obesity
- Rapid transition across growth percentiles in children
- Reports use of solid food as major food source before 5 months of age
- Sedentary lifestyle

Impaired Swallowing (00103)
(1986, 1998)

Domain 2: Nutrition
Class 1: Ingestion

Definition Abnormal functioning of the swallowing mechanism associated with deficits in oral, pharyngeal, or esophageal structure or function

Defining Characteristics

Esophageal Phase Impairment

- Abnormality in esophageal phase by swallow study
- Acidic-smelling breath
- Bruxism
- Epigastric pain
- Food refusal
- Heartburn
- Hematemesis
- Hyperextension of head (e.g., arching during or after meals)
- Nighttime awakening
- Nighttime coughing
- Observed evidence of difficulty in swallowing (e.g., stasis of food in oral cavity, coughing/choking)
- Odynophagia
- Regurgitation of gastric contents (wet burps)
- Repetitive swallowing
- Reports "something stuck"
- Unexplained irritability surrounding mealtimes
- Volume limiting
- Vomiting
- Vomitus on pillow

Oral Phase Impairment

- Abnormality in oral phase of swallow study
- Choking before a swallow
- Coughing before a swallow
- Drooling
- Food falls from mouth
- Food pushed out of mouth
- Gagging before a swallow
- Inability to clear oral cavity
- Incomplete lip closure
- Lack of chewing
- Lack of tongue action to form bolus
- Long meals with little consumption
- Nasal reflux
- Piecemeal deglutition
- Pooling in lateral sulci
- Premature entry of bolus
- Sialorrhea
- Slow bolus formation
- Weak suck resulting in inefficient nippling

Pharyngeal Phase Impairment

- Abnormality in pharyngeal phase by swallow study
- Altered head positions
- Choking
- Coughing
- Delayed swallow
- Food refusal
- Gagging

- Gurgly voice quality
- Inadequate laryngeal elevation
- Multiple swallows

- Nasal reflux
- Recurrent pulmonary infections
- Unexplained fevers

Related Factors

Congenital Deficits

- Behavioral feeding problems
- Conditions with significant hypotonia
- Congenital heart disease
- Failure to thrive
- History of tube feeding
- Mechanical obstruction (e.g., edema, tracheostomy tube, tumor)
- Neuromuscular impairment (e.g., decreased or absent gag reflex,

decreased strength or excursion of muscles involved in mastication, perceptual impairment, facial paralysis)
- Protein–energy malnutrition
- Respiratory disorders
- Self-injurious behavior
- Upper airway anomalies

Neurological Problems

- Achalasia
- Acquired anatomic defects
- Cerebral palsy
- Cranial nerve involvement
- Developmental delay
- Esophageal defects
- Gastroesophageal reflux disease
- Laryngeal abnormalities
- Laryngeal defects

- Nasal defects
- Nasopharyngeal cavity defects
- Oropharynx abnormalities
- Prematurity
- Tracheal defects
- Traumas
- Traumatic head injury
- Upper airway anomalies

Risk for Unstable Blood Glucose Level (00179)
(2006, LOE 2.1)

Domain 2: Nutrition
Class 4: Metabolism

Definition At risk for variation of blood glucose/sugar levels from the normal range that may compromise health

Risk Factors

- Deficient knowledge of diabetes management (e.g., action plan)
- Developmental level
- Dietary intake
- Inadequate blood glucose monitoring
- Lack of acceptance of diagnosis
- Lack of adherence to diabetes management plan (e.g., adhering to action plan)
- Lack of diabetes management (e.g., action plan)

- Medication management
- Mental health status
- Physical activity level
- Physical health status
- Pregnancy
- Rapid growth periods
- Stress
- Weight gain
- Weight loss

References

American Diabetes Association (2005). Standard of medical care in diabetes. *Diabetes Care, 29,* S1–S36.
Bierschbach, J., Cooper, L., & Liedl, J. (2004). Insulin pumps: What every school nurse needs to know. *Journal of School Nursing, 20*(2), 117–123.
US Department of Health & Human Services (2003). *Helping the student with diabetes succeed: A guide for school personnel.* Retrieved from http://ndep.nih.gov/resources/school.htm.

Neonatal Jaundice (00194)

(2008, 2010, LOE 2.1)

Domain 2: Nutrition
Class 4: Metabolism

Definition

The yellow–orange tint of the neonate's skin and mucous membranes that occurs after 24 hours of life as a result of unconjugated bilirubin in the circulation

Defining Characteristics

- Abnormal blood profile (e.g., hemolysis; total serum bilirubin >2 mg/dL; total serum bilirubin in the high-risk range on age in hour-specific nomogram)
- Abnormal skin bruising
- Yellow mucous membranes
- Yellow–orange skin
- Yellow sclera

Related Factors

- Abnormal weight loss (>7–8% in breastfeeding newborn, 15% in term infant)
- Feeding pattern not well established
- Infant experiences difficulty making the transition to extrauterine life
- Neonate age 1–7 days
- Stool (meconium) passage delayed

References

American Academy of Pediatrics (2004). Management of hyperbilirubinemia in the newborn infant 35 or more weeks of gestation. *Pediatrics, 114*(1), 297–316.

Beachy, J.M. (2007). Investigating jaundice in the newborn. *Neonatal Network, 26*(5), 327–333.

Bhutani, V.K., Johnson, L.H., Schwoebel, A., & Gennaro, S. (2006). A systems approach for neonatal hyperbilirubinemia in term and near-term newborns. *Journal of Obstetric, Gynecologic and Neonatal Nursing, 35*(4), 444–455.

Blackburn, S. (1995). Hyperbilirubinemia and neonatal jaundice. *Neonatal Network, 14*(7), 15–25.

Boyd, S. (2004). Treatment of physiological neonatal jaundice. *Nursing Times, 100*(13), 40–43.

Cohen, S.M. (2006). Jaundice in the full-term newborn. *Pediatric Nursing, 32*(3), 202–207.

Gartner, L., & Herschel, M. (2001). Jaundice and breastfeeding. *Pediatric Clinics of North America, 48*(2), 389–399.

Hillman, N. (2007). Hyperbilirubinemia in the late preterm infant. *Newborn and Infant Nursing Reviews, 7*(2), 91–94.

Porter M.L., & Dennis, B.L. (2003). Hyperbilirubinemia in the term newborn. *American Family Physician, 65*, 599–606, 613–614.

2. Nutrition

Risk for Neonatal Jaundice (00230)
(2010, LOE 2.1)

Domain 2: Nutrition
Class 4: Metabolism

Definition At risk for the yellow–orange tint of the neonate's skin and mucous membranes that occurs after 24 hours of life as a result of unconjugated bilirubin in the circulation

Risk Factors

- Abnormal weight loss (>7–8% in breastfeeding newborn, 15% in term infant)
- Feeding pattern not well established
- Infant experiences difficulty making the transition to extrauterine life
- Neonate aged 1–7 days
- Prematurity
- Stool (meconium) passage delayed

References

American Academy of Pediatrics (2004). Management of hyperbilirubinemia in the newborn infant 35 or more weeks of gestation. *Pediatrics, 114*(1), 297–316.

Beachy, J.M. (2007). Investigating jaundice in the newborn. *Neonatal Network, 26*(5), 327–333.

Bhutani, V.K., Johnson, L.H., Schwoebel, A., & Gennaro, S. (2006). A systems approach for neonatal hyperbilirubinemia in term and near-term newborns. *Journal of Obstetric, Gynecologic and Neonatal Nursing, 35*(4), 444–455.

Blackburn, S. (1995). Hyperbilirubinemia and neonatal jaundice. *Neonatal Network, 14*(7), 15–25.

Boyd, S. (2004). Treatment of physiological neonatal jaundice. *Nursing Times, 100*(13), 40–43.

Cohen, S.M. (2006). Jaundice in the full-term newborn. *Pediatric Nursing, 32*(3), 202–207.

Gartner, L., & Herschel, M. (2001). Jaundice and breastfeeding. *Pediatric Clinics of North America, 48*(2), 389–399.

Hillman, N. (2007). Hyperbilirubinemia in the late preterm infant. *Newborn and Infant Nursing Reviews, 7*(2), 91–94.

Porter, M.L., & Dennis, B.L. (2003). Hyperbilirubinemia in the term newborn. *American Family Physician, 65*, 599–606, 613–614.

Risk for Impaired Liver Function (00178)
(2006, 2008, LOE 2.1)

Domain 2: Nutrition
Class 4: Metabolism

Definition At risk for a decrease in liver function that may compromise health

Risk Factors

- Hepatotoxic medications (e.g., acetaminophen, statins)
- HIV coinfection
- Substance abuse (e.g., alcohol, cocaine)

- Viral infection (e.g., hepatitis A, hepatitis B, hepatitis C, Epstein–Barr)

References

AASLD Practice Guideline (2004). *Diagnosis, management, and treatment of hepatitis C.* Alexandria, VA: American Association for the Study of Liver Diseases.

Fontana, R.J., & Lok, S.F. (2002). Noninvasive monitoring of patients with chronic hepatitis C. *Hepatology, 36*(5 Suppl.), S57–S64.

Hoofnagle, J. (2002). Course and outcome of hepatitis C. *Hepatology, 36*(5 Suppl. 1): S21–S29.

Laboratory Medicine Practice Guidelines (2000). *Laboratory guidelines for screening, diagnosis and monitoring of hepatic injury.* Washington, DC: National Academy of Clinical Biochemistry.

National Institute of Diabetes and Digestive and Kidney Diseases (2003). *Chronic hepatitis C: Current disease management.* Washington, DC: US Department of Health and Human Services.

Palmer, M. (2000). *Hepatitis Liver Disease: What you need to know.* Garden City Park, NY: Avery Publishing Group, pp. 23, 26–31, 62–67, 72–73.

2. Nutrition

Risk for Electrolyte Imbalance (00195)
(2008, LOE 2.1)

Domain 2: Nutrition
Class 5: Hydration

Definition At risk for change in serum electrolyte levels that may compromise health

Risk Factors

- Deficient fluid volume
- Diarrhea
- Endocrine dysfunction
- Excess fluid volume
- Impaired regulatory mechanisms (e.g., diabetes insipidus, syndrome of inappropriate secretion of antidiuretic hormone)
- Renal dysfunction
- Treatment-related side effects (e.g., medications, drains)
- Vomiting

References

Elgart, H.N. (2004). Assessment of fluids and electrolytes. *ACCN Clinical Issues, 15*(4), 607–621.

Weglicki, W., Quamme, G., Tucker, K., Haigney, M., & Resnick, L. (2005). Potassium, magnesium, and electrolyte imbalance and complications in disease management. *Clinical and Experimental Hypertension, 27*(1), 95–112.

Readiness for Enhanced Fluid Balance (00160)

(2002, LOE 2.1)

Domain 2: Nutrition
Class 5: Hydration

Definition A pattern of equilibrium between the fluid volume and chemical composition of body fluids that is sufficient for meeting physical needs and can be strengthened

Defining Characteristics

- Expresses willingness to enhance fluid balance
- Good tissue turgor
- Intake adequate for daily needs
- Moist mucous membranes
- No evidence of edema
- No excessive thirst
- Risk for deficient fluid volume
- Specific gravity within normal limits
- Stable weight
- Straw-colored urine
- Urine output appropriate for intake

Deficient Fluid Volume (00027)
(1978, 1996)

Domain 2: Nutrition
Class 5: Hydration

Definition Decreased intravascular, interstitial, and/or intracellular fluid. This refers to dehydration, water loss alone without change in sodium

Defining Characteristics

- Change in mental status
- Decreased blood pressure
- Decreased pulse pressure
- Decreased pulse volume
- Decreased skin turgor
- Decreased tongue turgor
- Decreased urine output
- Decreased venous filling
- Dry mucous membranes
- Dry skin
- Elevated hematocrit
- Increased body temperature
- Increased pulse rate
- Increased urine concentration
- Sudden weight loss (except in third spacing)
- Thirst
- Weakness

Related Factors

- Active fluid volume loss
- Failure of regulatory mechanisms

Excess Fluid Volume (00026)
(1982, 1996)

Domain 2: Nutrition
Class 5: Hydration

Definition Increased isotonic fluid retention

Defining Characteristics

- Adventitious breath sounds
- Anasarca
- Anxiety
- Azotemia
- Blood pressure changes
- Change in mental status
- Changes in respiratory pattern
- Decreased hematocrit
- Decreased hemoglobin
- Dyspnea
- Edema
- Electrolyte imbalance
- Increased central venous pressure
- Intake exceeds output
- Jugular vein distension
- Oliguria
- Orthopnea
- Pleural effusion
- Positive hepatojugular reflex
- Pulmonary artery pressure changes
- Pulmonary congestion
- Restlessness
- Specific gravity changes
- S3 heart sound
- Weight gain over short period of time

Related Factors

- Compromised regulatory mechanism
- Excess fluid intake
- Excess sodium intake

Risk for Deficient Fluid Volume (00028)
(1978, 2010)

Domain 2: Nutrition
Class 5: Hydration

Definition   At risk for experiencing decreased intravascular, interstitial, and/ or intracellular fluid. This refers to a risk for dehydration, water loss alone without change in sodium

Risk Factors

- Active fluid volume loss
- Deficient knowledge
- Deviations affecting absorption of fluids
- Deviations affecting access of fluids
- Deviations affecting intake of fluids
- Excessive losses through normal routes (e.g., diarrhea)
- Extremes of age
- Extremes of weight
- Factors influencing fluid needs (e.g., hypermetabolic state)
- Failure of regulatory mechanisms
- Loss of fluid through abnormal routes (e.g., indwelling tubes)
- Pharmaceutical agents (e.g., diuretics)

Risk for Imbalanced Fluid Volume (00025)
(1998, 2008, LOE 2.1)

Domain 2: Nutrition
Class 5: Hydration

Definition At risk for a decrease, increase, or rapid shift from one to the other of intravascular, interstitial, and/or intracellular fluid that may compromise health. This refers to body fluid loss, gain, or both

Risk Factors

- Abdominal surgery
- Ascites
- Burns
- Intestinal obstruction
- Pancreatitis
- Receiving apheresis
- Sepsis
- Traumatic injury (e.g., fractured hip)

References

Batts, E., & Lazarus, H. (2007). Diagnosis and treatment of transplantation-associated thrombotic micro-angiopathy: Real progress or are we still waiting? *Bone Marrow Transplant*, *40*(8), 709–719 [Review].

Boctor, F. (2005). Red blood cell exchange transfusion as an adjunct treatment for severe pediatric falciparum malaria, using automated or manual procedures. *Pediatrics*, *116*(4), 592–595.

Burgstaler, E. (2003). Current instrumentation for apheresis. In B. McLeod, T. Price, & R. Weinstein (eds), *Apheresis: Principles and practice* (2nd ed.). Bethesda, MD: AABB Press, pp. 961–967.

Corbin, F., Cullis, H.M., Freireich, E.J., Ito, Y., Kellog, R.M., Latham, A., & McLeod, B.C. (2003). Development of apheresis instrumentation. In B. McLeod, T. Price, & R. Weinstein (eds), *Apheresis: Principles and practice* (2nd ed.). Bethesda, MD: AABB Press, pp. 1–3.

Crookston, K., & Simon, T. (2003). Physiology of apheresis. In B. McLeod, T. Price, & R. Weinstein (eds), *Apheresis: Principles and practice* (2nd ed.). Bethesda, MD: AABB Press, pp. 934–960.

Danielson, C. (2002). The role of red blood cell exchange transfusion in the treatment and prevention of complications of sickle cell disease. *Therapeutic Apheresis*, *6*(1), 24–31.

Fortenberry, J., & Paden, M. (2006). Extracorporeal therapies in the treatment of sepsis: experience and promise. *Seminars in Pediatric Infectious Diseases*, *17*(2), 72–79.

Gambro, B.C.T. (2005). *Spectra™ System Therapeutics Reference Book*. Denver: Gambro.

Hester, J. (1997). Therapeutic cell depletion. In B. McLeod, & D. Priceth (eds.), *Apheresis: Principles and practice*. Bethesda, MD: American Association of Blood Banks, pp. 254–259.

Kim, H. (2000). Therapeutic pediatric apheresis. *Journal of Clinical Apheresis*, *15*(1–2), 129–157.

Metheny, N.M. (ed.). (2000). *Fluid and Electrolyte Balance: Nursing considerations*, 4th ed. Philadelphia: Lippincott Williams & Wilkins.

Teruya, J., Styler, M., Verde, S., Topolsky, D., & Crilley, P. (2001). Questionable efficacy of plasma exchange for thrombotic thrombocytopenic purpura after bone marrow transplantation. *Journal of Clinical Apheresis*, *16*(4), 169–174.

Vucic, S., & Davies, L. (1998). Safety of plasmapheresis in the treatment of neurological disease. *Australian and New Zealand Journal of Medicine*, *28*(3), 301–305.

Woloskie, S., Armelagos, H., Meade, J., & Haas, D. (2001). Leukodepletion for acute lymphocytic leukemia in a three-week-old infant. *Journal of Clinical Apheresis*, *16*(1), 31–32.

Domain 3
Elimination and Exchange

NANDA International Nursing Diagnoses: Definitions & Classification 2012–2014, First Edition.
Edited by T. Heather Herdman.
© 2012 NANDA International. Published 2012 by Blackwell Publishing Ltd.

Functional Urinary Incontinence (00020)

(1986, 1998)

Domain 3: Elimination and Exchange
Class 1: Urinary Function

Definition Inability of a usually continent person to reach the toilet in time to avoid unintentional loss of urine

Defining Characteristics

- Able to completely empty bladder
- Amount of time required to reach toilet exceeds length of time between sensing the urge to void and uncontrolled voiding
- Loss of urine before reaching toilet
- May be incontinent only in the early morning
- Senses need to void

Related Factors

- Altered environmental factors
- Impaired cognition
- Impaired vision
- Neuromuscular limitations
- Psychological factors
- Weakened supporting pelvic structures

Overflow Urinary Incontinence (00176)
(2006, LOE 2.1)

Domain 3: Elimination and Exchange
Class 1: Urinary Function

Definition Involuntary loss of urine associated with overdistension of the bladder

Defining Characteristics

- Bladder distension
- High post-void residual volume
- Nocturia
- Observed involuntary leakage of small volumes of urine
- Reports involuntary leakage of small volumes of urine

Related Factors

- Bladder outlet obstruction
- Detrusor external sphincter dyssynergia
- Detrusor hypocontractility
- Fecal impaction
- Severe pelvic prolapse
- Side effects of anticholinergic medications
- Side effects of calcium channel blockers
- Side effects of decongestant medications
- Urethral obstruction

References

Agency for Health Care Policy and Research. (1992). *Clinical practice guideline: Urinary incontinence in adults*. AHCPR Pub. No. 92–0038. Rockville, MD: AHCPR.

National Institutes of Health. (1988). Urinary incontinence in adults. NIH consensus statement. Retrieved from http://consensus.nih.gov/cons/071/071_statement.htm.

National Kidney and Urologic Diseases Information Clearinghouse. (2004). Urinary incontinence in women. Retrieved from http://kidney.niddk.nih.gov/kudiseases/pubs/uiwomen/index.htm.

Noble, J. (ed.). (2001). *Textbook of primary care medicine*, 3rd ed. St. Louis, MO: Mosby.

Stenchever, M.A. (ed.). (2001). *Comprehensive gynecology*. St. Louis, MO: Mosby.

Walsh, P.C. (ed.). (2002). *Campbell's urology*, 8th ed. Philadelphia: Saunders.

Reflex Urinary Incontinence (00018)
(1986, 1998)

Domain 3: Elimination and Exchange
Class 1: Urinary Function

Definition   Involuntary loss of urine at somewhat predictable intervals when a specific bladder volume is reached

Defining Characteristics

- Inability to voluntarily inhibit voiding
- Inability to voluntarily initiate voiding
- Incomplete emptying with lesion above pontine micturition center
- Incomplete emptying with lesion above sacral micturition center
- No sensation of bladder fullness
- No sensation of urge to void
- No sensation of voiding
- Predictable pattern of voiding
- Sensation of urgency without voluntary inhibition of bladder contraction
- Sensations associated with full bladder (e.g., sweating, restlessness, abdominal discomfort)

Related Factors

- Neurological impairment above level of pontine micturition center
- Neurological impairment above level of sacral micturition center
- Tissue damage (e.g., due to radiation cystitis, inflammatory bladder conditions, radical pelvic surgery)

Stress Urinary Incontinence (00017)
(1986, 2006, LOE 2.1)

Domain 3: Elimination and Exchange
Class 1: Urinary Function

Definition Sudden leakage of urine with activities that increase intra-abdominal pressure

Defining Characteristics

- Observed involuntary leakage of small amounts of urine in the absence of detrusor contraction
- Observed involuntary leakage of small amounts of urine in the absence of an overdistended bladder
- Observed involuntary leakage of small amounts of urine on exertion
- Observed involuntary leakage of small amounts of urine with coughing
- Observed involuntary leakage of small amounts of urine with laughing
- Observed involuntary leakage of small amounts of urine with sneezing

- Reports involuntary leakage of small amounts of urine in the absence of detrusor contraction
- Reports involuntary leakage of small amounts of urine in the absence of an overdistended bladder
- Reports involuntary leakage of small amounts of urine on exertion
- Reports involuntary leakage of small amounts of urine with coughing
- Reports involuntary leakage of small amounts of urine with laughing
- Reports involuntary leakage of small amounts of urine with sneezing

Related Factors

- Degenerative changes in pelvic muscles
- High intra-abdominal pressure

- Intrinsic urethral sphincter deficiency
- Weak pelvic muscles

References

Abrams, P., Cardozo, L., Fall, M., Griffiths, D., Rosier, P., Ulmsten, U., Van Kerrebroeck, P., Victor, A., Wein, A.; Standardisation Sub-committee of the International Continence Society. (2002). The standardisation of terminology in lower urinary tract function: Report from the Standardisation Sub-committee of the International Continence Society. *Urology, 61*(1), 37–49.

Agency for Health Care Policy and Research. (1992). *Clinical practice guideline: Urinary incontinence in adults.* AHCPR Pub. No. 92–0038. Rockville, MD: AHCPR.

National Institutes of Health. (1988). Urinary incontinence in adults. NIH consensus statements. Retrieved from http://consensus.nih.gov/cons/071/071_statement.htm.

National Kidney and Urologic Diseases Information Clearinghouse. (2004). Urinary incontinence in women. Retrieved from http://kidney.niddk.nih.gov/kudiseases/pubs/uiwomen/index.htm.

Noble, J. (ed.) (2001). *Textbook of primary care medicine*, 3rd ed. St. Louis, MO: Mosby.

Sampselle, C.M. (2003). State of the science on urinary incontinence: Behavioral interventions in young and middle-age women. *American Journal of Nursing, 103*(3), 9–19.

Stenchever, M.A. (ed.) (2001). *Comprehensive gynecology*. St Louis, MO: Mosby.

Walsh, P.C. (ed.) (2002). *Campbell's urology*, 8th ed. Philadelphia: Saunders.

Domain 3: Elimination and Exchange
Class 1: Urinary Function

Definition Involuntary passage of urine occurring soon after a strong sense of urgency to void

Defining Characteristics

- Observed inability to reach toilet in time to avoid urine loss
- Reports inability to reach toilet in time to avoid urine loss
- Reports involuntary loss of urine with bladder contractions
- Reports involuntary loss of urine with bladder spasms
- Reports urinary urgency

Related Factors

- Alcohol intake
- Atrophic urethritis
- Atrophic vaginitis
- Bladder infection
- Caffeine intake
- Decreased bladder capacity
- Detrusor hyperactivity with impaired bladder contractility
- Diuretic use
- Fecal impaction

References

Abrams, P., Cardozo, L., Fall, M., Griffiths, D., Rosier, P., Ulmsten, U., Van Kerrebroeck, P., Victor, A., Wein, A.; Standardisation Sub-committee of the International Continence Society. (2002). The standardisation of terminology in lower urinary tract function: Report from the Standardisation Sub-committee of the International Continence Society. *Urology, 61*(1), 37–49.

Agency for Health Care Policy and Research. (1992). *Clinical practice guideline: Urinary incontinence in adults.* AHCPR Pub. No. 92–0038. Rockville, MD: AHCPR.

National Institutes of Health. (1988). Urinary incontinence in adults. NIH consensus statement. Retrieved from http://consensus.nih.gov/cons/071/071_statement.htm.

National Kidney and Urologic Diseases Information Clearinghouse. (2004). Urinary incontinence in women. Retrieved from http://kidney.niddk.nih.gov/kudiseases/pubs/uiwomen/index.htm.

Noble, J. (ed.). (2001). *Textbook of primary care medicine*, 3rd ed. St. Louis, MO: Mosby.

Sampselle, C.M. (2003). State of the science on urinary incontinence: Behavioral interventions in young and middle-age women. *American Journal of Nursing, 103*(3), 9–19.

Stenchever, M.A. (ed.). (2001). *Comprehensive gynecology*. St. Louis, MO: Mosby.

Walsh, P.C. (ed.). (2002). *Campbell's urology*, 8th ed. Philadelphia: Saunders.

Risk for Urge Urinary Incontinence (00022)
(1998; 2008, LOE 2.1)

Domain 3: Elimination and Exchange
Class 1: Urinary Function

Definition At risk for involuntary passage of urine occurring soon after a strong sensation of urgency to void

Risk Factors

- Atrophic urethritis
- Atrophic vaginitis
- Effects of alcohol
- Effects of caffeine
- Effects of pharmaceutical agents
- Detrusor hyperactivity with impaired bladder contractility
- Fecal impaction
- Impaired bladder contractility
- Ineffective toileting habits
- Involuntary sphincter relaxation
- Small bladder capacity

References

Abrams, P., Cardozo, L., Fall, M., Griffiths, D., Rosier, P., Ulmsten, U., Van Kerrebroeck, P., Victor, A., Wein, A.; Standardisation Sub-Committee of the International Continence Society. (2002). The standardisation of terminology in lower urinary tract function: Report from the Standardisation Sub-committee of the International Continence Society. *Urology, 61*(1), 37–49.

Agency for Health Care Policy and Research. (1992). *Clinical practice guideline: Urinary incontinence in adults.* AHCPR Pub. No. 92–0038. Rockville, MD: AHCPR.

National Institutes of Health. (1988). *Urinary incontinence in adults.* NIH consensus statement. Retrieved from http://consensus.nih.gov/cons/071/071_statement.htm.

National Kidney and Urologic Diseases Information Clearinghouse. (2004). *Urinary incontinence in women.* Retrieved from http://kidney.niddk.nih.gov/kudiseases/pubs/uiwomen/index.htm.

Noble, J. (ed.). (2001). *Textbook of primary care medicine,* 3rd ed. St. Louis, MO: Mosby.

Sampselle, C.M. (2003). State of the science on urinary incontinence: Behavioral interventions in young and middle-age women. *American Journal of Nursing, 103*(3), 9–19.

Stenchever, M.A. (ed.). (2001). *Comprehensive gynecology.* St. Louis, MO: Mosby.

Walsh, P.C. (ed.). (2002). *Campbell's urology,* 8th ed. Philadelphia: Saunders.

3. Elimination and Exchange

Impaired Urinary Elimination (00016)
(1973, 2006, LOE 2.1)

Domain 3: Elimination and Exchange
Class 1: Urinary Function

Definition Dysfunction in urine elimination

Defining Characteristics

- Dysuria
- Frequency
- Hesitancy
- Incontinence

- Nocturia
- Retention
- Urgency

Related Factors

- Anatomic obstruction
- Multiple causality

- Sensory motor impairment
- Urinary tract infection

References

Engberg, S., McDowell, B., Donovan, N., Brodak, I., & Weber, E. (1997). Treatment of urinary incontinence in homebound older adults: Interface between research and practice. *Ostomy/Wound Management, 48*(10), 18–26.

Fantl, J., Newman, D., & Colling, J. (1996). *Urinary incontinence in adults: Acute and chronic management.* Clinical practice guideline No. 2. Rockville, MD: US Department of Health and Human Services.

Messick, G. & Powe, C. (1997). Applying behavioral research to incontinence. *Ostomy/Wound management, 43*(10), 40–46, 48.

Readiness for Enhanced
Urinary Elimination (00166)
(2002, LOE 2.1)

Domain 3: Elimination and Exchange
Class 1: Urinary Function

Definition A pattern of urinary functions that is sufficient for meeting eliminatory needs and can be strengthened

Defining Characteristics

- Amount of output is within normal limits
- Expresses willingness to enhance urinary elimination
- Fluid intake is adequate for daily needs
- Positions self for emptying of bladder
- Specific gravity is within normal limits
- Urine is odorless
- Urine is straw colored

Urinary Retention (00023)
(1986)

Domain 3: Elimination and Exchange
Class 1: Urinary Function

Definition   Incomplete emptying of the bladder

Defining Characteristics

- Absence of urine output
- Bladder distension
- Dribbling
- Dysuria
- Frequent voiding
- Overflow incontinence
- Residual urine
- Sensation of bladder fullness
- Small voiding

Related Factors

- Blockage
- High urethral pressure
- Inhibition of reflex arc
- Strong sphincter

Constipation (00011)
(1975, 1998)

Domain 3: Elimination and Exchange
Class 2: Gastrointestinal Function

Definition Decrease in normal frequency of defecation accompanied by difficult or incomplete passage of stool and/or passage of excessively hard, dry stool

Defining Characteristics

- Abdominal pain
- Abdominal tenderness with palpable muscle resistance
- Abdominal tenderness without palpable muscle resistance
- Anorexia
- Atypical presentations in older adults (e.g., change in mental status, urinary incontinence, unexplained falls, elevated body temperature)
- Borborygmi
- Bright red blood with stool
- Change in bowel pattern
- Decreased frequency
- Decreased volume of stool
- Distended abdomen
- Feeling of rectal fullness
- Feeling of rectal pressure
- Generalized fatigue
- Hard, formed stool
- Headache
- Hyperactive bowel sounds
- Hypoactive bowel sounds
- Increased abdominal pressure
- Indigestion
- Nausea
- Oozing liquid stool
- Pain with defecation
- Palpable abdominal mass
- Palpable rectal mass
- Percussed abdominal dullness
- Presence of soft, paste-like stool in rectum
- Severe flatus
- Straining with defecation
- Unable to pass stool
- Vomiting

Related Factors

Functional

- Abdominal muscle weakness
- Habitual ignoring of urge to defecate
- Inadequate toileting (e.g., timeliness, positioning for defecation, privacy)
- Insufficient physical activity
- Irregular defecation habits
- Recent environmental changes

Psychological

- Depression
- Emotional stress
- Mental confusion

Pharmacological

- Aluminum-containing antacids
- Anticholinergics
- Anticonvulsants
- Antidepressants
- Antilipemic agents
- Bismuth salts
- Calcium carbonate
- Calcium channel blockers
- Diuretics
- Iron salts
- Laxative abuse
- Nonsteroidal anti-inflammatory agents
- Opiates
- Phenothiazines
- Sedatives
- Sympathomimetics

Mechanical

- Electrolyte imbalance
- Hemorrhoids
- Hirschsprung's disease
- Neurological impairment
- Obesity
- Postsurgical obstruction
- Pregnancy
- Prostate enlargement
- Rectal abscess
- Rectal anal fissures
- Rectal anal stricture
- Rectal prolapse
- Rectal ulcer
- Rectocele
- Tumors

Physiological

- Change in eating patterns
- Change in usual foods
- Decreased motility of gastrointestinal tract
- Dehydration
- Inadequate dentition
- Inadequate oral hygiene
- Insufficient fiber intake
- Insufficient fluid intake
- Poor eating habits

Perceived Constipation (00012)

(1988)

Domain 3: Elimination and Exchange
Class 2: Gastrointestinal Function

Definition
Self-diagnosis of constipation combined with abuse of laxatives, enemas, and/or suppositories to ensure a daily bowel movement

Defining Characteristics

- Expectation of a daily bowel movement
- Expectation of passage of stool at the same time every day
- Overuse of enemas
- Overuse of laxatives
- Overuse of suppositories

Related Factors

- Cultural health beliefs
- Family health beliefs
- Faulty appraisal
- Impaired thought processes

Risk for Constipation (00015)

(1998)

Domain 3: Elimination and Exchange
Class 2: Gastrointestinal Function

Definition At risk for a decrease in normal frequency of defecation accompanied by difficult or incomplete passage of stool and/or passage of excessively hard, dry stool

Risk Factors

Functional

- Abdominal muscle weakness
- Habitual ignoring of urge to defecate
- Inadequate toileting (e.g., timeliness, positioning for defecation, privacy)
- Insufficient physical activity
- Irregular defecation habits
- Recent environmental changes

Psychological

- Depression
- Emotional stress
- Mental confusion

Physiological

- Change in usual eating patterns
- Change in usual foods
- Decreased motility of gastrointestinal tract
- Dehydration
- Inadequate dentition
- Inadequate oral hygiene
- Insufficient fiber intake
- Insufficient fluid intake
- Poor eating habits

Pharmacological

- Aluminum-containing antacids
- Anticholinergics
- Anticonvulsants
- Antidepressants
- Antilipemic agents
- Bismuth salts
- Calcium carbonate
- Calcium channel blockers
- Diuretics
- Iron salts
- Laxative abuse
- Nonsteroidal anti-inflammatory agents
- Opiates
- Phenothiazines
- Sedatives
- Sympathomimetics

Mechanical

- Electrolyte imbalance
- Hemorrhoids
- Hirschsprung's disease
- Neurological impairment
- Obesity
- Postsurgical obstruction
- Pregnancy
- Prostate enlargement
- Rectal abscess
- Rectal anal fissures
- Rectal anal stricture
- Rectal prolapse
- Rectal ulcer
- Rectocele
- Tumors

Diarrhea (00013)
(1975, 1998)

Domain 3: Elimination and Exchange
Class 2: Gastrointestinal Function

Definition Passage of loose, unformed stools

Defining Characteristics

- Abdominal pain
- At least three loose liquid stools per day
- Cramping
- Hyperactive bowel sounds
- Urgency

Related Factors

Psychological

- Anxiety
- High stress levels

Situational

- Adverse effects of pharmaceutical agents
- Alcohol abuse
- Contaminants
- Laxative abuse
- Radiation
- Toxins
- Travel
- Tube feedings

Physiological

- Infectious processes
- Inflammation
- Irritation
- Malabsorption
- Parasites

Dysfunctional Gastrointestinal Motility (00196)
(2008, LOE 2.1)

Domain 3: Elimination and Exchange
Class 2: Gastrointestinal Function

Definition Increased, decreased, ineffective, or lack of peristaltic activity within the gastrointestinal system

Defining Characteristics

- Abdominal cramping
- Abdominal distension
- Abdominal pain
- Absence of flatus
- Accelerated gastric emptying
- Bile-colored gastric residual
- Change in bowel sounds (e.g., absent, hypoactive, hyperactive)
- Diarrhea
- Difficulty passing stool
- Dry stool
- Hard stool
- Increased gastric residual
- Nausea
- Regurgitation
- Vomiting

Related Factors

- Aging
- Anxiety
- Enteral feedings
- Food intolerance (e.g., gluten, lactose)
- Immobility
- Ingestion of contaminates (e.g., food, water)
- Malnutrition
- Pharmaceutical agents (e.g., narcotics/opiates, laxatives, antibiotics, anesthesia)
- Prematurity
- Sedentary lifestyle
- Surgery

References

Chial, H.J., & Camilleri, M. (2003). Motility disorders of the stomach and small intestine. In S.L. Friedman, K.R. McQuaid, & J.H. Grendell (eds), *Current diagnosis and treatment in gastroenterology*. New York: Lange Medical Books/McGraw Hill, pp. 355–367.

Holmes, H.N., Henry, K., Bilotta, K., Comerford, K., & Weinstock, D. (eds). (2007). *Professional guide to signs and symptoms*, 5th ed. Philadelphia, PA: Lippincott Williams & Wilkins, pp. 112–118.

Kahrilas, P.J. (2005). Esophageal motility disorders. In W.M. Weinstein, C.J. Hawkey, & J. Bosch (eds), *Clinical gastroenterology and hepatology*. St. Louis, MO: Elsevier Mosby, pp. 253–259.

Madsen, D., Sebolt T., Cullen, L., Folkedahl, B., Mueller, T., Richardson, C., & Titler, M. (2005). Listening to bowel sounds: An evidence-based practice project. *American Journal of Nursing*, 105(12), 40–49.

Ouyang, A., & Locke, G.R. (2007). Overview of neurogastroenterology – gastrointestinal motility and functional GI disorders: Classification, prevalence, and epidemiology. *Gastroenterology Clinics of North America*, 36(3), 485–498.

Quigley, E.M.M. (2006). Gastric motor and sensory function and motor disorders of the stomach. In M. Feldman, L.S. Friedman, L.J. Brandt, & M.H. Sleisenger (eds), *Sleisenger and Fordtran's gastrointestinal and liver disease pathophysiology/diagnosis/management*. St. Louis, MO: Saunders Elsevier, pp. 999–1028.

Tack, J. (2005). Gastric motility disorders. In: W.M. Weinstein, C.J. Hawkey, & J. Bosch (eds), *Clinical gastroenterology and hepatology*. St. Louis, MO: Elsevier Mosby, pp. 261–266.

Taylor, C., Lillis, C., LeMone, P., & Lynn, P. (2008). *Fundamentals of nursing: the art and science of nursing care*, 6th ed. Philadelphia, PA: Lippincott Williams & Wilkins, pp. 636–639.

Trinh, C., & Prabhakar, K. (2007). Diarrheal diseases in the elderly. *Clinics in Geriatric Medicine*, 23(4), 833–856.

Tursi, A. (2004). Gastrointestinal motility disturbances in celiac disease. *Journal of Clinical Gastroenterology*, 38(8), 642–645.

Watson, R.L. (2004). Gastrointestinal disorders. In: Verklan, M.T., & Walden, M. (eds), *Core curriculum for neonatal intensive care nursing*, 3rd ed. St. Louis, MO: Elsevier Saunders, pp. 654–683.

Wong, D., Hockenberry, M.J., Perry, S., Lowdermilk D., & Wilson, D. (2006). *Maternal child nursing care*, 3rd ed. St. Louis, MO: Mosby Elsevier, pp. 814–818, 859–860, 1531–1537.

Risk For Dysfunctional Gastrointestinal Motility (00197)
(2008, LOE 2.1)

Domain 3: Elimination and Exchange
Class 2: Gastrointestinal Function

Definition At risk for increased, decreased, ineffective, or lack of peristaltic activity within the gastrointestinal system

Risk Factors

- Abdominal surgery
- Aging
- Anxiety
- Change in food
- Change in water
- Decreased gastrointestinal circulation
- Diabetes mellitus
- Food intolerance (e.g., gluten, lactose)
- Gastroesophageal reflux disease (GERD)
- Immobility
- Infection (e.g., bacterial, parasitic, viral)
- Pharmaceutical agents (e.g., antibiotics, laxatives, narcotics/opiates, proton pump inhibitors)
- Prematurity
- Sedentary lifestyle
- Stress
- Unsanitary food preparation

References

Chial, H.J., & Camilleri, M. (2003). Motility disorders of the stomach and small intestine. In S.L. Friedman, K.R. McQuaid, & J.H. Grendell (eds), *Current diagnosis and treatment in gastroenterology*. New York: Lange Medical Books/McGraw Hill, pp. 355–367.

Holmes, H.N., Henry, K., Bilotta, K., Comerford, K., & Weinstock, D. (eds). (2007). *Professional guide to signs and symptoms*, 5th ed. Philadelphia, PA: Lippincott Williams & Wilkins, pp. 112–118.

Kahrilas, P.J. (2005). Esophageal motility disorders. In W.M. Weinstein, C.J. Hawkey, & J. Bosch (eds), *Clinical gastroenterology and hepatology*. St. Louis, MO: Elsevier Mosby, pp. 253–259.

Madsen, D., Sebolt T., Cullen, L., Folkedahl, B., Mueller, T., Richardson, C., & Titler, M. (2005). Listening to bowel sounds: An evidence-based practice project. *American Journal of Nursing*, 105(12), 40–49.

Ouyang, A., & Locke, G.R. (2007). Overview of neurogastroenterology – gastrointestinal motility and functional GI disorders: Classification, prevalence, and epidemiology. *Gastroenterology Clinics of North America*, 36(3), 485–498.

Quigley, E.M.M. (2006). Gastric motor and sensory function and motor disorders of the stomach. In M. Feldman, L.S. Friedman, L.J. Brandt, & M.H. Sleisenger (eds.), *Sleisenger and Fordtran's gastrointestinal and liver disease pathophysiology/diagnosis/management*. St. Louis, MO: Saunders Elsevier, pp. 999–1028.

Tack, J. (2005). Gastric motility disorders. In: W.M. Weinstein, C.J. Hawkey, & J. Bosch (eds), *Clinical gastroenterology and hepatology*. St. Louis, MO: Elsevier Mosby, pp. 261–266.

Taylor, C., Lillis, C. LeMone, P., & Lynn, P. (2008). *Fundamentals of nursing: the art and science of nursing care*, 6th ed. Philadelphia, PA: Lippincott Williams & Wilkins, pp. 636–639.

Trinh, C., & Prabhakar, K. (2007). Diarrheal diseases in the elderly. *Clinics in Geriatric Medicine*, 23(4), 833–856.

Tursi, A. (2004). Gastrointestinal motility disturbances in celiac disease. *Journal of Clinical Gastroenterology*, *38*(8), 642–645.

Watson, R.L. (2004). Gastrointestinal disorders. In: Verklan, M.T., & Walden, M. (eds), *Core curriculum for neonatal intensive care nursing*, 3rd ed. St. Louis, MO: Elsevier Saunders, pp. 654–683.

Wong, D., Hockenberry, M.J., Perry, S., Lowdermilk D., & Wilson, D. (2006). *Maternal child nursing care*, 3rd ed. St. Louis, MO: Mosby Elsevier, pp. 814–818, 859–860, 1531–1537.

Bowel Incontinence (00014)

(1975, 1998)

Domain 3: Elimination and exchange
Class 2: Gastrointestinal function

Definition Change in normal bowel habits characterized by involuntary passage of stool

Defining Characteristics

- Constant dribbling of soft stool
- Fecal odor
- Fecal staining of bedding
- Fecal staining of clothing
- Inability to delay defecation
- Inability to recognize urge to defecate
- Inattention to urge to defecate
- Recognizes rectal fullness but reports inability to expel formed stool
- Red perianal skin
- Self-report of inability to recognize rectal fullness
- Urgency

Related Factors

- Abnormally high abdominal pressure
- Abnormally high intestinal pressure
- Chronic diarrhea
- Colorectal lesions
- Dietary habits
- Environmental factors (e.g., inaccessible bathroom)
- General decline in muscle tone
- Immobility
- Impaction
- Impaired cognition
- Impaired reservoir capacity
- Incomplete emptying of bowel
- Laxative abuse
- Loss of rectal sphincter control
- Lower motor nerve damage
- Medications
- Rectal sphincter abnormality
- Stress
- Toileting self-care deficit
- Upper motor nerve damage

Impaired Gas Exchange (00030)
(1980, 1996, 1998)

Domain 3: Elimination and Exchange
Class 4: Respiratory Function

Definition Excess or deficit in oxygenation and/or carbon dioxide elimination at the alveolar–capillary membrane

Defining Characteristics

- Abnormal arterial blood gases
- Abnormal arterial pH
- Abnormal breathing (e.g., rate, rhythm, depth)
- Abnormal skin color (e.g., pale, dusky)
- Confusion
- Cyanosis (in neonates only)
- Decreased carbon dioxide
- Diaphoresis
- Dyspnea
- Headache upon awakening
- Hypercapnia
- Hypoxemia
- Hypoxia
- Irritability
- Nasal flaring
- Restlessness
- Somnolence
- Tachycardia
- Visual disturbances

Related Factors

- Alveolar–capillary membrane changes
- Ventilation–perfusion imbalance

Domain 4
Activity/Rest

NANDA International Nursing Diagnoses: Definitions & Classification 2012–2014, First Edition.
Edited by T. Heather Herdman.
© 2012 NANDA International. Published 2012 by Blackwell Publishing Ltd.

Insomnia (00095)

(2006, LOE 2.1)

Domain 4: Activity/Rest
Class 1: Sleep/Rest

Definition A disruption in amount and quality of sleep that impairs functioning

Defining Characteristics

- Increased absenteeism (e.g., work/school)
- Observed changes in affect
- Observed lack of energy
- Reports changes in mood
- Reports decreased health status
- Reports decreased quality of life
- Reports difficulty concentrating
- Reports difficulty falling asleep
- Reports difficulty staying asleep
- Reports dissatisfaction with sleep (current)
- Reports increased accidents
- Reports lack of energy
- Reports nonrestorative sleep
- Reports sleep disturbances that produce next-day consequences
- Reports waking up too early

Related Factors

- Activity pattern (e.g., timing, amount)
- Anxiety
- Depression
- Environmental factors (e.g., ambient noise, daylight/darkness exposure, ambient temperature/humidity, unfamiliar setting)
- Fear
- Frequent daytime naps
- Gender-related hormonal shifts
- Grief
- Impairment of normal sleep pattern (e.g., travel, shift work)
- Inadequate sleep hygiene (current)
- Intake of alcohol
- Intake of stimulants
- Interrupted sleep
- Parental responsibilities
- Pharmaceutical agents
- Physical discomfort (e.g., pain, shortness of breath, cough, gastroesophageal reflux, nausea, incontinence/urgency)
- Stress (e.g., ruminative pre-sleep pattern)

References

Attarian, H. (2000). Helping patients who say they cannot sleep. Practical ways to evaluate and treat insomnia. *Postgraduate Medicine, 107*(3), 127–130, 133–137, 140–142.

Becker, P., Dement, W., Erman, M., & Glazer, W. (2004). Poor sleep: The impact on the health of our patients. Retrieved from http://www.medscape.com/viewarticle/475291_1

Buysse, D.J., Reynolds, C.F. III, Monk, T.H., Berman, S.R., & Kupfer, D.J. (1989). The Pittsburgh Sleep Quality Index: A new instrument for psychiatric practice and research. *Psychiatry Research, 28*(2), 193–213.

Cochran, H. (2003). Diagnose and treat primary insomnia. *Nurse Practitioner, 28*(9), 13–27.

4. Activity/Rest

Doran, C.M. (2003). *Prescribing mental health medication*. New York: Routledge.

First, M.B. (ed.). (2000). *Diagnostic and statistical manual – text revision (DSM-IV-TR, 2000)*. Washington, DC: American Psychiatric Association.

Fogel, J. (2003). Behavioral treatments for insomnia in primary care settings. *Advanced Practice Nursing e journal*, 3(4), 1–8. Retrieved from http://www.medscape.com/viewarticle/462938 .

Hoffman, S. (2003). Sleep in the older adult: Implications for nurses. *Geriatric Nursing*, 24(4), 210–214; quiz 215–216.

Krahn, L. (2003). Sleep disorders. *Seminars in Neurology*, 23(3), 307–314.

Linton, S., & Bryngelsson, I. (2000). Insomnia and its relationship to work and health in a working age population. *Journal of Occupational Rehabilitation*, 10(2), 169–183.

Lippmann, S.L., Mazour, I., & Shahab, H. (2001). Insomnia: Therapeutic approach. *Southern Medical Journal*, 94(9), 866–873.

McCall, V., & Rakel, R. (1999). *A practical guide to insomnia*. Minneapolis, MN: McGraw-Hill.

Mahowald, M. (2000). What is causing excessive daytime sleepiness? *Postgraduate Medicine*, 107(3), 108–110, 115–118, 123.

Medscape (2004). Understanding sleep problems – the basics. Retrieved from http://www.medscape.com/viewarticle/474122.

Merriam-Webster Online (2004). Insomnia. Retrieved from http://www.m-w.com/cgi-bin/dictionary?book=Dictionary&va=insomnia.

Sateia, M., & Nowell, P. (2004). Insomnia. *Lancet*, 364(9449), 1959–1973.

Simon, R. (1999). Diagnosis of insomnia: A primary care perspective. *Family Practice Recertification*, 21(10), 12–19.

Sleep Health. (2004). Ineffective activity planning. Are you resting easy? *Nursing*, 2004, 34(4), 74.

Smith, M., Perlis, M., Park, A., et al. (2002). Comparative meta-analysis of pharmacotherapy and behavior therapy for persistent insomnia. *American Journal of Psychiatry*, 159(1), 5–11.

Walsh, J. (1999). Insomnia: Prevalence and clinical and public health considerations. *Family Practice Recertification*, 21(10), 4–11.

Sleep Deprivation (00096)
(1998)

Domain 4: Activity/Rest
Class 1: Sleep/Rest

Definition Prolonged periods of time without sleep (sustained natural, periodic suspension of relative consciousness)

Defining Characteristics

- Acute confusion
- Agitation
- Anxiety
- Apathy
- Combativeness
- Daytime drowsiness
- Decreased ability to function
- Fatigue
- Fleeting nystagmus
- Hallucinations
- Hand tremors
- Heightened pain sensitivity
- Inability to concentrate
- Irritability
- Lethargy
- Listlessness
- Malaise
- Perceptual disorders (e.g., disturbed body sensation, delusions, feeling afloat)
- Restlessness
- Slowed reaction
- Transient paranoia

Related Factors

- Aging-related sleep stage shifts
- Dementia
- Familial sleep paralysis
- Idiopathic central nervous system hypersomnolence
- Inadequate daytime activity
- Narcolepsy
- Nightmares
- Nonsleep-inducing parenting practices
- Periodic limb movement (e.g., restless leg syndrome, nocturnal myoclonus)
- Prolonged discomfort (e.g., physical, psychological)
- Prolonged use of dietary antisoporifics
- Prolonged use of pharmacological agents
- Sleep apnea
- Sleep-related enuresis
- Sleep-related painful erections
- Sleep terror
- Sleep walking
- Sundowner's syndrome
- Sustained circadian asynchrony
- Sustained environmental stimulation
- Sustained inadequate sleep hygiene
- Sustained uncomfortable sleep environment

Readiness for Enhanced Sleep (00165)
(2002, LOE 2.1)

Domain 4: Activity/Rest
Class 1: Sleep/Rest

Definition A pattern of natural, periodic suspension of consciousness that provides adequate rest, sustains a desired lifestyle, and can be strengthened

Defining Characteristics

- Amount of sleep is congruent with developmental needs
- Expresses willingness to enhance sleep
- Follows sleep routines that promote sleep habits
- Occasional use of pharmaceutical agents to induce sleep
- Reports being rested after sleep

Disturbed Sleep Pattern (00198)
(1980, 1998, 2006, LOE 2.1)

Domain 4: Activity/Rest
Class 1: Sleep/Rest

Definition Time-limited interruptions of sleep amount and quality due to external factors

Defining Characteristics

- Change in normal sleep pattern
- Decreased ability to function
- Dissatisfaction with sleep
- Reports being awakened
- Reports no difficulty falling asleep
- Reports not feeling well rested

Related Factors

- Ambient humidity
- Ambient temperature
- Caregiving responsibilities
- Change in daylight–darkness exposure
- Interruptions (e.g., for therapeutics, monitoring, lab tests)
- Lack of sleep control
- Lack of sleep privacy
- Lighting
- Noise
- Noxious odors
- Physical restraint
- Sleep partner
- Unfamiliar sleep furnishings

4. Activity/Rest

Risk for Disuse Syndrome (00040)
(1988)

Domain 4: Activity/Rest
Class 2: Activity/Exercise

Definition   At risk for deterioration of body systems as the result of prescribed or unavoidable musculoskeletal inactivity

Risk Factors

- Altered level of consciousness
- Mechanical immobilization
- Paralysis
- Prescribed immobilization
- Severe pain

Note: Complications from immobility can include pressure ulcer, constipation, stasis of pulmonary secretions, thrombosis, urinary tract infection and/or retention, decreased strength or endurance, orthostatic hypotension, decreased range of joint motion, disorientation, body-image disturbance, and powerlessness.

Impaired Bed Mobility (00091)
(1998, 2006, LOE 2.1)

Domain 4: Activity/Rest
Class 2: Activity/Exercise

Definition   Limitation of independent movement from one bed position to another

Defining Characteristics

- Impaired ability to move from long sitting to supine
- Impaired ability to move from prone to supine
- Impaired ability to move from sitting to supine
- Impaired ability to move from supine to long sitting
- Impaired ability to move from supine to prone
- Impaired ability to move from supine to sitting
- Impaired ability to reposition self in bed
- Impaired ability to turn from side to side

Related Factors

- Cognitive impairment
- Deconditioning
- Deficient knowledge
- Environmental constraints (e.g., bed size, bed type, treatment equipment, restraints)
- Insufficient muscle strength
- Musculoskeletal impairment
- Neuromuscular impairment
- Obesity
- Pain
- Sedating pharmaceutical agents

References

Brouwer, K., Nysseknabm, J., & Culham, E. (2004). Physical function and health status among seniors with and without fear of falling. *Gerontology, 50*(3), 135–141.

Goldstein, S. (1993). The biology of aging: Looking to defuse the time bomb. *Geriatrics, 48*(9), 76–82.

Lewis, C.L., Moutoux, M., Slaughter, M., & Bailey, S.P. (2004). Characteristics of individuals who fell while receiving home health services. *Physical Therapy, 84*(1), 23–32.

Matsouka, O., Harahousou, Y., Kabiatis, C., & Trigonis, I. (2003). Effects of a physical activity program: The study of selected physical abilities among elderly women. *Journal of Gerontological Nursing, 29*(7), 50–55.

Tinetti, M.E., & Ginter, S.F. (1988). Identifying mobility dysfunction in elderly persons. *Journal of American Medical Association, 259*(8), 1190–1193.

Note: Specify level of independence using a standardized functional scale.

Impaired Physical Mobility (00085)
(1973, 1998)

Domain 4: Activity/Rest
Class 2: Activity/Exercise

Definition   Limitation in independent, purposeful physical movement of the body or of one or more extremities

Defining Characteristics

- Decreased reaction time
- Difficulty turning
- Engages in substitutions for movement (e.g., increased attention to other's activity, controlling behavior, focus on pre-illness disability/activity)
- Exertional dyspnea
- Gait changes
- Jerky movements
- Limited ability to perform fine motor skills
- Limited ability to perform gross motor skills
- Limited range of motion
- Movement-induced tremor
- Postural instability
- Slowed movement
- Uncoordinated movements

Related Factors

- Activity intolerance
- Altered cellular metabolism
- Anxiety
- Body mass index above 75th age-appropriate percentile
- Cognitive impairment
- Contractures
- Cultural beliefs regarding age-appropriate activity
- Deconditioning
- Decreased endurance
- Decreased muscle control
- Decreased muscle mass
- Decreased muscle strength
- Deficient knowledge regarding value of physical activity
- Depressive mood state
- Developmental delay
- Discomfort
- Disuse
- Joint stiffness
- Lack of environmental supports (e.g., physical or social)
- Limited cardiovascular endurance
- Loss of integrity of bone structures
- Malnutrition
- Musculoskeletal impairment
- Neuromuscular impairment
- Pain
- Pharmaceutical agents
- Prescribed movement restrictions
- Reluctance to initiate movement
- Sedentary lifestyle
- Sensoriperceptual impairments

Note: Specify level of independence using a standardized functional scale.

Impaired Wheelchair Mobility (00089)

(1998, 2006, LOE 2.1)

Domain 4: Activity/Rest
Class 2: Activity/Exercise

Definition
Limitation of independent operation of wheelchair within environment

Defining Characteristics

- Impaired ability to operate manual wheelchair on a decline
- Impaired ability to operate manual wheelchair on an incline
- Impaired ability to operate manual wheelchair on curbs
- Impaired ability to operate manual wheelchair on even surface
- Impaired ability to operate manual wheelchair on uneven surface

- Impaired ability to operate power wheelchair on a decline
- Impaired ability to operate power wheelchair on an incline
- Impaired ability to operate power wheelchair on curbs
- Impaired ability to operate power wheelchair on even surface
- Impaired ability to operate power wheelchair on uneven surface

Related Factors

- Cognitive impairment
- Deconditioning
- Deficient knowledge
- Depressed mood
- Environmental constraints (e.g., stairs, inclines, uneven surfaces, unsafe obstacles, distances, lack of assistive devices or person, wheelchair type)

- Impaired vision
- Insufficient muscle strength
- Limited endurance
- Musculoskeletal impairment (e.g., contractures)
- Neuromuscular impairment
- Obesity
- Pain

References

Brouwer, K., Nysseknabm, J., & Culham, E. (2004). Physical function and health status among seniors with and without fear of falling. *Gerontology, 50*(3), 135–141.

Goldstein, S. (1993). The biology of aging: Looking to defuse the time bomb. *Geriatrics, 48*(9), 76–82.

Lewis, C.L., Moutoux, M., Slaughter, M., & Bailey, S.P. (2004). Characteristics of individuals who fell while receiving home health services. *Physical Therapy, 84*(1), 23–32.

Matsouka, O., Harahousou, Y., Kabiatis, C., & Trigonis, I. (2003). Effects of a physical activity program: The study of selected physical abilities among elderly women. *Journal of Gerontological Nursing, 29*(7), 50–55.

Tinetti., M.E., & Ginter, S.F. (1988). Identifying mobility dysfunction in elderly persons. *Journal of American Medical Association, 259*(8), 1190–1193.

Note: Specify level of independence using a standardized functional scale.

Impaired Transfer Ability (00090)
(1998, 2006, LOE 2.1)

Domain 4: Activity/Rest
Class 2: Activity/Exercise

Definition Limitation of independent movement between two nearby surfaces

Defining Characteristics

- Inability to transfer between uneven levels
- Inability to transfer from bed to chair
- Inability to transfer from bed to standing
- Inability to transfer from car to chair
- Inability to transfer from chair to bed
- Inability to transfer from chair to car
- Inability to transfer from chair to floor
- Inability to transfer from chair to standing
- Inability to transfer from floor to chair
- Inability to transfer from floor to standing
- Inability to transfer from standing to bed
- Inability to transfer from standing to chair
- Inability to transfer from standing to floor
- Inability to transfer in or out of bath tub
- Inability to transfer in or out of shower
- Inability to transfer on or off a commode
- Inability to transfer on or off a toilet

Related Factors

- Cognitive impairment
- Deconditioning
- Deficient knowledge
- Environmental constraints (e.g., bed height, inadequate space, wheelchair type, treatment equipment, restraints)
- Impaired balance
- Impaired vision
- Insufficient muscle strength
- Musculoskeletal impairment (e.g., contractures)
- Neuromuscular impairment
- Obesity
- Pain

References

Brouwer, K., Nysseknabm, J., & Culham, E. (2004). Physical function and health status among seniors with and without fear of falling. *Gerontology, 50*(3), 135–141.

Lewis, C.L., Moutoux, M., Slaughter, M., & Bailey, S.P. (2004). Characteristics of individuals who fell while receiving home health services. *Physical Therapy, 84*(1), 23–32.

Tinetti., M.E., & Ginter, S.F. (1988). Identifying mobility dysfunction in elderly persons. *Journal of American Medical Association, 259*(8), 1190–1193.

Note: Specify level of independence using a standardized functional scale.

Impaired Walking (00088)

(1998, 2006, LOE 2.1)

Domain 4: Activity/Rest
Class 2: Activity/Exercise

Definition   Limitation of independent movement within the environment on foot

Defining Characteristics

- Impaired ability to climb stairs
- Impaired ability to navigate curbs
- Impaired ability to walk on a decline
- Impaired ability to walk on an incline
- Impaired ability to walk on uneven surfaces
- Impaired ability to walk required distances

Related Factors

- Cognitive impairment
- Deconditioning
- Depressed mood
- Environmental constraints (e.g., stairs, inclines, uneven surfaces, unsafe obstacles, distances, lack of assistive devices or person, restraints)
- Fear of falling
- Impaired balance
- Impaired vision
- Insufficient muscle strength
- Lack of knowledge
- Limited endurance
- Musculoskeletal impairment (e.g., contractures)
- Neuromuscular impairment
- Obesity
- Pain

References

Brouwer, K., Nysseknabm, J., & Culham, E. (2004). Physical function and health status among seniors with and without fear of falling. *Gerontology, 50*(3), 135–141.

Lewis, C.L., Moutoux, M., Slaughter, M., & Bailey, S.P. (2004). Characteristics of individuals who fell while receiving home health services. *Physical Therapy, 84*(1), 23–32.

Tinetti., M.E., & Ginter, S.F. (1988). Identifying mobility dysfunction in elderly persons. *Journal of American Medical Association, 259*(8), 1190–1193.

Note: Specify level of independence using a standardized functional scale.

4. Activity/Rest

Disturbed Energy Field (00050)
(1994, 2004, LOE 2.1)

Domain 4: Activity/Rest
Class 3: Energy Balance

Definition Disruption of the flow of energy surrounding a person's being that results in disharmony of the body, mind, and/or spirit

Defining Characteristics

- Perceptions of changes in patterns of energy flow, such as:
  - Movement (wave, spike, tingling, dense, flowing)
  - Sounds (tone, words)
  - Temperature change (warmth, coolness)
- Visual changes (image, color)
- Disruption of the field (deficit, hole, spike, bulge, obstruction, congestion, diminished flow in energy field)

Related Factors

Slowing or blocking of energy flows secondary to:

Maturational factors

- Age-related developmental crisis
- Age-related developmental difficulties

Pathophysiological factors

- Illness
- Injury
- Pregnancy

Situational factors

- Anxiety
- Fear
- Grieving
- Pain

Treatment-related factors

- Chemotherapy
- Immobility
- Labor and delivery
- Perioperative experience

Fatigue (00093)
(1988, 1998)

Domain 4: Activity/Rest
Class 3: Energy Balance

Definition An overwhelming sustained sense of exhaustion and decreased capacity for physical and mental work at the usual level

Defining Characteristics

- Compromised concentration
- Compromised libido
- Decreased performance
- Disinterest in surroundings
- Drowsy
- Increase in physical complaints
- Increase in rest requirements
- Introspection
- Lack of energy
- Lethargic
- Listless
- Perceived need for additional energy to accomplish routine tasks
- Reports an overwhelming lack of energy
- Reports an unremitting lack of energy
- Reports feeling tired
- Reports guilt over not keeping up with responsibilities
- Reports inability to maintain usual level of physical activity
- Reports inability to maintain usual routines
- Reports inability to restore energy even after sleep

Related Factors

Psychological

- Anxiety
- Depression
- Reports boring lifestyle
- Stress

Physiological

- Anemia
- Disease states
- Increased physical exertion
- Malnutrition
- Poor physical condition
- Pregnancy
- Sleep deprivation

Environmental

- Humidity
- Lights
- Noise
- Temperature

Situational

- Negative life events
- Occupation

Wandering (00154)
(2000)

Domain 4: Activity/Rest
Class 3: Energy Balance

Definition Meandering, aimless, or repetitive locomotion that exposes the individual to harm; frequently incongruent with boundaries, limits, or obstacles

Defining Characteristics

- Continuous movement from place to place
- Frequent movement from place to place
- Fretful locomotion
- Getting lost
- Haphazard locomotion
- Hyperactivity
- Inability to locate significant landmarks in a familiar setting
- Locomotion into unauthorized/ private spaces
- Locomotion resulting in unintended leaving of a premises
- Locomotion that cannot be easily dissuaded
- Long periods of locomotion without an apparent destination
- Pacing
- Periods of locomotion interspersed with periods of nonlocomotion (e.g., sitting, standing, sleeping)
- Persistent locomotion in search of something
- Scanning behaviors
- Searching behaviors
- Shadowing a caregiver's locomotion
- Trespassing

Related Factors

- Cognitive impairment (e.g., memory and recall deficits, disorientation, poor visuoconstructive or visuospatial ability, language defects)
- Cortical atrophy
- Emotional state (e.g., frustration, anxiety, boredom, depression, agitation)
- Overstimulating environment
- Physiological state or need (e.g., hunger, thirst, pain, urination, constipation)
- Premorbid behavior (e.g., outgoing, sociable personality, premorbid dementia)
- Sedation
- Separation from familiar environment
- Time of day

Activity Intolerance (00092)
(1982)

Domain 4: Activity/Rest
Class 4: Cardiovascular/Pulmonary Responses

Definition Insufficient physiological or psychological energy to endure or complete required or desired daily activities

Defining Characteristics

- Abnormal blood pressure response to activity
- Abnormal heart rate response to activity
- EKG changes reflecting arrhythmias
- EKG changes reflecting ischemia
- Exertional discomfort
- Exertional dyspnea
- Reports fatigue
- Reports feeling weak

Related Factors

- Bed rest
- Generalized weakness
- Imbalance between oxygen supply/ demand
- Immobility
- Sedentary lifestyle

Risk for Activity Intolerance (00094)
(1982)

Domain 4: Activity/Rest
Class 4: Cardiovascular/Pulmonary Responses

Definition At risk for experiencing insufficient physiological or psychological energy to endure or complete required or desired daily activities

Risk Factors

- Circulatory problems
- Deconditioned status
- History of previous activity intolerance
- Inexperience with an activity
- Respiratory problems

Ineffective Breathing Pattern (00032)
(1980, 1996, 1998, 2010, LOE 2.1)

Domain 4: Activity/Rest
Class 4: Cardiovascular/Pulmonary Responses

Definition Inspiration and/or expiration that does not provide adequate ventilation

Defining Characteristics

- Alterations in depth of breathing
- Altered chest excursion
- Assumption of three-point position
- Bradypnea
- Decreased expiratory pressure
- Decreased inspiratory pressure
- Decreased minute ventilation
- Decreased vital capacity
- Dyspnea
- Increased anterior–posterior diameter
- Nasal flaring
- Orthopnea
- Prolonged expiration phase
- Pursed-lip breathing
- Tachypnea
- Use of accessory muscles to breathe

Related Factors

- Anxiety
- Body position
- Bony deformity
- Chest wall deformity
- Fatigue
- Hyperventilation
- Hypoventilation syndrome
- Musculoskeletal impairment
- Neurological damage
- Neurological immaturity
- Neuromuscular dysfunction
- Obesity
- Pain
- Respiratory muscle fatigue
- Spinal cord injury

References

Amaral, A.C.S., Coeli, C.M., Costa, M.C.E., Cardoso, V.S., Toledo, A.L.A., & Fernandes, C.R. (2004). Perfil de morbidade e de mortalidade de pacientes idosos hospitalizados. *Cadernos de Saúde Pública*, 20(6), 1617–1626.

Andrade, L.H.S.G., & Gorensteins C. (1998). Aspectos gerais das escalas de avaliação de ansiedade. *Revista de Psiquiatria Clínica*, 25(6), 285–290. Retrieved from http://www.hcnet.usp.br.

Andrade, L.T. (2007). *Validação das Intervenções de Enfermagem para o Diagnóstico de mobilidade física prejudicada em lesados medulares*. Master's dissertation, Faculdade de Enfermagem, Universidade Federal de Minas Gerais, Belo Horizonte, Brazil.

Argimon, I.I.L., Bica, M., Timm, L.M., & Vivan, A. (2006). Funções executivas e a avaliação de flexibilidade de pensamento em idosos. *Revista Brasileira de Ciências do Envelhecimento Humano*, Jul/Dec, 35–42.

Atkinson, L.D., & Murray, M.E. (1989). *Fundamentos de enfermagem. Introdução ao processo de enfermagem*. Rio de Janeiro: Guanabara-Koogan.

Barros, A.L.B.L. (2006). *Anamnese e exame físico* (5th ed.). Porto Alegre: Artmed.

Bickley, L.S.B. (2005). *Propedêutica Médica* (7th ed.). Rio de Janeiro: Guanabara Koogan.

Cafer, C.R., Barros, A.L.B.L., Lucena, A.F., Mahl, M.L.S., & Michel, J.L.M. (2005). Diagnóstico de enfermagem e proposta de intervenção para pacientes com lesão medular. *Acta Paulista de Enfermagem*, *18*(4), 347–353.

Cavalcante, A.M.R.Z. (2009). *Nursing intervention of "ineffective breathing pattern" in elderly people*. Dissertation, Faculty of Nursing/UFG, Goiânia.

Charchat-Fichman, H., Caramelli, P., Sameshima, K., & Nitrini, R. (2005). Declínio da capacidade cognitiva durante o envelhecimento. *Revista Brasileira de Psiquiatria*, *27*(1), 79–82.

Corrêa, C.G. (1997). *Dor: Validação clínica no pós-operatório de cirurgia cardíaca*. Dissertation, Universidade de São Paulo, Brazil.

Cotran, R.S., Kumar, V., Collins, T. (2000). *Robbins Patologia estrutural e functional* (6th ed.). [Robbins Pathologic Basis of Disease, 6th Ed.] Rio de Janeiro: Guanabara Koogan.

Dellaroza, M.S., Pimenta, C.A.M., & Matsuo, T. (2007). Prevalência e caracterização da dor crônica em idosos não institucionalizados. *Cadernos de Saúde Pública*, *23*(5), 1151–1160.

D'Ottaviano, E.J. (2001). Sistema nervoso e 3ª idade. *Revista Argumento*, *III*(5), 29–46.

Dourado, V.Z., Tanni, S.E., Vale, A.S., Faganello, M.M., Sanchez, F.F., & Godoy, I. (2006). Manifestações sistêmicas na doença pulmonar obstrutiva crônica. *Jornal Brasileiro de Pneumologia*, *32*(2), 161–171.

Ferrantin, A.C., Borges, C.F., Morelli, J.G.S., & Rebelatto, J.R. (2005). Qualidade da execução de AVDs em idosos institucionalizados e não-institucionalizados que permaneciam sem sair de suas residências por mais de 6 meses. *Revista Brasileira de Fisioterapia*, *6*(5), 372–375.

Freitas, E.V., Py, L., Cançado, F.A.X., & Gorzoni, M.L. (2002). *Tratado de geriatria e gerontologia* (2nd ed.). Rio de Janeiro: Guanabara Koogan.

Gardner, W.N. (1996). The pathophysiology of hyperventilation disorders. *Chest Journal*, *109*(2), 516–534.

Gonçalves, M.P. (2007). *Influência de um programa de treinamento muscular respiratório no desempenho cognitivo e na qualidade de vida do idoso*. Thesis, Universidade de Brasília, Brazil.

Guyton, A.C., & Hall, J.E. (2002). *Tratado de fisiologia médica* (10th ed.). Rio de Janeiro: Guanabara Koogan.

Hudak, C.M., & Gallo, B.M. (1997). *Cuidados intensivos de enfermagem. Uma abordagem holística* (6th ed.). Rio de Janeiro: Guanabara Koogan.

Kauffman, T.L. (2001). *Manual de reabilitação geriátrica*. Rio de Janeiro: Guanabara Koogan.

Kim, M.J., & Larson, J. (1987). Ineffective airway clearance and ineffective breathing patterns: Theoretical and research base for nursing diagnosis. *Nursing Clinics of North America*, *22*(1), 12–34.

Loyola Filho, A.I., Matos, D.L., Giatti, L., Afradique, M.E., Peixoto, S.V., & Lima-Costa, M.F. (2004). Causas de internações hospitalares entre idosos brasileiros no âmbito do Sistema Único de Saúde. *Epidemiologia e Serviços de Saúde*, *13*(4), 229–238.

Matsudo, S.M., Matsudo, V.K.R., & Barros, N.T.L. (2000). Impacto do envelhecimento nas variáveis antropométricas, neuromotoras e metabólicas da aptidão física. *Revista Brasileira de Ciência e Movimento*, *8*(4), 21–32.

Paiva, K.C.A., & Beppu, O.S. (2005). Posição prona. *Jornal Brasileiro de Pneumologia*, *31*(4), 332–340.

Papaléo Netto, M. (2007). *Gerontologia: A velhice e o envelhecimento em visão globalizada*. São Paulo: Atheneu.

Paulin, E., Brunetto, A.F., & Carvalho, C.R.F. (2003). Efeitos de programa de exercícios físicos direcionado ao aumento da mobilidade torácica em pacientes portadores de doença pulmonar obstrutiva crônica. *Jornal de Pneumologia*, *29*(5), 287–294.

Pereira, A.L.S. (2005). *Construção de um protocolo de tratamento para o transtorno de ansiedade generalizada*. Dissertation, Instituto de Psicologia, Rio de Janeiro.

Porto, C.C. (2005). *Semiologia Médica* (5th ed.). Rio de Janeiro: Guanabara Koogan.

Rasslan, Z., Junior, R.S., Stirbulov, R., Fabbri, R.M.A., & Lima, C.A.C. (2004). Avaliação da função pulmonar na obesidade graus I e II. *Jornal Brasileiro de Pneumologia*, *30*(6), 508–514.

Rigatto, A.M., Alvez, S.C.C., Gonçalves, C.B., Firmo, J.F., & Provin, L.M. (2005). Performance ventilatória na obesidade. *Saúde em Revista*, *7*(17), 57–62.

Scanlan, C.L., Wilkins, R.L., & Stoller, J.K. (2000). *Fundamentos da terapia respiratória de Egan* (7th ed.). São Paulo: Manole.

Silva, G.A. (2006). Síndrome obesidade-hipoventilação alveolar. *Medicina, Ribeirão Preto*, *39*(2), 195–204.

Simpson, H. (2006). Respiratory assessment. *British Journal of Nursing*, *15*(9), 484–488.

Smeltzer, S.C., & Bare, B.G. (2005). *Tratado de enfermagem médico-cirúrgico* (9th ed.). Rio de Janeiro: Guanabara Koogan.

Decreased Cardiac Output (00029)
(1975, 1996, 2000)

Domain 4: Activity/Rest
Class 4: Cardiovascular/Pulmonary Responses

Definition Inadequate blood pumped by the heart to meet the metabolic demands of the body

Defining Characteristics

Altered Heart Rate/Rhythm

- Arrhythmias
- Bradycardia
- EKG changes
- Palpitations
- Tachycardia

Altered Preload

- Decreased central venous pressure (CVP)
- Decreased pulmonary artery wedge pressure (PAWP)
- Edema
- Fatigue
- Increased CVP
- Increased PAWP
- Jugular vein distension
- Murmurs
- Weight gain

Altered Afterload

- Clammy skin
- Decreased peripheral pulses
- Decreased pulmonary vascular resistance (PVR)
- Decreased systemic vascular resistance (SVR)
- Dyspnea
- Increased PVR
- Increased SVR
- Oliguria
- Prolonged capillary refill
- Skin color changes
- Variations in blood pressure readings

Altered Contractility

- Cough
- Crackles
- Decreased cardiac index
- Decreased ejection fraction
- Decreased left ventricular stroke work index (LVSWI)
- Decreased stroke volume index (SVI)
- Orthopnea
- Paroxysmal nocturnal dyspnea
- S3 sounds
- S4 sounds

Behavioral/Emotional

- Anxiety
- Restlessness

Related Factors

- Altered afterload
- Altered contractility
- Altered heart rate
- Altered preload
- Altered rhythm
- Altered stroke volume

Risk for Ineffective Gastrointestinal Perfusion* (00202)
(2008, LOE 2.1)

Domain 4: Activity/Rest
Class 4: Cardiovascular/Pulmonary Responses

Definition At risk for decrease in gastrointestinal circulation that may compromise health

Risk Factors

- Abdominal aortic aneurysm
- Abdominal compartment syndrome
- Abnormal partial thromboplastin time
- Abnormal prothrombin time
- Acute gastrointestinal hemorrhage
- Age >60 years
- Anemia
- Coagulopathy (e.g., sickle cell anemia)
- Diabetes mellitus
- Disseminated intravascular coagulation
- Female gender
- Gastroesophageal varices
- Gastrointestinal disease (e.g., duodenal or gastric ulcer, ischemic colitis, ischemic pancreatitis)
- Hemodynamic instability
- Liver dysfunction
- Myocardial infarction
- Poor left ventricular performance
- Renal failure
- Smoking
- Stroke
- Trauma
- Treatment-related side effects (e.g., cardiopulmonary bypass, pharmaceutical agents, gastric surgery)
- Vascular disease (e.g., peripheral vascular disease, aortoiliac occlusive disease)

References

McSweeney, M.E., Garwood, S., Levin, J., Marino, M., Wang, S., Kardatzke, D., Mangano, D.T., & Wolman, R. Investigators of the Ischemia Research and Education Foundation of the Multicenter Study of Perioperative Ischemia Research Group (2004). Adverse gastrointestinal complications after cardiopulmonary bypass: Can outcome be predicted from preoperative risk factors? *Anesthesia and Analgesia*, *98*(6), 1610–1617.

O'Donnell, J.M., & N'acul, F. (eds) (2001). *Surgical intensive care medicine*. Boston: Kluwer Academic.

Scott-Conner, C.E.H., & Ballinger, B. (2005). Abdominal angina. Retrieved from http://www.emedicine.com/med/topic2.htm.

Swearingen, P.L., & Hicks Keen, J. (eds) (2001). *Manual of critical care nursing: Nursing interventions and collaborative management* (4th ed.). St. Louis, MO: Mosby.

*This diagnosis formerly held the label *Ineffective Tissue Perfusion (Specify type: Gastrointestinal)*.

Risk for Ineffective Renal Perfusion* (00203)

(2008, LOE 2.1)

Domain 4: Activity/Rest
Class 4: Cardiovascular/Pulmonary Responses

Definition At risk for a decrease in blood circulation to the kidney that may compromise health

Risk Factors

- Abdominal compartment syndrome
- Advanced age
- Bilateral cortical necrosis
- Burns
- Cardiac surgery
- Cardiopulmonary bypass
- Diabetes mellitus
- Exposure to nephrotoxins
- Female gender
- Glomerulonephritis
- Hypertension
- Hypovolemia
- Hypoxemia
- Hypoxia
- Infection (e.g., sepsis, localized infection)
- Interstitial nephritis
- Malignancy
- Malignant hypertension
- Metabolic acidosis
- Multitrauma
- Polynephritis
- Renal artery stenosis
- Renal disease (polycystic kidney)
- Smoking
- Substance abuse
- Systemic inflammatory response syndrome
- Treatment-related side effects (e.g., pharmaceutical agents, surgery)
- Vascular embolism
- Vasculitis

References

O'Donnell, J.M., & N'acul, F. (eds) (2001). *Surgical intensive care medicine*. Boston: Kluwer Academic.

Spinowitz, B., & Rodriguez, J. (2006). Renal artery stenosis. Retrieved from http://www.emedicine.com/med/topic2001.htm .

Swearingen, P.L., & Hicks Keen, J. (eds) (2001). *Manual of critical care nursing: Nursing interventions and collaborative management* (4th ed.). St. Louis, NO: Mosby.

*This diagnosis formerly held the label *Ineffective Tissue Perfusion (Specify type: Renal)*.

Impaired Spontaneous Ventilation (00033)
(1992)

Domain 4: Activity/Rest
Class 4: Cardiovascular/Pulmonary Responses

Definition Decreased energy reserves resulting in an inability to maintain independent breathing that is adequate to support life

Defining Characteristics

- Decreased cooperation
- Decreased Po_2
- Decreased Sao_2
- Decreased tidal volume
- Dyspnea
- Increased heart rate
- Increased metabolic rate
- Increased Pco_2
- Increased restlessness
- Increased use of accessory muscles
- Reports apprehension

Related Factors

- Metabolic factors
- Respiratory muscle fatigue

Ineffective Peripheral Tissue Perfusion*

(00204)

(2008, 2010, LOE 2.1)

Domain 4: Activity/Rest
Class 4: Cardiovascular/Pulmonary Responses

Definition Decrease in blood circulation to the periphery that may compromise health

Defining Characteristics

- Absent pulses
- Altered motor function
- Altered skin characteristics (color, elasticity, hair, moisture, nails, sensation, temperature)
- Ankle-brachial index < 0.90
- Blood pressure changes in extremities
- Capillary refill time > 3 seconds
- Claudication
- Color does not return to leg on lowering it
- Delayed peripheral wound healing
- Diminished pulses
- Edema
- Extremity pain
- Femoral bruit
- Shorter total distances achieved in the six-minute walk test
- Shorter pain free distances achieved in the six-minute walk test
- Paresthesia
- Skin color pale on elevation

Related Factors

- Deficient knowledge of aggravating factors (e.g., smoking, sedentary lifestyle, trauma, obesity, salt intake, immobility)
- Deficient knowledge of disease process (e.g., diabetes, hyperlipidemia)
- Diabetes mellitus
- Hypertension
- Sedentary lifestyle
- Smoking

References

Cournot, M., Boccalon, H. Cambou, J-P., Guilloux, J., Taraszkiewicz, D., Hanaire-Broutin, H., Chamontin, B., et al. (2007). Accuracy of the screening physical examination to identify subclinical atherosclerosis and peripheral arterial disease in asymptomatic subjects. *Journal of Vascular Surgery, 46*(6), 1215–1221. DOI: 10.1016/j.jvs.2007.08.022)

Lewis, C.D. (2001). Peripheral arterial disease of the lower extremity. *Journal of Cardiovascular Nursing, 15*(4), 45–63.

Hernando, F.J.S. & Conejero, A.M. (2007). Enfermedad arterial periferica: aspectos fisiopatologicos, clinicos y terapeuticos. *Revista Española de Cardiología, 60*(9), 969–982.

Khan, N.A., Rahim, S.A., Anand, S.S., Simel, D.L. & Panju, A. (2006). Does the clinical examination predict lower extremity peripheral arterial disease? *Journal of the American Medical Association, 295*(5), 536–546.

*This diagnosis formerly held the label *Ineffective Tissue Perfusion (Specify type: Peripheral)*.

Kruidenier, L.M., Nicolaï, S.P.A., Willigendael, E.M., de Bie, R.A. Prins, M.H., & Teijink, J.A.W. (2009). Functional claudication distance: a reliable and valid measurement to assess functional limitation in patients with intermittent claudication. *BMC Cardiovascular Disorders, 9*(9). doi:10.1186/1471-2261-9-9

Lopez Rowe, V. (2005). Peripheral arterial occlusive disease. Retrieved from http://www.emedicine.com/med/topic391.htm .

McDermott, M.M., Ades, P.A., Dyer, A., Guralnik, J.M., Kibbe, M., Criqui, M.H. (2008). Corridor-based functional performance measures correlate better with physical activity during daily life than treadmill measures in persons with peripheral arterial disease. *Journal of Vascular Surgery, 48*(5), 1231–1237.e1, DOI: 10.1016/j.jvs.2008.06.050)

Maffei, F.H.A., Lastoria, S., Yoshida, W.B., Rollo, H.A. (eds.) (2002). *Doenças vasculares periféricas*. Rio de Janeiro: Medsi.

O'Donnell, J.M., & N'acul, F. (eds.) (2001). *Surgical intensive care medicine*. Boston: Kluwer Academic.

Silva, R.C.G. (2010). Validação das características definidoras do diagnóstico de enfermagem: perfusão tissular periférica ineficaz em pacientes com doença arterial obstrutiva periférica sintomática. [Validation of defining characteristics of the nursing diagnosis ineffective peripheral tissue perfusion in patients with peripheral arterial disease in the lower limbs.] Doctoral dissertation. Universidade de São Paulo. Faculdade de Medicina, 191p.

Silva, R.C.G., Cruz, D.A.L.M., Bortolotto, L.A., Irigoyen, M.C.C., Krieger, E.M., Palomo, J.S.H.P., & Consolim-Colombo, F.M. (2006). Ineffective peripheral tissue perfusion: Clinical validation in patients with hypertensive cardiomyopathy. *International Journal of Nursing Terminologies and Classifications, 17*(2), 97–107.

Stephens, E. (2005). Peripheral vascular disease. Retrieved from http://www.emedicine.com/emerg/topic862.htm.

Swearingen, P.L., & Hicks Keen, J. (eds). (2001). *Manual of critical care nursing: Nursing interventions and collaborative management* (4th ed.). St. Louis, MO: Mosby.

Risk for Decreased Cardiac Tissue Perfusion*
(00200)
(2008, LOE 2.1)

Domain 4: Activity/Rest
Class 4: Cardiovascular/Pulmonary Responses

Definition   At risk for a decrease in cardiac (coronary) circulation that may compromise health

Risk Factors

- Birth control pills
- Cardiac surgery
- Cardiac tamponade
- Coronary artery spasm
- Deficient knowledge of modifiable risk factors (e.g., smoking, sedentary lifestyle, obesity)
- Diabetes mellitus
- Elevated C-reactive protein
- Family history of coronary artery disease
- Hyperlipidemia
- Hypertension
- Hypovolemia
- Hypoxemia
- Hypoxia
- Substance abuse

References

Alzamora, M.T., Baena-Díez, J.M., Sorribes, M., Forés, R., Toran, P., Vicheto, M. et al., (2007). PERART study. Peripheral Arterial Disease study (PERART): Prevalence and predictive values of asymptomatic peripheral arterial occlusive disease related to cardiovascular morbidity and mortality. *BMC Public Health, 7*, 348. doi:10.1186/1471-2458-7-348.

Dogan, A., Ozgul, M., Ozaydin, M., Aslan, S., Gedikli, O., & Altinbas, A. (2005). Effect of clopidogrel plus aspirin on tissue perfusion and coronary flow in patients with ST-segment elevation myocardial infarction: A new reperfusion strategy. *American Heart Journal, 149*(6), 1037–1042.

Hung, J., Knuiman, M., Divitini, M., Davis, T., & Beiby, J. (2008). Prevalence and risk factor correlates of elevated C-reactive protein in an adult Australian population. *American Journal of Cardiology, 101*(2), 193–198.

O'Donnell, J.M., & N'acul, F. (eds.) (2001). *Surgical intensive care medicine.* Boston: Kluwer Academic.

Sharma, S. (2006). Pulmonary embolism. Retrieved from http://www.emedicine.com/med/TOPIC1958. HTM.

Steen, H., Lehrke, S., Wiegand, U.K.H., Merten, C., Schuster, L., Richardt, G, et al. (2005). Very early cardiac magnetic resonance imaging for quantification of myocardial tissue perfusion in patients receiving tirofiban before percutaneous coronary intervention for ST-elevation myocardial infarction. *American Heart Journal, 149*(3), 564.e1–564.e7.

Swearingen, P.L., & Hicks Keen, J. (eds.) (2001). *Manual of critical care nursing: Nursing interventions and collaborative management* (4th ed.). St. Louis, MO: Mosby.

*This diagnosis formerly held the label *Ineffective Tissue Perfusion (Specify type: Cardiopulmonary)*.

Risk for Ineffective Cerebral Tissue Perfusion* (00201)
(2008, LOE 2.1)

Domain 4: Activity/Rest
Class 4: Cardiovascular/Pulmonary Responses

Definition At risk for a decrease in cerebral tissue circulation that may compromise health

Risk Factors

- Abnormal partial thromboplastin time
- Abnormal prothrombin time
- Akinetic left ventricular segment
- Aortic atherosclerosis
- Arterial dissection
- Atrial fibrillation
- Atrial myxoma
- Brain tumor
- Carotid stenosis
- Cerebral aneurysm
- Coagulopathy (e.g., sickle cell anemia)
- Dilated cardiomyopathy
- Disseminated intravascular coagulation
- Embolism
- Head trauma
- Hypercholesterolemia
- Hypertension
- Infective endocarditis
- Mechanical prosthetic valve
- Mitral stenosis
- Neoplasm of the brain
- Recent myocardial infarction
- Sick sinus syndrome
- Substance abuse
- Thrombolytic therapy
- Treatment-related side effects (cardiopulmonary bypass, pharmaceutical agents)

References

Asante-Siaw, J., Tyrrell, J., & Hoschtitzky, A. (2006). Does the use of a centrifugal pump offer any additional benefit for patients having open heart surgery? *Best BETS*, Record 01148. Retrieved from http://www.bestbets.org/cgi-bin/bets.pl?record=01148 .

Barnard, J., Musleh, G., & Bitta, M. (2004). In aortic arch surgery is there any benefit in using antegrade cerebral perfusion or retrograde cerebral perfusion as an adjunct to hypothermic circulatory arrest? *BestBETS*, Record 00690. Retrieved from http://www.bestbets.org/cgi-bin/bets.pl?record=00690 .

O'Donnell, J.M., & N'acul, F. (eds.) (2001). *Surgical intensive care medicine*. Boston: Kluwer Academic.

Sharma, M., Clark, H., Armour, T., Stotts, G., Coté, R., Hill, M.D. et al. (2005). *Acute stroke: Evaluation and treatment*. Evidence Report/Technology Assessment No. 127. Rockville, MD: Agency for Healthcare Research and Quality.

Swearingen, P.L., & Hicks Keen, J., (weds.) (2001). *Manual of critical care nursing: Nursing interventions and collaborative management* (4th ed.). St. Louis, MO: Mosby.

*This diagnosis formerly held the label Ineffective Tissue Perfusion (Specify type: Cerebral).

Risk for Ineffective Peripheral Tissue Perfusion* (00228)
(2010, LOE 2.1)

Domain 4: Activity/Rest
Class 4: Cardiovascular/Pulmonary Responses

Definition At risk for a decrease in blood circulation to the periphery that may compromise health

Risk Factors

- Age >60 years
- Deficient knowledge of aggravating factors (e.g., smoking, sedentary lifestyle, trauma, obesity, salt intake, immobility)
- Deficient knowledge of disease process (e.g., diabetes, hyperlipidemia)
- Diabetes mellitus
- Endovascular procedures
- Hypertension
- Sedentary lifestyle
- Smoking

References

Cournot, M., Boccalon, H. Cambou, J-P., Guilloux, J., Taraszkiewicz, D., Hanaire-Broutin, H., Chamontin, B., et al. (2007). Accuracy of the screening physical examination to identify subclinical atherosclerosis and peripheral arterial disease in asymptomatic subjects. *Journal of Vascular Surgery, 46*(6), 1215–1221. DOI: 10.1016/j.jvs.2007.08.022)

Hernando, F.J.S. & Conejero, A.M. (2007). Enfermedad arterial periferica: aspectos fisiopatologicos, clinicos y terapeuticos. *Revista Española de Cardiología, 60*(9), 969–982.

Khan, N.A., Rahim, S.A., Anand, S.S., Simel, D.L. & Panju, A. (2006). Does the clinical examination predict lower extremity peripheral arterial disease? *Journal of the American Medical Association, 295*(5), 536–546.

Kruidenier, L.M., Nicolaï, S.P.A., Willigendael, E.M., de Bie, R.A. Prins, M.H., & Teijink, J.A.W. (2009). Functional claudication distance: a reliable and valid measurement to assess functional limitation in patients with intermittent claudication. *BMC Cardiovascular Disorders, 9*(9). doi:10.1186/1471-2261-9-9

Lewis, C.D. (2001). Peripheral arterial disease of the lower extremity. *Journal of Cardiovascular Nursing, 15*(4), 45–63.

Lopez Rowe, V. (2005). Peripheral arterial occlusive disease. Retrieved from http://www.emedicine.com/med/topic391.htm.

McDermott, M.M., Ades, P.A., Dyer, A., Guralnik, J.M., Kibbe, M., Criqui, M.H. (2008). Corridor-based functional performance measures correlate better with physical activity during daily life than treadmill measures in persons with peripheral arterial disease. *Journal of Vascular Surgery, 48*(5), 1231–1237.e1, DOI: 10.1016/j.jvs.2008.06.050)

Maffei, F.H.A., Lastoria, S., Yoshida, W.B., Rollo, H.A. (eds.) (2002). *Doenças vasculares periféricas.* Rio de Janeiro: Medsi.

O'Donnell, J.M., & N'acul, F. (eds.) (2001). *Surgical intensive care medicine.* Boston: Kluwer Academic.

Silva, R.C.G. (2010). Validação das características definidoras do diagnóstico de enfermagem: perfusão tissular periférica ineficaz em pacientes com doença arterial obstrutiva periférica sintomática. [Validation of defining characteristics of the nursing diagnosis ineffective peripheral tissue perfusion

*This diagnosis formerly held the label Ineffective Tissue Perfusion (Specify type: Peripheral).

in patients with peripheral arterial disease in the lower limbs.] Doctoral dissertation. Universidade de São Paulo. Faculdade de Medicina, 191p.

Silva, R.C.G., Cruz, D.A.L.M., Bortolotto, L.A., Irigoyen, M.C.C., Krieger, E.M., Palomo, J.S.H.P., & Consolim-Colombo, F.M. (2006). Ineffective peripheral tissue perfusion: Clinical validation in patients with hypertensive cardiomyopathy. *International Journal of Nursing Terminologies and Classifications*, *17*(2), 97–107.

Stephens, E. (2005). Peripheral vascular disease. Retrieved from http://www.emedicine.com/emerg/topic862.htm.

Swearingen, P.L., & Hicks Keen, J. (eds). (2001). *Manual of critical care nursing: Nursing interventions and collaborative management* (4th ed.). St. Louis, MO: Mosby.

Dysfunctional Ventilatory Weaning Response (00034)
(1992)

Domain 4: Activity/Rest
Class 4: Cardiovascular/Pulmonary Responses

Definition   Inability to adjust to lowered levels of mechanical ventilator support that interrupts and prolongs the weaning process

Defining Characteristics

Mild

- Breathing discomfort
- Fatigue
- Increased concentration on breathing
- Queries about possible machine malfunction
- Reports feelings of increased need for oxygen
- Restlessness
- Slight increase of respiratory rate from baseline
- Warmth

Moderate

- Baseline increase in respiratory rate (<5 breaths/min)
- Color changes
- Decreased air entry on auscultation
- Diaphoresis
- Hypervigilance to activities
- Inability to cooperate
- Inability to respond to coaching
- Minimal respiratory accessory muscle use
- Pale
- Reports apprehension
- Slight cyanosis
- Slight increase from baseline blood pressure (<20 mmHg)
- Slight increase from baseline heart rate (<20 beats/min)
- Wide-eyed look

Severe

- Adventitious breath sounds
- Agitation
- Asynchronized breathing with the ventilator
- Audible airway secretions
- Cyanosis
- Decreased level of consciousness
- Deterioration in arterial blood gases from current baseline
- Full respiratory accessory muscle use
- Gasping breaths
- Increase from baseline blood pressure (≥20 mmHg)
- Increase from baseline heart rate (≥20 breaths/min)
- Paradoxical abdominal breathing
- Profuse diaphoresis
- Respiratory rate increases significantly from baseline
- Shallow breaths

Related Factors

Physiological

- Inadequate nutrition
- Ineffective airway clearance
- Sleep pattern disturbance
- Uncontrolled pain

Psychological

- Anxiety
- Decreased motivation
- Decreased self-esteem
- Deficient knowledge of the weaning process
- Fear
- Hopelessness
- Insufficient trust in healthcare providers
- Perceived inefficacy about ability to wean
- Powerlessness

Situational

- Adverse environment (e.g., noisy, active environment, negative events in the room, low nurse:patient ratio, unfamiliar nursing staff)
- History of multiple unsuccessful weaning attempts
- History of ventilator dependence >4 days
- Inadequate social support
- Inappropriate pacing of diminished ventilator support
- Uncontrolled episodic energy demands

4. Activity/Rest

Impaired Home Maintenance (00098)
(1980)

Domain 4: Activity/Rest
Class 5: Self-Care

Definition Inability to independently maintain a safe growth-promoting immediate environment

Defining Characteristics

Objective

- Disorderly surroundings
- Inappropriate household temperature
- Insufficient clothes
- Insufficient linen
- Lack of clothes
- Lack of linen
- Lack of necessary equipment
- Offensive odors
- Overtaxed family members
- Presence of vermin
- Repeated unhygienic disorders
- Repeated unhygienic infections
- Unavailable cooking equipment
- Unclean surroundings

Subjective

- Household members report difficulty in maintaining their home in a comfortable fashion
- Household members report financial crises
- Household members report outstanding debts
- Household members request assistance with home maintenance

Related Factors

- Deficient knowledge
- Disease
- Illness
- Impaired functioning
- Inadequate support systems
- Injury
- Insufficient family organization
- Insufficient family planning
- Insufficient finances
- Lack of role modeling
- Unfamiliarity with neighborhood resources

Readiness for Enhanced Self-Care (00182)
(2006, LOE 2.1)

Domain 4: Activity/Rest
Class 5: Self-Care

Definition A pattern of performing activities for oneself that helps to meet health-related goals and can be strengthened

Defining Characteristics

- Expresses desire to enhance independence in maintaining health
- Expresses desire to enhance independence in maintaining life
- Expresses desire to enhance independence in maintaining personal development
- Expresses desire to enhance independence in maintaining well-being
- Expresses desire to enhance knowledge of strategies for self-care
- Expresses desire to enhance responsibility for self-care
- Expresses desire to enhance self-care

References

Artinian, N.T., Magnan, M., Sloan, M., & Lange, M.P. (2002). Self care behaviors among patients with heart failure. *Heart and Lung, 31*(3), 161–172.

Backscheider, J.E. (1974). Self care requirements, self care capabilities and nursing systems in the diabetic nurse management clinic. *American Journal of Public Health, 64*(12), 1138–1146.

Becker, G., Gates, R.J., & Newsom, E. (2004). Self-care among chronically ill African Americans: Culture, health disparities, and health insurance status. *American Journal of Public Health, 94*(12), 2066–2073.

Biggs, A.J. (1990). Family caregiver versus nursing assessments of elderly self-care abilities. *Journal of Gerontological Nursing, 16*(8), 11–16.

Conn, V. (1991). Self care actions taken by older adults for influenza and colds. *Nursing Research, 40*(3), 176–181.

Dashiff, C., Bartolucci, A., Wallander, J., & Abdullatif, H. (2005). The relationship of family structure, maternal employment, and family conflict with self-care adherence of adolescents with type 1 diabetes. *Families, Systems, and Health, 23*(1), 66–79.

Harris, J.L., & Williams, L.K. (1991). Universal self-care requisites as identified by homeless elderly men. *Journal of Gerontological Nursing, 17*(6), 39–43.

Hartweg, D.L. (1993). Self-care actions of healthy middle-aged women to promote well-being. *Nursing Research, 42*(4), 221–227.

Moore, J.B., & Beckwitt, A.E. (2004). Children with cancer and their parents: Self care and dependent care practices. *Issues in Comprehensive Pediatric Nursing, 27*(1), 1–17.

Oliver, M. (2005). Reaching positive outcomes by assessing and teaching patient self efficacy. *Home Healthcare Nurse, 23*(9), 559–562.

Orem, D.E. (2001). *Nursing: Concepts and practice* (6th ed.). St. Louis, MO: Mosby.

Richardson, A., & Ream, E.K. (1997). Self-care behaviours initiated by chemotherapy patients in response to fatigue. *International Journal of Nursing Studies, 34*(1), 35–43.

Smits, M.W., & Kee, C.C. (1992). Correlates of self-care among the independent elderly: Self care affects well-being. *Journal of Gerontological Nursing, 18*(9), 13–18.

Weston-Eborn, R. (2004). Home care and the adult learner. *Home Healthcare Nurse, 22*(8), 522–523.

Bathing Self-Care Deficit* (00108)
(1980, 1998, 2008)

Domain 4: Activity/Rest
Class 5: Self-Care

Definition Impaired ability to perform or complete bathing activities for self

Defining Characteristics

- Inability to access bathroom
- Inability to dry body
- Inability to get bath supplies

- Inability to obtain water source
- Inability to regulate bath water
- Inability to wash body

Related Factors

- Cognitive impairment
- Decreased motivation
- Environmental barriers
- Inability to perceive body part
- Inability to perceive spatial relationship

- Musculoskeletal impairment
- Neuromuscular impairment
- Pain
- Perceptual impairment
- Severe anxiety
- Weakness

Note: Specify level of independence using a standardized functional scale.

*This diagnosis formerly held the label *Bathing/Hygiene Self-care Deficit.*

Dressing Self-Care Deficit* (00109)
(1980, 1998, 2008)

Domain 4: Activity/Rest
Class 5: Self-Care

Definition
Impaired ability to perform or complete dressing activities for self

Defining Characteristics

- Impaired ability to fasten clothing
- Impaired ability to obtain clothing
- Impaired ability to put on necessary items of clothing
- Impaired ability to put on shoes
- Impaired ability to put on socks
- Impaired ability to take off necessary items of clothing
- Impaired ability to take off shoes
- Impaired ability to take off socks
- Inability to choose clothing
- Inability to maintain appearance at a satisfactory level
- Inability to pick up clothing
- Inability to put clothing on lower body
- Inability to put clothing on upper body
- Inability to put on shoes
- Inability to put on socks
- Inability to remove clothes
- Inability to remove shoes
- Inability to remove socks
- Inability to use assistive devices
- Inability to use zippers

Related Factors

- Cognitive impairment
- Decreased motivation
- Discomfort
- Environmental barriers
- Fatigue
- Musculoskeletal impairment
- Neuromuscular impairment
- Pain
- Perceptual impairment
- Severe anxiety
- Weakness

Note: Specify level of independence using a standardized functional scale.

*This diagnosis formerly held the label *Dressing/Grooming Self-care Deficit*.

Feeding Self-Care Deficit (00102)
(1980, 1998)

Domain 4: Activity/Rest
Class 5: Self-Care

Definition Impaired ability to perform or complete self-feeding activities

Defining Characteristics

- Inability to bring food from a receptacle to the mouth
- Inability to chew food
- Inability to complete a meal
- Inability to get food onto utensil
- Inability to handle utensils
- Inability to ingest food in a socially acceptable manner
- Inability to ingest food safely
- Inability to ingest sufficient food
- Inability to manipulate food in the mouth
- Inability to open containers
- Inability to pick up cup or glass
- Inability to prepare food for ingestion
- Inability to swallow food
- Inability to use assistive device

Related Factors

- Cognitive impairment
- Decreased motivation
- Discomfort
- Environmental barriers
- Fatigue
- Musculoskeletal impairment
- Neuromuscular impairment
- Pain
- Perceptual impairment
- Severe anxiety
- Weakness

Note: Specify level of independence using a standardized functional scale.

Toileting Self-Care Deficit (00110)
(1980, 1998, 2008)

Domain 4: Activity/Rest
Class 5: Self-Care

Definition   Impaired ability to perform or complete toileting activities for self

Defining Characteristics

- Inability to carry out proper toilet hygiene
- Inability to flush toilet or commode
- Inability to get to toilet or commode
- Inability to manipulate clothing for toileting
- Inability to rise from toilet or commode
- Inability to sit on toilet or commode

Related Factors

- Cognitive impairment
- Decreased motivation
- Environmental barriers
- Fatigue
- Impaired mobility status
- Impaired transfer ability
- Musculoskeletal impairment
- Neuromuscular impairment
- Pain
- Perceptual impairment
- Severe anxiety
- Weakness

Note: Specify level of independence using a standardized functional scale.

Domain 4: Activity/Rest
Class 5: Self-Care

Definition A constellation of culturally framed behaviors involving one or more self-care activities in which there is a failure to maintain a socially accepted standard of health and well-being (Gibbons, Lauder & Ludwick, 2006)

Defining Characteristics

- Inadequate environmental hygiene
- Inadequate personal hygiene
- Nonadherence to health activities

Related Factors

- Capgras syndrome
- Cognitive impairment (e.g., dementia)
- Depression
- Executive processing ability
- Fear of institutionalization
- Frontal lobe dysfunction
- Functional impairment
- Learning disability
- Lifestyle choice
- Maintaining control
- Major life stressor
- Malingering
- Obsessive–compulsive disorder
- Paranoid personality disorders
- Schizotypal personality disorders
- Substance abuse

References

Abrams, R.C., Lachs, M., McAvay, G., Keohane, D.J., & Bruce, M.L. (2002). Predictors of self-neglect in community-dwelling elders. *American Journal of Psychiatry, 159*(10), 1724–1730.

Adams, J., & Johnson, J. (1998). Nurses' perceptions of gross self-neglect amongst older people living in the community. *Journal of Clinical Nursing, 7*(6), 547–552.

Al-Adwani, A., & Nabi, W. (2001). Coexisting Diogenes and Capgras syndromes. *International Journal of Psychiatry in Clinical Practice, 5*(1), 75–76.

Barocka, A., Seehuber, D., & Schone, D. (2004.) Messy house syndrome. *MMW Fortschritte der Medizin, 146*(45), 36–39.

Blondell, R.D. (1999). Alcohol abuse and self-neglect in the elderly. *Journal of Elder Abuse and Neglect, 11*(2), 55–75.

Bozinovski, S.D. (2000). Older self-neglecters: Interpersonal problems and the maintenance of self-continuity. *Journal of Elder Abuse and Neglect, 12*(1), 37–56.

Branch, L. (2002). The epidemiology of elder abuse and neglect. *Public Policy and Aging Report, 12*(2), 19–22.

Chang, B., Uman, G., & Hirsch, M. (1998). Predictive power of clinical indicators for self-care deficit. *Nursing Diagnosis, 9*(2), 71–82.

Clark, A.N.G., Mankikar, G.D., & Gray, I. (1975). Diogenes syndrome: A clinical study of gross neglect in old age. *Lancet, 305*(7903), 366–368.

Daly, J.M., & Jogerst, G. (2001). Statute definitions of elder abuse. *Journal of Elder Abuse and Neglect, 13*(4), 39–57.

Drummond, L.M., Turner, J., & Reid, S. (1997). Diogenes' syndrome: A load of old rubbish? *Irish Journal of Psychological Medicine, 14*(3), 99–102.

Dyer, C.B., Pavlik, V.N., Murphy, K.P., & Hyman, D.J. (2000). The high prevalence of depression and dementia in elder abuse or neglect. *Journal of the American Geriatrics Society, 48*(2), 205–208.

Esposito, D., Rouillon, F., & Limosin, F. (2003). Diogenes syndrome in a pair of siblings. *Canadian Journal of Psychiatry, 48*(8), 571–572.

Finkel, S.I. (2003). Cognitive screening in the primary care setting: The role of physicians at the first point of entry. *Geriatrics,* (6), 43–44.

Gee, A., Jones, J.S., & Brown, M.D. (1998). Self-neglect in the elderly: Emergency department assessment and crisis intervention. *Annals of Emergency Medicine, 32*(30 Suppl. Part 2): S42.

Gibbons, S. (2007). Characteristics and behaviors of self-neglect in community-dwelling older adults. Doctoral dissertation. Retrieved from Dissertation Abstracts International, UMI No. 3246949.

Gibbons, S., Lauder, W., & Ludwick, R. (2006). Self-neglect: A proposed new NANDA diagnosis. *International Journal of Nursing Terminologies and Classification, 17*(1), 10–18.

Greve, K.W., Curtis, K.L., Bianchini, K.J., & Collins, B.T. (2004). Personality disorder masquerading as dementia: A case of apparent Diogenes syndrome. *International Journal of Geriatric Psychiatry, 19*(7), 703–705.

Gruman, C.A., Stern, A.S., & Caro, F.G. (1997). Self-neglect among the elderly: A distinct phenomenon. *Journal of Mental Health and Aging, 3*(3), 309–323.

Gunstone, S. (2003). Risk assessment and management of patients whom self-neglect: A grey area for mental health workers. *Journal of Psychiatric and Mental Health Nursing, 10*(3), 287–296.

Halliday, G., Banerjee, S., Philpot, M., & Macdonald, A. (2000). Community study of people who live in squalor. *Lancet, 355*(9207), 882–886.

Jackson, G.A. (1997). Diogenes syndrome: How should we manage it? *Journal of Mental Health, 6*(2), 113–116.

Jurgens, A. (2000). Refuse hoarding syndrome. *Psychiatrische Praxis, 27*(1), 42–46.

Lachs, M.S., Williams, C.S., O'Brien, S., Pillemer, K.A., & Charlson, M.E. (1998). The mortality of elder mistreatment. *Journal of the American Medical Association, 280*(5), 428–432.

Lachs, M.S., Williams, C.S., O'Brien, S., & Pillemer, K.A. (2002). Adult protective services use and nursing home placement. *Gerontologist, 42*(6), 734–739.

Lauder, W. (1999a). A survey of self-neglect in patients living in the community. *Journal of Clinical Nursing, 8*(1), 95–102.

Lauder, W. (1999b). Constructions of self-neglect: A multiple case study design. *Nursing Inquiry, 6*(1), 48–57.

Lauder, W. (2001). The utility of self-care theory as a theoretical basis for self-neglect. *Journal of Advanced Nursing, 34*(4), 345–351.

Lauder, W., Scott, P.A., & Whyte, A. (2001). Nurses' judgments of self-neglect: A factorial survey. *International Journal of Nursing Studies, 38*(5), 601–608.

Lauder, W., Anderson, I., & Barclay, A. (2002). Housing and self-neglect: Clients' and carers' perspectives. Report to the Economic and Social Research Council. Award No. R000223387.

Lauder, W., Anderson, I., & Barclay, A. (2005). Guidelines for good practice in self-neglect. *Journal of Psychiatric and Mental Health Nursing, 12*(2), 192–198.

Longres, J.F. (1995). Self-neglect among the elderly. *Journal of Elder Abuse and Neglect, 7*(1), 69–86.

Macmillan, D., & Shaw, P. (1966). Senile breakdown in standards of personal and environmental cleanliness. *British Medical Journal, 2*(5521), 1032–1037.

National Centre on Elder Abuse. (1998). National Elder Abuse Incidence Study. Washington, DC: Administration for Children and Families and the Administration on Aging, US Department of Health and Human Services.

O'Brien, J.G., Thibault, J.M., Turner, L.C., & Laird-Fick, H.S. (1999). Self-neglect: An overview. *Journal of Elder Abuse and Neglect, 11*(2), 1–19.

Orem, D.E. (1995). *Nursing: Concepts of practice* (5th edn.). St. Louis, MO: Mosby-Yearbook.

Orrell, M.W., Sahakin, B.J., & Bergmann, K. (1989). Self-neglect and frontal lobe dysfunction. *British Journal of Psychiatry, 155*, 101–105.

Pavlik, V.N., Hyman, D.J., Festa, N.A., & Dyer, C.B. (2001). Quantifying the problem of abuse and neglect in adults – analysis of a statewide database. *Journal of the American Geriatrics Society, 49*(1), 45–48.

Radebaugh, T.S., Hooper, F.J., & Gruenberg, E.M. (1987). The social breakdown syndrome in the elderly population living in the community: The helping study. *British Journal of Psychiatry, 151*, 341–346.

4. Activity/Rest

Rathbone-McCuan, E., & Bricker-Jenkins, M. (1992). A general framework for elder self-neglect. In E. Rathbone-McCuan & D.R. Fabian (eds.). *Self-neglecting elders: A clinical dilemma*. Westport, CT: Auburn House.

Reifler, B. (1996). Diogenes syndrome: Of omelettes and souffles. *Journal of the American Geriatrics Society*, 44(12), 1484–1485.

Reyes-Ortiz, C.A. (2001). Diogenes syndrome: The self-neglect elderly. *Comprehensive Therapy*, 27(2), 117–121.

Roby, J.L., & Sullivan, R. (2000). Adult protection service laws: a comparison of state statutes from definition to case closure. *Journal of Elder Abuse and Neglect*, 12(3/4), 17–51.

Roe, P.F. (1987). Self-neglect or chosen lifestyle? *British Journal of Hospital Medicine*, 37(1), 83–84 [Letter].

Sengstock, M.C., Thibault, J.M., & Zaranek, R. (1999). Community dimensions of elderly self-neglect. *Journal of Elder Abuse and Neglect*, 11(2), 77–93.

Snowdon, J. (1987). Uncleanliness among persons seen by community health workers. *Hospital and Community Psychiatry*, 38(5), 491–494.

Tierney, M.C., Charles, J., Naglie, G., Jaglal, S., Kiss, A., & Fisher, R.H. (2004). Risk for harm in cognitively impaired seniors who live alone: A prospective study. *Journal of the American Geriatrics Society*, 52(9), 1576–1577.

Ungvari, G.S., & Hantz, P.M. (1991). Social breakdown in the elderly. I Case studies and management. *Comprehensive Psychiatry*, 32(5), 440–444.

Vostanis, P., & Dean, C. (1992). Self-neglect in adult life. *British Journal of Psychiatry*, 161, 265–267.

Domain 5
Perception/Cognition

NANDA International Nursing Diagnoses: Definitions & Classification 2012–2014, First Edition.
Edited by T. Heather Herdman.
© 2012 NANDA International. Published 2012 by Blackwell Publishing Ltd.

Unilateral Neglect (00123)
(1986, 2006, LOE 2.1)

Domain 5: Perception/Cognition
Class 1: Attention

Definition   Impairment in sensory and motor response, mental representation, and spatial attention of the body, and the corresponding environment, characterized by inattention to one side and overattention to the opposite side. Left-side neglect is more severe and persistent than right-side neglect

Defining Characteristics

- Appears unaware of positioning of neglected limb
- Difficulty remembering details of internally represented familiar scenes that are on the neglected side
- Displacement of sounds to the non-neglected side
- Distortion of drawing on the half of the page on the neglected side
- Failure to cancel lines on the half of the page on the neglected side
- Failure to dress neglected side
- Failure to eat food from portion of the plate on the neglected side
- Failure to groom neglected side
- Failure to move eyes in the neglected hemispace despite being aware of a stimulus in that space
- Failure to move head in the neglected hemispace despite being aware of a stimulus in that space
- Failure to move limbs in the neglected hemispace despite being aware of a stimulus in that space
- Failure to move trunk in the neglected hemispace despite being aware of a stimulus in that space
- Failure to notice people approaching from the neglected side
- Lack of safety precautions with regard to the neglected side
- Marked deviation* of the eyes to the non-neglected side to stimuli and activities on that side
- Marked deviation* of the head to the non-neglected side to stimuli and activities on that side
- Marked deviation* of the trunk to the non-neglected side to stimuli and activities on that side
- Omission of drawing on the half of the page on the neglected side
- Perseveration of visual motor tasks on the non-neglected side
- Substitution of letters to form alternative words that are similar to the original in length when reading
- Transfer of pain sensation to the non-neglected side
- Use of only vertical half of page when writing

*As if drawn magnetically to stimuli and activities on that side.

Related Factors

- Brain injury from cerebrovascular problems
- Brain injury from neurological illness
- Brain injury from trauma

- Brain injury from tumor
- Hemianopsia
- Left hemiplegia from cerebrovascular accident (CVA) of the right hemisphere

References

Bartolomeo, P., & Chokron, S. (1999). Left unilateral neglect or right hyperattention? *Neurology, 53*(9), 2023–2027.

Bartolomeo, P., & Chokron, S. (2002). Orienting of neglect in left unilateral neglect. *Neuroscience and Behavioral Reviews, 26*(2), 217–234.

Halligan, P.W., & Marshall J.C. (1993). The history and clinical presentation of neglect. In I. H. Robertson, & J. C. Marshall (eds), *Unilateral neglect: Clinical and experimental studies*. Hove: Lawrence Erlbaum Associates, pp. 3–19.

Rizzolati, G., & Berti, A. (1993). Neural mechanisms of spatial neglect. In: I. H. Robertson, & J. C. Marshall (eds), *Unilateral neglect: Clinical and experimental studies*. Hove: Lawrence Erlbaum Associates, pp. 87–102.

Rusconi, M.L., Maravita, A., Bottini, G., & Vallar, G. (2002). Is the intact side really intact? Perseverative responses in patients with unilateral neglect: A productive manifestation. *Neuropsychologia, 40*(6), 594–604.

Stone, S.P., Halligan, P.W, Marshall, J.C., & Greenwood, R.J. (1998). Unilateral neglect a common but heterogeneous syndrome. *Neurology, 50*(6), 1902–1905.

Swan, L. (2001). Unilateral spatial neglect. *Physical Therapy, 81*(9), 1572–1580.

Weitzel, E.A. (2001). Unilateral neglect. In: M. Maas, K. Buckwalter, M. Hardy, T. Tripp-Reimer, M. Titler, & J. Specht (eds), *Nursing care of older adults: Diagnosis, outcomes, and interventions*. St. Louis, MO: Mosby, pp. 492–502.

Impaired Environmental Interpretation Syndrome* (00127)
(1994)

Domain 5: Perception/Cognition
Class 2: Orientation

Definition Consistent lack of orientation to person, place, time, or circumstances over more than 3–6 months necessitating a protective environment

Defining Characteristics

- Chronic confusional states
- Consistent disorientation
- Inability to concentrate
- Inability to follow simple directions
- Inability to reason
- Loss of occupation
- Loss of social functioning
- Slow in responding to questions

Related Factors

- Dementia
- Depression
- Huntington's disease

This diagnosis will retire from the NANDA-I Taxonomy in the 2015–2017 edition unless additional work is completed to bring it into compliance with the definition of syndrome diagnoses (requires two or more nursing diagnoses as defining characteristics/risk factors).

5. Perception/Cognition

Acute Confusion (00128)
(1994, 2006, LOE 2.1)

Domain 5: Perception/Cognition
Class 4: Cognition

Definition
Abrupt onset of reversible disturbances of consciousness, attention, cognition, and perception that develop over a short period of time

Defining Characteristics

- Fluctuation in cognition
- Fluctuation in level of consciousness
- Fluctuation in psychomotor activity
- Hallucinations
- Increased agitation
- Increased restlessness
- Lack of motivation to follow through with goal-directed behavior
- Lack of motivation to follow through with purposeful behavior
- Lack of motivation to initiate goal-directed behavior
- Lack of motivation to initiate purposeful behavior
- Misperceptions

Related Factors

- Delirium
- Dementia
- Fluctuation in sleep–wake cycle
- Over 60 years of age
- Substance abuse

References

Agostini, J.V., Leo-Summers, L.S., & Inouye, S.K. (2001). Cognitive and other adverse effects of diphenhydramine use in hospitalized older patients. *Archives of Internal Medicine, 161*(17), 2091–2097.

Alciati, A., Scaramelli, B., Fusi, A., Butteri, E., Cattameo, M.L., & Mellado, C. (1999). Three cases of delirium after "ecstasy" ingestion. *Journal of Psychoactive Drugs, 31*(2), 167–170.

Aldemir, M., Ozen, S., Kara, I.H., Sir, A., & Bac, B. (2001). Predisposing factors for delirium in the surgical intensive care unit. *Critical Care, 5*(5), 265–270.

Bowman, A.M. (1997). Sleep satisfaction, perceived pain and acute confusion in elderly clients undergoing orthopaedic procedures. *Journal of Advanced Nursing, 26*(3), 550–564.

Brauer, C., Morrison, R.S., Silberzweig, S.B., & Sui, A.L. (2000). The cause of delirium in patients with hip fracture. *Archives of Internal Medicine, 160*(12), 1856–1860.

Coyle, N., Breitbart, W., Weaver, S., & Portenoy, R. (1994). Delirium as a contributing factor to "crescendo" pain: Three case reports. *Journal of Pain and Symptom Management, 9*(1), 44–47.

Edlund, A., Lundstrom, M., Brannstrom, B., Bucht, G., & Gustafson, Y. (2001). Delirium before and after operation for femoral neck fracture. *Journal of the American Geriatrics Society, 49*(10), 1335–1340.

Elie, M., Cole, M.G., Primeau, F. J., & Bellavance, F. (1998). Delirium risks factors in elderly hospitalized patients. *Journal of General Internal Medicine, 13*(3), 204–212.

Erkinjuntti, T., Wikstrom, J., Palo, J., & Autio, L. (1986). Dementia among medical inpatients: Evaluation of 2000 consecutive admissions. *Archives of Internal Medicine, 146*(10), 1923–1926.

Fisher, B.W. & Flowerdew, G. (1995). A simple model for predicting postoperative delirium in older patients undergoing elective orthopedic surgery. *Journal of the American Geriatric Society, 43*(2), 175–178.

Foreman, M. (1989). Confusion in the hospitalized elderly: Incidence, onset, and associated factors. *Research in Nursing and Health, 12*(1), 21–29.

Francis, J., Martin, D., & Kapoor, W. (1990). A prospective study of delirium in hospitalized elderly. *Journal of the American Medical Association, 263*(8), 1097–1101.

Grandberg, A.I., Malmros, C.W., Bergborn, I.L., & Lundberg, D.B. (2002) Intensive care syndrome/ delirium is associated with anemia, drug therapy and duration of ventilation treatment. *Acta Anaesthesiologica Scandinavica, 46*(6), 726–731.

Gustafson, Y., Berggren, D., Brannstrom, B., Bucht, G., et al. (1988). Acute confusional state in elderly patients treated for femoral neck fracture. *Journal of the American Geriatric Association, 36*(6), 525–530.

Han, L., McCusher, J., Cole, M., Abrahamowiz, M., Primeau, F., & Elie, M. (2001). Use of medications with anticholinergic effect predicts clinical severity of delirium symptoms in older medical inpatients. *Archives of Internal Medicine, 161*(8), 1099–1105.

Haynes, C. (1999). Emergence delirium: A literature review. *British Journal of Theatre Nursing, 9*(11), 502–510.

Inouye, S.K., & Charpentier, P.A. (1996). Precipitating factors for delirium in hospitalized elderly persons: Predictive model and interrelationship with baseline vulnerability. *Journal of the American Medical Association, 275*(11), 852–857.

Jitapunkul, S., Pillay, I., & Ebrahim, S. (1992). Delirium in newly admitted elderly patients: A prospective study. *Quarterly Journal of Medicine, 83*(300), 307–314.

Kelly, M. (1997). The best is yet to be. Postoperative delirium in the elderly. *Today's Surgical Nurse, 19*(5), 10–12.

Koponen, H., Stenback, U., Mattila, E., Soininen, H., Reinikainen, K., & Riekkinen, P. (1989). Delirium among elderly persons admitted to a psychiatric hospital: clinical course during the acute state and one-year follow-up. *Acta Psychiatrica Scandinavica, 79*(6), 579–585.

Korevaar, J.C., van Munster, B.C., & de Rooij, S.E. (2005). Risk factors for delirium in acutely admitted elderly patients: A prospective cohort study. Retrieved from http://www.biomedcentral.com/1471-2318/5/6.

Lawlor, P.G., Gagnon, B., Mancini, I.L., Pereira, J.L., Hanson, J., Suarez-Almazor, M.E., & Bruera, E.D. (2000). Occurrence, causes, and outcome of delirium in patients with advanced cancer. *Archives of Internal Medicine, 160*(6), 786–794.

Levkoff, S.E., Safran, C., Cleary, P.D., Gallop, J., & Phillips, R.S. (1988). Identification of factors associated with the diagnosis of delirium in elderly hospitalized patients. *Journal of the American Geriatrics Society, 36*(12), 1099–1104.

Lipov, E.G. (1991). Emergence delirium in the PACU. *Critical Care Nursing Clinics of North America, 3*(1), 145–149.

Lynch, E.P., Lazor, M.A., Gellis, J.E., Orav, J., Goldman, L., & Marcantonioa, E.R. (1998). The impact of postoperative pain on the development of post operative delirium. *Anesthesia and Analgesia, 86*(4), 781–785.

McCuster, J., Cole, M., Abrahamowica, M., Han, L., Podoba, J., & Ramman-Haddad, L. (2001). Environmental risk factors for delirium in hospitalized older people. *Journal of the American Geriatrics Society, 49*(10), 1327–1334.

Marcantonio, E.R., Goldman, L., Mangione, C.M., et al. (1994). A clinical prediction rule for delirium after elective noncardiac surgery. *Journal of the American Medical Association, 271*(2), 134–139.

Marcantonio, E.R., Simon, S.E., Bergmann, M.A., Jones, R.N., Murphy, K.M., & Morris, J.N. (2003). Delirium symptoms in post-acute care: Prevalent, persistent, and associated with poor functional recovery. *Journal of the American Geriatrics Society, 51*(1), 4–9.

Massie, M.J. & Holland, J.C. (1992). The cancer patient with pain: Psychiatric complications and their management. *Journal of Pain and Symptom Management, 7*(2), 99–109.

Mentes, J., Culp, J., Maas, M., & Rantz, M. (1999). Acute confusion indicators: Risk factors and prevalence using MDS data. *Research in Nursing and Health, 22*(2), 95–105.

Morita, T., Tei, Y., Tsunoda, J., Inouye, S., & Chihara, S. (2001). Underlying pathologies and their associations with clinical features in terminal delirium of cancer patients. *Journal of Pain and Symptom Management, 22*(6), 997–1006.

Morrison, R.S., Magaziner, J., Gilbert, M., Koval, K. J., McLaughlin, M.A., Orosz, G., Strauss, E., & Siu, A. (2003). Relationship between pain and opioid analgesics on the development of delirium following hip fracture. *Journal of Gerontology Series A – A Biological Sciences and Medical Sciences, 58*(1), 76–81.

Nishikawa, K., Nakayama, M., Omote, K., & Namiki, A. (2004). Recovery characteristics and post operative delirium after long-duration laparoscope-assisted surgery in elderly patients: Propofol-based vs. sevoflurane-based anesthesia. *Acta Anaesthesiologica Scandinavica, 48*(2), 162–168.

O'Brien, D. (2002). Acute postoperative delirium: definitions, incidence, recognition, and interventions. *Journal of Peri-Anesthesia Nursing, 17*, 384–92.

Pompei, P., Foreman, M., Rudberg, M., Inouye, S., Braund, V., & Cassel, C. (1994). Delirium in hospitalized older persons: Outcomes and predictors. *Journal of the American Geriatrics Society, 42*, 809–15.

Praticò, C., Quattrone, D., Lucanto, T., Amato, A., Penna, O., Riscitano, C., & Fodale, V. (2005). Drugs of anesthesia acting on central cholinergic system may cause post operative cognitive dysfunction and delirium. *Medical Hypotheses, 65*, 972–82.

Rockwood, K. (1989). Acute confusion in elderly medical patients. *Journal of the American Geriatrics Society, 37*, 150–4.

Rolfson, D.B., McElhaney, J.E., Rockwood, K., Finnegan, B.A., Entwistle, L.M., Wong, J.F., & Suarez-Almazor, M.E. (1999). Incidence and risk factors for delirium and other adverse outcomes in older adults after coronary artery bypass graft surgery. *Canadian Journal of Cardiology, 15*, 771–776.

Ross, D.L. (1998). Factors associated with excited delirium, deaths in police custody. *Modern Pathology, 11*, 1127–1137.

Ruttenber, A.J., Lawler-Heavner, J., Yin, M., Wetli, C.V., Hearn, W.L., & Mash, D.C. (1997). Fatal excited delirium following cocaine use: Epidemiological findings provide new evidence for mechanisms of cocaine toxicity. *Journal of Forensic Sciences, 42*(1), 25–31.

Ruttenber, A.J., McAnally, H.B., & Wetli, C.V. (1999). Cocaine-associated rhabdomyolysis and excited delirium: different stages of the same syndrome. *American Journal of Forensic Medicine and Pathology, 20*(2), 120–127.

Schor, J.D., Levkoff, S.E., Lipsitz, L.A., Reilly, C.H., Cleary, P.D., Rowe, J.W., & Evans, D.A. (1992). Risk factors for delirium in hospitalized elderly. *Journal of the American Medical Association, 267*(6), 827–831.

Schururmans, M.J., Duursma, S.A., Shortridge-Baggett, L.M., Clevers, G., & Pel-Little, R. (2003). Elderly patients with hip fracture: The risk for delirium. *Applied Nursing Research, 16*(2), 75–84.

Seaman, J.S., Schillerstrom, J., Carroll, D., & Brown, T.M. (2006). Impaired oxidative metabolism precipitates delirium: A study of 101 ICU patients. *Psychosomatics, 47*(1), 56–61.

Seymour, D.G., & Vaz, F.G. (1989). A prospective study of elderly general surgical patients. II: Post operative complications. *Age and Ageing, 18*(5), 316–326.

Seymour, D.G., Henschke, P.J., Cape, R.D., & Campbell, A.J. (1980). Acute confusional states and dementia in the elderly: The role of dehydration/volume depletion, physical illness and age. *Age and Ageing, 9*(3), 137–146.

Williams, M.A., Holloway, J.R., Winn, M.C., Wolanin, M.O., Lawler, M.L., Westwick, C.R., & Chin, M.H. (1979). Nursing activities and acute confusional states in elderly hip-fractured patients. *Nursing Research, 28*(1), 25–35.

Williams-Russo, P., Urquhart, B.L., Sharrock, N.E., & Charlson, M.E. (1992). Post-operative delirium: Prognosis in elderly orthopedic patients. *Journal of the American Geriatrics Society, 40*(8), 759–767.

Wilson, L.M. (1972). Intensive care delirium. *Archives of Internal Medicine, 130*(2), 225–226.

Chronic Confusion (00129)

(1994)

Domain 5: Perception/Cognition
Class 4: Cognition

Definition   Irreversible, longstanding, and/or progressive deterioration of intellect and personality characterized by decreased ability to interpret environmental stimuli and decreased capacity for intellectual thought processes, and manifested by disturbances of memory, orientation, and behavior

Defining Characteristics

- Altered interpretation
- Altered personality
- Altered response to stimuli
- Clinical evidence of organic impairment
- Impaired long-term memory

- Impaired short-term memory
- Impaired socialization
- Longstanding cognitive impairment
- No change in level of consciousness
- Progressive cognitive impairment

Related Factors

- Alzheimer's disease
- Cerebral vascular attack
- Head injury

- Korsakoff's psychosis
- Multi-infarct dementia

Risk for Acute Confusion (00173)

(2006, LOE 2.2)

Domain 5: Perception/Cognition
Class 4: Cognition

Definition   At risk for reversible disturbances of consciousness, attention, cognition, and perception that develop over a short period of time

Risk Factors

- Decreased mobility
- Decreased restraints
- Dementia
- Fluctuation in sleep–wake cycle
- History of stroke
- Impaired cognition
- Infection
- Male gender
- Metabolic abnormalities:
  - Azotemia
  - Decreased hemoglobin
  - Dehydration
  - Electrolyte imbalances
  - Increased blood urea nitrogen (BUN)/creatinine
  - Malnutrition
- Over 60 years of age
- Pain
- Pharmaceutical agents:
  - Anesthesia
  - Anticholinergics
  - Diphenhydramine
  - Multiple medications
  - Opioids
  - Psychoactive drugs
- Sensory deprivation
- Substance abuse
- Urinary retention

References

Agostini, J.V., Leo-Summers, L.S., & Inouye, S.K. (2001). Cognitive and other adverse effects of diphen-hydramine use in hospitalized older patients. *Archives of Internal Medicine, 161*(17), 2091–2097.

Alciati, A., Scaramelli, B., Fusi, A., Butteri, E., Cattameo, M.L., & Mellado, C. (1999). Three cases of delirium after "ecstasy" ingestion. *Journal of Psychoactive Drugs, 31*(2), 167–170.

Aldemir, M., Ozen, S., Kara, I.H., Sir, A., & Bac, B. (2001). Predisposing factors for delirium in the surgical intensive care unit. *Critical Care, 5*(5), 265–270.

Bowman, A.M. (1997). Sleep satisfaction, perceived pain and acute confusion in elderly clients undergoing orthopaedic procedures. *Journal of Advanced Nursing, 26*(3), 550–564.

Brauer, C., Morrison, R.S., Silberzweig, S.B., & Sui, A.L. (2000). The cause of delirium in patients with hip fracture. *Archives of Internal Medicine, 160*(12), 1856–1860.

Coyle, N., Breitbart, W., Weaver, S., & Portenoy, R. (1994). Delirium as a contributing factor to "crescendo" pain: Three case reports. *Journal of Pain and Symptom Management, 9*(1), 44–47.

Edlund, A., Lundstrom, M., Brannstrom, B., Bucht, G., & Gustafson, Y. (2001). Delirium before and after operation for femoral neck fracture. *Journal of the American Geriatrics Society, 49*(10), 1335–1340.

Elie, M., Cole, M.G., Primeau, F. J., & Bellavance, F. (1998). Delirium risks factors in elderly hospitalized patients. *Journal of General Internal Medicine, 13*(3), 204–212.

Erkinjuntti, T., Wikstrom, J., Palo, J., & Autio, L. (1986). Dementia among medical inpatients: Evaluation of 2000 consecutive admissions. *Archives of Internal Medicine, 146*(10), 1923–1926.

Fisher, B.W. & Flowerdew, G. (1995). A simple model for predicting postoperative delirium in older patients undergoing elective orthopedic surgery. *Journal of the American Geriatric Society, 43*(2), 175–178.

Foreman, M. (1989). Confusion in the hospitalized elderly: Incidence, onset, and associated factors. *Research in Nursing and Health*, *12*(1), 21–29.

Francis, J., Martin, D., & Kapoor, W. (1990). A prospective study of delirium in hospitalized elderly. *Journal of the American Medical Association*, *263*(8), 1097–1101.

Grandberg, A.I., Malmros, C.W., Bergborn, I.L., & Lundberg, D.B. (2002) Intensive care syndrome/delirium is associated with anemia, drug therapy and duration of ventilation treatment. *Acta Anaesthesiologica Scandinavica*, *46*(6), 726–731.

Gustafson, Y., Berggren, D., Brannstrom, B., Bucht, G., et al. (1988). Acute confusional state in elderly patients treated for femoral neck fracture. *Journal of the American Geriatric Association*, *36*(6), 525–530.

Han, L., McCusher, J., Cole, M., Abrahamowiz, M., Primeau, F., & Elie, M. (2001). Use of medications with anticholinergic effect predicts clinical severity of delirium symptoms in older medical inpatients. *Archives of Internal Medicine*, *161*(8), 1099–1105.

Haynes, C. (1999). Emergence delirium: A literature review. *British Journal of Theatre Nursing*, *9*(11), 502–510.

Inouye, S.K., & Charpentier, P.A. (1996). Precipitating factors for delirium in hospitalized elderly persons: Predictive model and interrelationship with baseline vulnerability. *Journal of the American Medical Association*, *275*(11), 852–857.

Jitapunkul, S., Pillay, I., & Ebrahim, S. (1992). Delirium in newly admitted elderly patients: A prospective study. *Quarterly Journal of Medicine*, *83*(300), 307–314.

Kelly, M. (1997). The best is yet to be. Postoperative delirium in the elderly. *Today's Surgical Nurse*, *19*(5), 10–12.

Koponen, H., Stenback, U., Mattila, E., Soininen, H., Reinikainen, K., & Riekkinen, P. (1989). Delirium among elderly persons admitted to a psychiatric hospital: clinical course during the acute state and one-year follow-up. *Acta Psychiatrica Scandinavica*, *79*(6), 579–585.

Korevaar, J.C., van Munster, B.C., & de Rooij, S.E. (2005). Risk factors for delirium in acutely admitted elderly patients: A prospective cohort study. Retrieved from http://www.biomedcentral.com/1471-2318/5/6.

Lawlor, P.G., Gagnon, B., Mancini, I.L., Pereira, J.L., Hanson, J., Suarez-Almazor, M.E., & Bruera, E.D. (2000). Occurrence, causes, and outcome of delirium in patients with advanced cancer. *Archives of Internal Medicine*, *160*(6), 786–794.

Levkoff, S.E., Safran, C., Cleary, P.D., Gallop, J., & Phillips, R.S. (1988). Identification of factors associated with the diagnosis of delirium in elderly hospitalized patients. *Journal of the American Geriatrics Society*, *36*(12), 1099–1104.

Lipov, E.G. (1991). Emergence delirium in the PACU. *Critical Care Nursing Clinics of North America*, *3*(1), 145–149.

Lynch, E.P., Lazor, M.A., Gellis, J.E., Orav, J., Goldman, L., & Marcantonioa, E.R. (1998). The impact of postoperative pain on the development of post operative delirium. *Anesthesia and Analgesia*, *86*(4), 781–785.

McCuster, J., Cole, M., Abrahamowica, M., Han, L., Podoba, J., & Ramman-Haddad, L. (2001). Environmental risk factors for delirium in hospitalized older people. *Journal of the American Geriatrics Society*, *49*(10), 1327–1334.

Marcantonio, E.R., Goldman, L., Mangione, C.M., et al. (1994). A clinical prediction rule for delirium after elective noncardiac surgery. *Journal of the American Medical Association*, *271*(2), 134–139.

Marcantonio, E.R., Simon, S.E., Bergmann, M.A., Jones, R.N., Murphy, K.M., & Morris, J.N. (2003). Delirium symptoms in post-acute care: Prevalent, persistent, and associated with poor functional recovery. *Journal of the American Geriatrics Society*, *51*(1), 4–9.

Massie, M.J. & Holland, J.C. (1992). The cancer patient with pain: Psychiatric complications and their management. *Journal of Pain and Symptom Management*, *7*(2), 99–109.

Mentes, J., Culp, J., Maas, M., & Rantz, M. (1999). Acute confusion indicators: Risk factors and prevalence using MDS data. *Research in Nursing and Health*, *22*(2), 95–105.

Morita, T., Tei, Y., Tsunoda, J., Inouye, S., & Chihara, S. (2001). Underlying pathologies and their associations with clinical features in terminal delirium of cancer patients. *Journal of Pain and Symptom Management*, *22*(6), 997–1006.

Morrison, R.S., Magaziner, J., Gilbert, M., Koval, K. J., McLaughlin, M.A., Orosz, G., Strauss, E., & Siu, A. (2003). Relationship between pain and opioid analgesics on the development of delirium following hip fracture. *Journal of Gerontology Series A – A Biological Sciences and Medical Sciences*, *58*(1), 76–81.

Nishikawa, K., Nakayama, M., Omote, K., & Namiki, A. (2004). Recovery characteristics and post operative delirium after long-duration laparoscope-assisted surgery in elderly patients: Propofol-based vs. sevoflurane-based anesthesia. *Acta Anaesthesiologica Scandinavica*, *48*(2), 162–168.

O'Brien, D. (2002). Acute postoperative delirium: definitions, incidence, recognition, and interventions. *Journal of Peri-Anesthesia Nursing, 17*, 384–92.

Pompei, P., Foreman, M., Rudberg, M., Inouye, S., Braund, V., & Cassel, C. (1994). Delirium in hospitalized older persons: Outcomes and predictors. *Journal of the American Geriatrics Society, 42*, 809–15.

Praticò, C., Quattrone, D., Lucanto, T., Amato, A., Penna, O., Riscitano, C., & Fodale, V. (2005). Drugs of anesthesia acting on central cholinergic system may cause post operative cognitive dysfunction and delirium. *Medical Hypotheses, 65*, 972–82.

Rockwood, K. (1989). Acute confusion in elderly medical patients. *Journal of the American Geriatrics Society, 37*, 150–4.

Rolfson, D.B., McElhaney, J.E., Rockwood, K., Finnegan, B.A., Entwistle, L.M., Wong, J.F., & Suarez-Almazor, M.E. (1999). Incidence and risk factors for delirium and other adverse outcomes in older adults after coronary artery bypass graft surgery. *Canadian Journal of Cardiology, 15*, 771–776.

Ross, D.L. (1998). Factors associated with excited delirium, deaths in police custody. *Modern Pathology, 11*, 1127–1137.

Ruttenber, A.J., Lawler-Heavner, J., Yin, M., Wetli, C.V., Hearn, W.L., & Mash, D.C. (1997). Fatal excited delirium following cocaine use: Epidemiological findings provide new evidence for mechanisms of cocaine toxicity. *Journal of Forensic Sciences, 42*(1), 25–31.

Ruttenber, A.J., McAnally, H.B., & Wetli, C.V. (1999). Cocaine-associated rhabdomyolysis and excited delirium: different stages of the same syndrome. *American Journal of Forensic Medicine and Pathology, 20*(2), 120–127.

Schor, J.D., Levkoff, S.E., Lipsitz, L.A., Reilly, C.H., Cleary, P.D., Rowe, J.W., & Evans, D.A. (1992). Risk factors for delirium in hospitalized elderly. *Journal of the American Medical Association, 267*(6), 827–831.

Schururmans, M.J., Duursma, S.A., Shortridge-Baggett, L.M., Clevers, G., & Pel-Little, R. (2003). Elderly patients with hip fracture: The risk for delirium. *Applied Nursing Research, 16*(2), 75–84.

Seaman, J.S., Schillerstrom, J., Carroll, D., & Brown, T.M. (2006). Impaired oxidative metabolism precipitates delirium: A study of 101 ICU patients. *Psychosomatics, 47*(1), 56–61.

Seymour, D.G., & Vaz, F.G. (1989). A prospective study of elderly general surgical patients. II: Post operative complications. *Age and Ageing, 18*(5), 316–326.

Seymour, D.G., Henschke, P.J, Cape, R.D., & Campbell, A.J. (1980). Acute confusional states and dementia in the elderly: The role of dehydration/volume depletion, physical illness and age. *Age and Ageing, 9*(3), 137–146.

Williams, M.A., Holloway, J.R., Winn, M.C., Wolanin, M.O., Lawler, M.L., Westwick, C.R., & Chin, M.H. (1979). Nursing activities and acute confusional states in elderly hip-fractured patients. *Nursing Research, 28*(1), 25–35.

Williams-Russo, P., Urquhart, B.L., Sharrock, N.E., & Charlson, M.E. (1992). Post-operative delirium: Prognosis in elderly orthopedic patients. *Journal of the American Geriatrics Society, 40*(8), 759–767.

Wilson, L.M. (1972). Intensive care delirium. *Archives of Internal Medicine, 130*(2), 225–226.

Ineffective Impulse Control (00222)
(2010, LOE 2.1)

Domain 5: Perception/Cognition
Class 4: Cognition

Definition   A pattern of performing rapid, unplanned reactions to internal or external stimuli without regard for the negative consequences of these reactions to the impulsive individual or to others

Defining Characteristics

- Acting without thinking
- Asking personal questions of others despite their discomfort
- Inability to save money or regulate finances
- Irritability
- Pathological gambling
- Sensation seeking
- Sexual promiscuity
- Sharing personal details inappropriately
- Temper outbursts
- Too familiar with strangers
- Violence

Related Factors

- Anger
- Chronic low self-esteem
- Co-dependency
- Compunction
- Delusion
- Denial
- Disorder of cognition
- Disorder of development
- Disorder of mood
- Disorder of personality
- Disturbed body image
- Economically disadvantaged
- Environment that might cause frustration
- Environment that might cause irritation
- Fatigue
- Hopelessness
- Ineffective coping
- Insomnia
- Organic brain disorders
- Smoker
- Social isolation
- Stress vulnerability
- Substance abuse
- Suicidal feeling
- Unpleasant physical symptoms

References

American Psychiatric Association. (2000). *Diagnostic and statistical manual of mental disorders*, 4th ed., Text-Revision. Washington, DC: American Psychiatric Association.

Barkley, R.A., Edwards, G., Laneri, M., Fletcher, K., & Metevia, L. (2001). Executive functioning, temporal discounting, and sense of time in adolescents with attention deficit hyperactivity disorder (ADHD) and oppositional defiant disorder (ODD). *Journal of Abnormal Child Psychology*, 29(6), 541–556.

Baron-Cohen, S. (1988). An assessment of violence in young man with Asperger's syndrome. *Journal of Child Psychology and Psychiatry*, 29(3), 351–360.

Bradley, E.A., & Isaacs, B.J. (2006). Inattention, hyperactivity, and impulsivity in teenagers with intellectual disabilities, with and without autism. *Canadian Journal of Psychiatry*, 51(9), 598–606.

Brain Injury Association of Queensland (2009. July 2). Impulsivity – Fact Sheet. Retrieved from http://braininjury.org.au/portal/behavioural/impulsivity—fact-sheet.html.

Cloninger, C.R. (1987). A systematic method for clinical description and classification of personality variants. A proposal. *Archives of General Psychiatry*, 44(6), 573–588.

Coffey, S.F., Gudleski, G.D., Saladin, M.E., & Brady, K.T. (2003). Impulsivity and rapid discounting of delayed hypothetical rewards in cocaine-dependent individuals. *Experimental and Clinical Psychopharmacology*, 11(1), 18–25.

Conner, K.R., & Duberstein, P.R. (2004). Predisposing and precipitating factors for suicide among alcoholic: Empirical review and conceptual integration. *Alcoholism, Clinical and Experimental Research*, 28(5 Suppl.), 6S–17S.

Hare, R.D. (2008). Hare Psychopathy Checklist-Revised (2nd Edition) (PCL-R). In B. Cutler (Ed.), *Encyclopedia of psychology and law*. Thousand Oaks, CA: Sage Publications.

Madden, G.J., Petry, N.M., Bader, G.J., & Bickel, W.K. (1997) Impulsive and self-control choices in opioid-dependent patients and non-drug-using control participants: drug and monetary rewards. *Experimental and Clinical Psychopharmacology*, 5(3), 256–262.

Moeller, F.G., Barratt, E.S., Dougherty, D.M., Schmitz, J.M., & Swann A.C. (2001). Psychiatric aspects of impulsivity. *American Journal of Psychiatry*, 158(11), 1783–1793.

Petry, N.M., & Casarella, T. (1999). Excessive discounting of delayed rewards in substance abusers with gambling problem. *Drug and Alcohol Dependence*, 56(1), 25–32.

Reynolds, B., Karraker, K., Horn, K., & Richards, J.B. (2003). Delay and probability discounting as related to different stages of adolescent smoking and non- smoking. *Behavioural Processes*, 64(3), 333–344.

Verdejo-García, A, Bechara, A., Recknor, E.C., & Pérez-Garcia, M. (2007). Negative emotion-driven impulsivity predicts substance dependence problems. *Drug and Alcohol Dependence*, 91(2–3), 213–219.

Vuchinich, R.E., & Simpson, C.A. (1998). Hyperbolic temporal discounting in social drinkers and problem drinkers. *Experimental and Clinical Psychopharmacology*, 6(3), 292–305.

Deficient Knowledge (00126)
(1980)

Domain 5: Perception/Cognition
Class 4: Cognition

Definition
Absence or deficiency of cognitive information related to a specific topic

Defining Characteristics

- Exaggerated behaviors
- Inaccurate follow-through of instruction
- Inaccurate performance of test
- Inappropriate behaviors (e.g., hysterical, hostile, agitated, apathetic)
- Reports the problem

Related Factors

- Cognitive limitation
- Information misinterpretation
- Lack of exposure
- Lack of interest in learning
- Lack of recall
- Unfamiliarity with information resources

Readiness for Enhanced Knowledge (00161)
(2002, LOE 2.1)

Domain 5: Perception/Cognition
Class 4: Cognition

Definition   A pattern of cognitive information related to a specific topic, or its acquisition, that is sufficient for meeting health-related goals and can be strengthened

Defining Characteristics

- Behaviors congruent with expressed knowledge
- Describes previous experiences pertaining to the topic
- Explains knowledge of the topic
- Expresses an interest in learning

5. Perception/Cognition

Impaired Memory (00131)
(1994)

Domain 5: Perception/Cognition
Class 4: Cognition

Definition   Inability to remember or recall bits of information or behavioral skills

Defining Characteristics

- Forgets to perform a behavior at a scheduled time
- Inability to learn new information
- Inability to learn new skills
- Inability to perform a previously learned skill
- Inability to recall events
- Inability to recall factual information
- Inability to recall if a behavior was performed
- Inability to retain new information
- Inability to retain new skills
- Reports experience of forgetting

Related Factors

- Anemia
- Decreased cardiac output
- Electrolyte imbalance
- Excessive environmental disturbances
- Fluid imbalance
- Hypoxia
- Neurological disturbances

Readiness for Enhanced Communication (00157)

(2002, LOE 2.1)

Domain 5: Perception/Cognition
Class 5: Communication

Definition A pattern of exchanging information and ideas with others that is sufficient for meeting one's needs and life's goals, and can be strengthened

Defining Characteristics

- Able to speak a language
- Able to write a language
- Expresses feelings
- Expresses satisfaction with ability to share ideas with others
- Expresses satisfaction with ability to share information with others
- Expresses thoughts
- Expresses willingness to enhance communication
- Forms phrases
- Forms sentences
- Forms words
- Interprets nonverbal cues appropriately
- Uses nonverbal cues appropriately

Impaired Verbal Communication (00051)
(1983, 1996, 1998)

Domain 5: Perception/Cognition
Class 5: Communication

Definition   Decreased, delayed, or absent ability to receive, process, transmit, and/or use a system of symbols

Defining Characteristics

- Absence of eye contact
- Cannot speak
- Difficulty expressing thoughts verbally (e.g., aphasia, dysphasia, apraxia, dyslexia)
- Difficulty forming sentences
- Difficulty forming words (e.g., aphonia, dyslalia, dysarthria)
- Difficulty in comprehending usual communication pattern
- Difficulty in maintaining usual communication pattern
- Difficulty in selective attending
- Difficulty in use of body expressions
- Difficulty in use of facial expressions
- Disorientation to person
- Disorientation to space
- Disorientation to time
- Does not speak
- Dyspnea
- Inability to speak language of caregiver
- Inability to use body expressions
- Inability to use facial expressions
- Inappropriate verbalization
- Partial visual deficit
- Slurring
- Speaks with difficulty
- Stuttering
- Total visual deficit
- Verbalizes with difficulty
- Willful refusal to speak

Related Factors

- Absence of significant others
- Alteration in self-concept
- Alteration of central nervous system
- Altered perceptions
- Anatomic defect (e.g., cleft palate, alteration of the neuromuscular visual system, auditory system, phonatory apparatus)
- Brain tumor
- Chronic low self-esteem
- Cultural differences
- Decreased circulation to brain
- Differences related to developmental age
- Emotional conditions
- Environmental barriers
- Lack of information
- Physical barrier (e.g., tracheostomy, intubation)
- Physiological conditions
- Psychological barriers (e.g., psychosis, lack of stimuli)
- Situational low self-esteem
- Stress
- Treatment-related side effects (e.g., pharmacological agents)
- Weakened musculoskeletal system

Domain 6
Self-Perception

NANDA International Nursing Diagnoses: Definitions & Classification 2012–2014, First Edition.
Edited by T. Heather Herdman.
© 2012 NANDA International. Published 2012 by Blackwell Publishing Ltd.

Hopelessness (00124)
(1986)

Domain 6: Self-Perception
Class 1: Self-Concept

Definition Subjective state in which an individual sees limited or no alternatives or personal choices available and is unable to mobilize energy on own behalf

Defining Characteristics

- Closing eyes
- Decreased affect
- Decreased appetite
- Decreased response to stimuli
- Decreased verbalization
- Lack of initiative
- Lack of involvement in care
- Passivity
- Shrugging in response to speaker
- Sleep pattern disturbance
- Turning away from speaker
- Verbal cues (e.g., despondent content, "I can't," sighing)

Related Factors

- Abandonment
- Deteriorating physiological condition
- Long-term stress
- Lost belief in spiritual power
- Lost belief in transcendent values
- Prolonged activity restriction
- Social isolation

6. Self-Perception

Risk for Compromised Human Dignity (00174)
(2006, LOE 2.1)

Domain 6: Self-Perception
Class 1: Self-Concept

Definition   At risk for perceived loss of respect and honor

Risk Factors

- Cultural incongruity
- Disclosure of confidential information
- Exposure of the body
- Inadequate participation in decision-making
- Loss of control of body functions
- Perceived dehumanizing treatment
- Perceived humiliation
- Perceived intrusion by clinicians
- Perceived invasion of privacy
- Stigmatizing label
- Use of undefined medical terms

References

Haddock, J. (1996). Towards further clarification of the concept "dignity". *Journal of Advanced Nursing*, 24(5), 924–931.

Mairis, E. (1994). Concept clarification of professional practice dignity. *Journal of Advanced Nursing*, 19(5), 947–953.

Shotton, L., & Seedhouse, D. (1998). Practical dignity in caring. *Nursing Ethics*, 5(3), 246–255.

Walsh, K., & Kowanko, I. (2002). Nurses' and patients' perceptions of dignity. *International Journal of Nursing Practice*, 8(3), 143–151.

Watson, J. (1995). *Nursing and the philosophy and science of caring*. Niwot, CO: University of Colorado Press.

Risk for Loneliness (00054)

(1994, 2006, LOE 2.1)

Domain 6: Self-Perception
Class 1: Self-Concept

Definition At risk for experiencing discomfort associated with a desire or need for more contact with others

Risk Factors

- Affectional deprivation
- Cathectic deprivation
- Physical isolation
- Social isolation

References

Leiderman, P.H. (1969). Loneliness: A psychodynamic interpretation. In: E.S Scheidman, & M.J. Ortega (eds), *Aspects of depression*. International Psychiatry Clinics, Vol. 6. Boston: Little, Brown, pp. 155, 174.

Lien-Gieschen, T. (1993). Validation of social isolation related to maturational age: Elderly. *Nursing Diagnosis*, 4(1), 37–44.

Warren, B.J. (1993). Explaining social isolation through concept analysis. *Archives of Psychiatric Nursing*, 7(5), 270–276.

6. Self-Perception

Disturbed Personal Identity (00121)
(1978, 2008, LOE 2.1)

Domain 6: Self-Perception
Class 1: Self-Concept

Definition
Inability to maintain an integrated and complete perception of self

Defining Characteristics

- Contradictory personal traits
- Delusional description of self
- Disturbed body image
- Gender confusion
- Ineffective coping
- Ineffective relationships
- Ineffective role performance
- Reports feelings of emptiness
- Reports feelings of strangeness
- Reports fluctuating feelings about self
- Unable to distinguish between inner and outer stimuli
- Uncertainty about cultural values (e.g., beliefs, religion, moral questions)
- Uncertainty about goals
- Uncertainty about ideological values (e.g., beliefs, religion, moral questions)

Related Factors

- Chronic low self-esteem
- Cult indoctrination
- Cultural discontinuity
- Discrimination
- Dysfunctional family processes
- Ingestion of toxic chemicals
- Inhalation of toxic chemicals
- Manic states
- Multiple personality disorder
- Organic brain syndromes
- Perceived prejudice
- Psychiatric disorders (e.g., psychoses, depression, dissociative disorder)
- Situational crises
- Situational low self-esteem
- Social role change
- Stages of development
- Stages of growth
- Use of psychoactive pharmaceutical agents

References

Bender, D., & Skodol, A. (2007). Borderline personality as a self-other representational disturbance. *Journal of Personality Disorders*, 21(5), 500–517.

Bergh, S., & Erling, A. (2005). Adolescent identity formation: A Swedish study of identity status using the EOM-EIS-II. *Adolescence*, 40(158), 377–396.

Erikson, E.H. (1982). *Identitet: Ungdom og kriser* [*Identity: Youth and crisis*]. Denmark: Hans Reitzel.

Evang, A. (2003). *Utvikling, personlighet og borderline* [*Development, personality and borderline*]. Norway: Cappelen Akademisk Forlag.

Fuchs, T. (2007). Fragmented selves: Temporality and identity in borderline personality disorder. *Psychopathology*, 40(6), 379–388.

Mitchell, A. (1985). The borderline diagnosis and integration of self. *American Journal of Psychoanalysis*, 45, 234–250.

Stuart, G.W., & Laraia, M.T. (2001). *Principles and practice of psychiatric nursing*. St. Louis, MO: Mosby.

Risk for Disturbed Personal Identity (00225)
(2010, LOE 2.1)

Domain 6: Self-Perception
Class 1: Self-Concept

Definition Risk for the inability to maintain an integrated and complete perception of self

Risk Factors

- Chronic low self-esteem
- Cult indoctrination
- Cultural discontinuity
- Discrimination
- Dysfunctional family processes
- Ingestion of toxic chemicals
- Inhalation of toxic chemicals
- Manic states
- Multiple personality disorder
- Organic brain syndromes
- Perceived prejudice
- Psychiatric disorders (e.g., psychoses, depression, dissociative disorder)
- Situational crises
- Situational low self-esteem
- Social role change
- Stages of development
- Stages of growth
- Use of psychoactive pharmaceutical agents

References

Bender, D., & Skodol, A. (2007). Borderline personality as a self-other representational disturbance. *Journal of Personality Disorders, 21*(5), 500–517.

Bergh, S., & Erling, A. (2006). Adolescent identity formation: a Swedish study of identity status using the EOM-EIS-II. *Adolescence, 40*(158): 377–396.

Erikson, E.H. (1982). *Identitet: Ungdom og kriser* [*Identity: Youth and crisis*]. Denmark: Hans Reitzel.

Evang, A. (2003). *Utvikling, personlighet og borderline* [*Development, personality and borderline*]. Norway: Cappelen Akademisk Forlag.

Fuchs, T. (2007). Fragmented selves: Temporality and identity in borderline personality disorder. *Psychopathology, 40*(6), 379–388.

Mitchell A. (1985). The borderline diagnosis and integration of self. *American Journal of Psychoanalysis, 45*, 234–250.

Stuart, G.W., & Laraia, M.T. (2001) *Principles and practice of psychiatric nursing*. St. Louis, MO: Mosby.

6. Self-Perception

Readiness for Enhanced Self-Concept (00167)

(2002, LOE 2.1)

Domain 6: Self-Perception
Class 1: Self-Concept

Definition A pattern of perceptions or ideas about the self that is sufficient for well-being and can be strengthened

Defining Characteristics

- Accepts limitations
- Accepts strengths
- Actions are congruent with verbal expression
- Expresses confidence in abilities
- Expresses satisfaction with body image
- Expresses satisfaction with personal identity
- Expresses satisfaction with role performance
- Expresses satisfaction with sense of worthiness
- Expresses satisfaction with thoughts about self
- Expresses willingness to enhance self-concept

Chronic Low Self-Esteem (00119)
(1988, 1996, 2008, LOE 2.1)

Domain 6: Self-Perception
Class 2: Self-Esteem

Definition
Longstanding negative self-evaluating/feelings about self or self-capabilities

Defining Characteristics

- Dependent on others' opinions
- Evaluation of self as unable to deal with events
- Exaggerates negative feedback about self
- Excessively seeks reassurance
- Frequent lack of success in life events
- Hesitant to try new situations
- Hesitant to try new things
- Indecisive behavior
- Lack of eye contact
- Nonassertive behavior
- Overly conforming
- Passive
- Rejects positive feedback about self
- Reports feelings of guilt
- Reports feelings of shame

Related Factors

- Ineffective adaptation to loss
- Lack of affection
- Lack of approval
- Lack of membership in group
- Perceived discrepancy between self and cultural norms
- Perceived discrepancy between self and spiritual norms
- Perceived lack of belonging
- Perceived lack of respect from others
- Psychiatric disorder
- Repeated failures
- Repeated negative reinforcement
- Traumatic event
- Traumatic situation

References

Bredeholf, D. (1990). An evaluation study of the self-esteem: a family affair program with risk abuse parents. *Transactional Analysis Journal*, *20*(2), 111–117.

Brown, J., & Dutton, K. (1995). The thrill of victory, the complexity of defeat: Self-esteem and people's emotional reactions to success and failure. *Journal of Personality and Social Psychology*, *68*(4), 712–722.

Buckner, J., Mezzacappa, E., & Beardslee, W. (2003). Characteristics of resilient youths living in poverty: The role of self-regulatory processes. *Developmental Psychopathology*, *15*(1), 139–162.

Buckner, J., Beardslee, W., Bassuk, E., & Ray, S. (2004). Exposure to violence and low-income children's mental health: Direct, moderated, and mediated relations. *American Journal of Orthopsychiatry*, *74*(4), 413–423.

Byers, P., Raven, L., Hill, J., & Robyak, J. (1990). Enhancing self-esteem of inpatient alcoholics. *Issues in Mental Health Nursing*, *11*(4), 337–346.

Consoli, S.M. (2003). Dépression et maladies organiques associées, une comorbidité encore sous-estimée. Résultat de l'enquête [Depression and associated organic pathologies. A still under-estimated comorbidity. Results of the DIALOGUE study]. *Presse Médicale*, *32*(1), 10–21.

Crowe, M. (2004). Never good enough. II: Clinical implications. *Journal of Psychiatric Mental Health Nursing, 11*(3), 335–340.

Dumas, D., & Pelletier, L. (1997). La perception de soi: La clé de voûte des interventions de l'infirmière auprès de l'enfant hyperactive [Self perception: The key stone of nursing interventions with hyperactive children]. *L'infirmière du Québec, 4*(4), 28–36.

Fitts, W. (1972). *The self-concept and psychopathology.* Nashville, TN: Counselor Recordings and Tests.

Gary, F., Baker, M., & Grandbois, D. (2005). Perspectives on suicide prevention among American Indian and Alaska native children and adolescents: A call for help. *Online Journal of Issues in Nursing, 10*(2), 6.

Hall, P., & Tarrier, N. (2003). The cognitive-behavioural treatment of low self-esteem in psychotic patients: A pilot study. *Behavior Research and Therapy, 41*(3), 317–332.

Heap, J. (2004). Enuresis in children and young people: A public health nurse approach in New Zealand. *Journal of Child Health Care, 8*(2), 92–101 [Review].

Leblanc, L., & Ouellet, N. (2004). Dépistage de la violence conjugale: Le role de l'infirmière. [Screening for spousal abuse: The nurse's role]. *Perspective Infirmière: Revue Officielle De l'Ordre Des Infirmières et Infirmiers du Québec, 5*, 39–43.

Maslow, A. (1970). *Motivation and personality*, 2nd ed. New York: Harper & Row.

Meridith, P., Strong J., & Feeney, J. (2006). The relationship of adult attachment to emotion, catastrophizing, control, threshold and tolerance, in experimentally-induced pain. *Pain, 120*(1–2), 44–52.

Mozley, P. (1976). Psychophysiologic infertility: An overview. *Clinical Obstetrics and Gynecology, 19*(2), 407–417.

Nishina, A., & Juvonen, J. (2005). Daily reports of witnessing and experiencing peer harassment in middle school. *Child Development, 76*(2), 435–450.

Page, C. (1995). Intervenir auprès des femmes présentant un trouble dépressif [Helping women with a depressive disease]. *L'infirmière Du Québec: Revue Officielle De L'ordre Des Infirmières Et Infirmiers Du Québec, 2*(5), 26–33.

Ray, S., & Heap, J. (2001). Male survivors' perspectives of incest/sexual abuse. *Perspectives on Psychiatric Care, 37*(2), 49–59.

Rodin, J. (1993). Cultural and psychosocial determinants of weight concerns. *Annals in Internal Medicine, 119*(7 Pt 2), 643–645.

Rotheram-Borus, M.J. (1990). Adolescents' reference group choices, self-esteem, and judgment. *Journal of Personality and Social Psychology, 59*(5), 1075–1081.

Sharma, V., & Mavi, J. (2001). Self-esteem and performance on word tasks. *Journal of Social Psychology, 141*(6), 723–729.

Sloman, L., Gilbert, P., & Hasey, G. (2003). Evolved mechanisms in depression: The role and interaction of attachment and social rank in depression. *Journal of Affective Disorders, 74*(2), 107–121.

Talf, L. (1985). Self-esteem in later life: A nursing perspective. *Advances in Nursing Science, 8*(1), 77–84.

Thorne, A., & Michaelieu, Q. (1996). Situating adolescent gender and self-esteem personal memories. *Child Development, 67*(4), 1374–1390.

Trabut, P.C. (2000). Les abus sexuels chez les enfants en bas âge [Sexual abuse of young children]. *L'infirmière Du Québec: Revue Officielle De L'ordre Des Infirmières et Infirmiers du Québec, 8*(1), 27–32.

Westermeyer, J. (1989). Cross-cultural care for PTSD: Research, training and service needs for the future. *Journal of Traumatic Stress, 2*(4), 515–536.

Situational Low Self-Esteem (00120)

(1988, 1996, 2000)

Domain 6: Self-Perception
Class 2: Self-Esteem

Definition Development of a negative perception of self-worth in response to a current situation

Defining Characteristics

- Evaluation of self as unable to deal with events
- Evaluation of self as unable to deal with situations
- Indecisive behavior
- Nonassertive behavior
- Reports current situational challenge to self-worth
- Reports helplessness
- Reports uselessness
- Self-negating verbalizations

Related Factors

- Behavior inconsistent with values
- Developmental changes
- Disturbed body image
- Failures
- Functional impairment
- Lack of recognition
- Loss
- Rejections
- Social role changes

6. Self-Perception

Risk for Chronic Low Self-Esteem (00224)
(2010, LOE 2.1)

Domain 6: Self-Perception
Class 2: Self-Esteem

Definition At risk for longstanding negative self-evaluating/feelings about self or self-capabilities

Risk Factors

- Ineffective adaptation to loss
- Lack of affection
- Lack of membership in group
- Perceived discrepancy between self and cultural norms
- Perceived discrepancy between self and spiritual norms
- Perceived lack of belonging
- Perceived lack of respect from others
- Psychiatric disorder
- Repeated failures
- Repeated negative reinforcement
- Traumatic event
- Traumatic situation

References

Bredeholf, D. (1990). An evaluation study of the self-esteem: a family affair program with risk abuse parents. *Transactional Analysis Journal, 20*(2), 111–117.

Brown, J., & Dutton, K. (1995). The thrill of victory, the complexity of defeat: Self-esteem and people's emotional reactions to success and failure. *Journal of Personality and Social Psychology, 68*(4), 712–722.

Buckner, J., Mezzacappa, E., & Beardslee, W. (2003). Characteristics of resilient youths living in poverty: The role of self-regulatory processes. *Developmental Psychopathology, 15*(1), 139–162.

Buckner, J., Beardslee, W., Bassuk, E., & Ray, S. (2004). Exposure to violence and low-income children's mental health: Direct, moderated, and mediated relations. *American Journal of Orthopsychiatry, 74*(4), 413–423.

Byers, P., Raven, L., Hill, J., & Robyak, J. (1990). Enhancing self-esteem of inpatient alcoholics. *Issues in Mental Health Nursing, 11*(4), 337–346.

Consoli, S.M. (2003). Dépression et maladies organiques associées, une comorbidité encore sous-estimée. Résultat de l'enquête [Depression and associated organic pathologies. A still under-estimated comorbidity. Results of the DIALOGUE study]. *Presse Médicale, 32*(1), 10–21.

Crowe, M. (2004). Never good enough. II: Clinical implications. *Journal of Psychiatric Mental Health Nursing, 11*(3), 335–340.

Dumas, D., & Pelletier, L. (1997). La perception de soi: La clé de voûte des interventions de l'infirmière auprès de l'enfant hyperactive [Self perception: The key stone of nursing interventions with hyperactive children]. *L'infirmière du Québec, 4*(4), 28–36.

Fitts, W. (1972). *The self-concept and psychopathology*. Nashville, TN: Counselor Recordings and Tests.

Gary, F., Baker, M., & Grandbois, D. (2005). Perspectives on suicide prevention among American Indian and Alaska native children and adolescents: A call for help. *Online Journal of Issues in Nursing, 10*(2), 6.

Hall, P., & Tarrier, N. (2003). The cognitive-behavioural treatment of low self-esteem in psychotic patients: A pilot study. *Behavior Research and Therapy, 41*(3), 317–332.

Heap, J. (2004). Enuresis in children and young people: A public health nurse approach in New Zealand. *Journal of Child Health Care, 8*(2), 92–101 [Review].

Leblanc, L., & Ouellet, N. (2004). Dépistage de la violence conjugale: Le role de l'infirmière. [Screening for spousal abuse: The nurse's role]. *Perspective Infirmière: Revue Officielle De l'Ordre Des Infirmières et Infirmiers du Québec, 5*, 39–43.

Maslow, A. (1970). *Motivation and personality*, 2nd ed. New York: Harper & Row.

Meridith, P., Strong J., & Feeney, J. (2006). The relationship of adult attachment to emotion, catastrophizing, control, threshold and tolerance, in experimentally-induced pain. *Pain*, *120*(1–2), 44–52.

Mozley, P. (1976). Psychophysiologic infertility: An overview. *Clinical Obstetrics and Gynecology*, *19*(2), 407–417.

Nishina, A., & Juvonen, J. (2005). Daily reports of witnessing and experiencing peer harassment in middle school. *Child Development*, *76*(2), 435–450.

Page, C. (1995). Intervenir auprès des femmes présentant un trouble dépressif [Helping women with a depressive disease]. *L'infirmière Du Québec: Revue Officielle De L'ordre Des Infirmières Et Infirmiers Du Québec*, *2*(5), 26–33.

Ray, S., & Heap, J. (2001). Male survivors' perspectives of incest/sexual abuse. *Perspectives on Psychiatric Care*, *37*(2), 49–59.

Rodin, J. (1993). Cultural and psychosocial determinants of weight concerns. *Annals in Internal Medicine*, *119*(7 Pt 2), 643–645.

Rotheram-Borus, M.J. (1990). Adolescents' reference group choices, self-esteem, and judgment. *Journal of Personality and Social Psychology*, *59*(5), 1075–1081.

Sharma, V., & Mavi, J. (2001). Self-esteem and performance on word tasks. *Journal of Social Psychology*, *141*(6), 723–729.

Sloman, L., Gilbert, P., & Hasey, G. (2003). Evolved mechanisms in depression: The role and interaction of attachment and social rank in depression. *Journal of Affective Disorders*, *74*(2), 107–121.

Talf, L. (1985). Self-esteem in later life: A nursing perspective. *Advances in Nursing Science*, *8*(1), 77–84.

Thorne, A., & Michaelieu, Q. (1996). Situating adolescent gender and self-esteem personal memories. *Child Development*, *67*(4), 1374–1390.

Trabut, P.C. (2000). Les abus sexuels chez les enfants en bas âge [Sexual abuse of young children]. *L'infirmière Du Québec: Revue Officielle De L'ordre Des Infirmières et Infirmiers du Québec*, *8*(1), 27–32.

Westermeyer, J. (1989). Cross-cultural care for PTSD: Research, training and service needs for the future. *Journal of Traumatic Stress*, *2*(4), 515–536.

6. Self-Perception

Risk for Situational Low Self-Esteem (00153)
(2000)

Domain 6: Self-Perception
Class 2: Self-Esteem

Definition At risk for developing a negative perception of self-worth in response to a current situation

Risk Factors

- Behavior inconsistent with values
- Decreased control over environment
- Developmental changes
- Disturbed body image
- Failures
- Functional impairment
- History of abandonment
- History of abuse
- History of learned helplessness
- History of neglect
- Lack of recognition
- Loss
- Physical illness
- Rejections
- Social role changes
- Unrealistic self-expectations

Disturbed Body Image (00118)
(1973, 1998)

Domain 6: Perception/Cognition
Class 3: Body Image

Definition Confusion in mental picture of one's physical self

Defining Characteristics

- Behaviors of acknowledgment of one's body
- Behaviors of avoidance of one's body
- Behaviors of monitoring one's body
- Nonverbal response to actual change in body (e.g., appearance, structure, function)
- Nonverbal response to perceived change in body (e.g., appearance, structure, function)
- Reports feelings that reflect an altered view of one's body (e.g., appearance, structure, function)
- Reports perceptions that reflect an altered view of one's body in appearance

Objective

- Actual change in function
- Actual change in structure
- Behaviors of acknowledging one's body
- Behaviors of monitoring one's body
- Change in ability to estimate spatial relationship of body to environment
- Change in social involvement
- Extension of body boundary to incorporate environmental objects
- Intentional hiding of body part
- Intentional overexposure of body part
- Missing body part
- Not looking at body part
- Not touching body part
- Trauma to nonfunctioning part
- Unintentional hiding of body part
- Unintentional overexposing of body part

Subjective

- Depersonalization of loss by use of impersonal pronouns
- Depersonalization of part by use of impersonal pronouns
- Emphasis on remaining strengths
- Focus on past appearance
- Focus on past function
- Focus on past strength
- Heightened achievement
- Personalization of loss by name
- Personalization of body part by name
- Preoccupation with change
- Preoccupation with loss
- Refusal to verify actual change
- Reports change in lifestyle
- Reports fear of reaction by others
- Reports negative feelings about body (e.g., feelings of helplessness, hopelessness, powerlessness)

Related Factors

- Biophysical
- Cognitive
- Cultural
- Developmental changes
- Illness
- Injury

- Perceptual
- Psychosocial
- Spiritual
- Surgery
- Trauma
- Treatment regimen

Domain 7
Role Relationships

NANDA International Nursing Diagnoses: Definitions & Classification 2012–2014, First Edition.
Edited by T. Heather Herdman.
© 2012 NANDA International. Published 2012 by Blackwell Publishing Ltd.

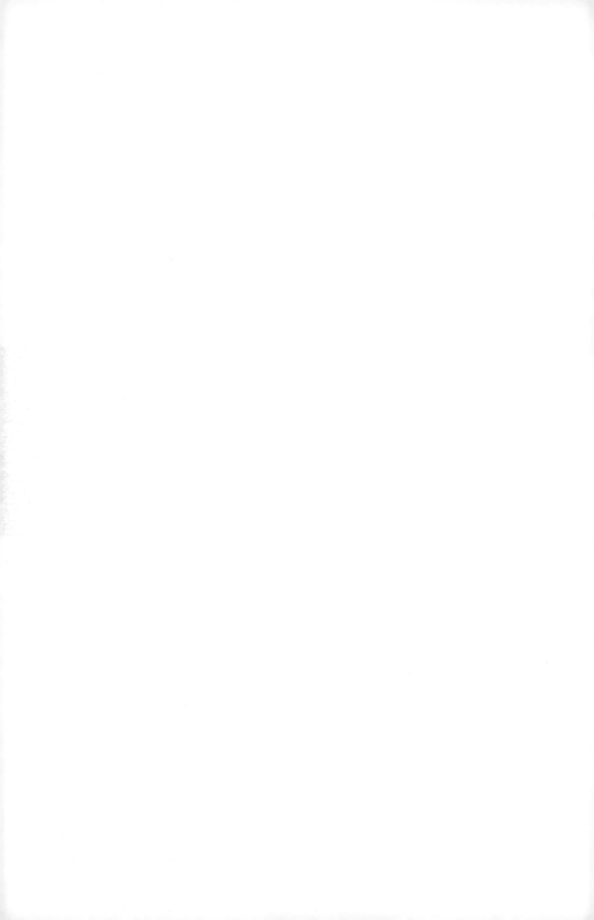

Ineffective Breastfeeding (00104)
(1988, 2010)

Domain 7: Role Relationships
Class 1: Caregiving Roles

Definition Dissatisfaction or difficulty a mother, infant, or child experiences with the breastfeeding process

Defining Characteristics

- Inadequate milk supply
- Infant arching at the breast
- Infant crying at the breast
- Infant crying within the first hour after breastfeeding
- Infant exhibiting fussiness within the first hour after breastfeeding
- Infant inability to latch on to maternal breast correctly
- Infant resisting latching on
- Infant unresponsive to other comfort measures
- Insufficient emptying of each breast per feeding
- Insufficient opportunity for suckling at the breast
- Lack of infant weight gain
- No observable signs of oxytocin release
- Perceived inadequate milk supply
- Persistence of sore nipples beyond first week of breastfeeding
- Sustained infant weight loss
- Unsatisfactory breastfeeding process
- Unsustained suckling at the breast

Related Factors

- Deficient knowledge
- Infant anomaly
- Infant receiving supplemental feedings with artificial nipple
- Interrupted breastfeeding
- Maternal ambivalence
- Maternal anxiety
- Maternal breast anomaly
- Nonsupportive family
- Nonsupportive partner
- Poor infant sucking reflex
- Prematurity
- Previous breast surgery
- Previous history of breastfeeding failure

Interrupted Breastfeeding (00105)
(1992)

Domain 7: Role Relationships
Class 1: Caregiving Roles

Definition Break in the continuity of the breastfeeding process as a result of inability or inadvisability to put baby to breast for feeding

Defining Characteristics

- Deficient knowledge about expression of breast milk
- Deficient knowledge about storage of breast milk
- Infant receives no nourishment at the breast for some or all feedings
- Maternal desire to provide breast milk for child's nutritional needs
- Maternal desire to maintain breastfeeding for child's nutritional needs
- Mother–child separation

Related Factors

- Contraindications to breastfeeding (e.g., certain pharmaceutical agents)
- Infant illness
- Infant prematurity
- Maternal employment
- Maternal illness
- Need to abruptly wean infant

Readiness for Enhanced Breastfeeding* (00106)
(1990, 2010)

Domain 7: Role Relationships
Class 1: Caregiving Roles

Definition A pattern of proficiency and satisfaction of the mother–infant dyad that is sufficient to support the breastfeeding process and can be strengthened

Defining Characteristics

- Adequate infant elimination patterns for age
- Appropriate infant weight pattern for age
- Eagerness of infant to nurse
- Effective mother–infant communication patterns
- Infant content after feeding
- Mother able to position infant at breast to promote a successful latching-on response
- Mother reports satisfaction with the breastfeeding process
- Regular suckling at the breast
- Regular swallowing at the breast
- Signs of oxytocin release are present
- Sustained suckling at the breast
- Sustained swallowing at the breast
- Symptoms of oxytocin release are present

*This diagnosis previously held the label, Effective Breastfeeding

Caregiver Role Strain (00061)
(1992, 1998, 2000)

Domain 7: Role Relationships
Class 1: Caregiving Roles

Definition Difficulty in performing family/significant other caregiver role

Defining Characteristics

Caregiving Activities

- Apprehension about care receiver's care if caregiver unable to provide care
- Apprehension about the future regarding caregiver's ability to provide care
- Apprehension about the future regarding care receiver's health
- Apprehension about possible institutionalization of care receiver
- Difficulty completing required tasks
- Difficulty performing required tasks
- Dysfunctional change in caregiving activities
- Preoccupation with care routine

Caregiver Health Status

Physical

- Cardiovascular disease
- Diabetes
- Fatigue
- Gastrointestinal upset
- Headaches
- Hypertension
- Rash
- Weight change

Emotional

- Anger
- Disturbed sleep pattern
- Frustration
- Impatience
- Increased emotional lability
- Increased nervousness
- Ineffective coping
- Lack of time to meet personal needs
- Reports feeling depressed
- Sleep deprivation
- Somatization
- Stress

Socioeconomic

- Changes in leisure activities
- Low work productivity
- Refuses career advancement
- Withdraws from social life

Caregiver–Care Receiver Relationship

- Reports difficulty watching care receiver go through the illness
- Reports grief regarding changed relationship with care receiver
- Reports uncertainty regarding changed relationship with care receiver

Family Processes

- Reports concerns about family members
- Family conflict

Related Factors

Care Receiver Health Status

- Addiction
- Co-dependency
- Cognitive problems
- Dependency
- Illness chronicity
- Illness severity
- Increasing care needs
- Instability of care receiver's health
- Problem behaviors
- Psychological problems
- Substance abuse
- Unpredictability of illness course

Caregiver Health Status

- Co-dependency
- Cognitive problems
- Inability to fulfill one's own expectations
- Inability to fulfill other's expectations
- Marginal coping patterns
- Physical problems
- Psychological problems
- Substance abuse
- Unrealistic expectations of self

Caregiver–Care Receiver Relationship

- History of poor relationship
- Mental status of elder inhibiting conversation
- Presence of abuse
- Presence of violence
- Unrealistic expectations of caregiver by care receiver

Caregiving Activities

- 24-hour care responsibilities
- Amount of activities
- Complexity of activities
- Discharge of family members to home with significant care needs
- Ongoing changes in activities
- Unpredictability of care situation
- Years of caregiving

Family Processes

- History of family dysfunction
- History of marginal family coping

Resources

- Caregiver is not developmentally ready for caregiver role
- Deficient knowledge about community resources
- Difficulty accessing community resources
- Difficulty accessing formal assistance
- Difficulty accessing formal support
- Emotional strength
- Inadequate community resources (e.g., respite services, recreational resources)
- Inadequate equipment for providing care
- Inadequate informal assistance
- Inadequate informal support
- Inadequate physical environment for providing care (e.g., housing, temperature, safety)
- Inadequate transportation
- Inexperience with caregiving
- Insufficient finances
- Insufficient time
- Lack of caregiver privacy
- Lack of support
- Physical energy

Socioeconomic

- Alienation from others
- Competing role commitments
- Insufficient recreation
- Isolation from others

Risk for Caregiver Role Strain (00062)
(1992, 2010)

Domain 7: Role Relationships
Class 1: Caregiving Roles

Definition At risk for caregiver vulnerability for felt difficulty in performing the family caregiver role

Risk Factors

- Amount of caregiving tasks
- Care receiver exhibits bizarre behavior
- Care receiver exhibits deviant behavior
- Caregiver health impairment
- Caregiver is female
- Caregiver is spouse
- Caregiver isolation
- Caregiver not developmentally ready for caregiver role
- Caregiver's competing role commitments
- Co-dependency
- Cognitive problems in care receiver
- Complexity of caregiving tasks
- Congenital defect
- Developmental delay of caregiver
- Developmental delay of care receiver
- Discharge of family member with significant home care needs
- Duration of caregiving required
- Family dysfunction before the caregiving situation
- Family isolation
- Illness severity of the care receiver
- Inadequate physical environment for providing care (e.g., housing, transportation, community services, equipment)
- Inexperience with caregiving
- Instability in the care receiver's health
- Lack of recreation for caregiver
- Lack of respite for caregiver
- Marginal caregiver's coping patterns
- Marginal family adaptation
- Past history of poor relationship between caregiver and care receiver
- Premature birth
- Presence of abuse
- Presence of situational stressors that normally affect families (e.g., significant loss, disaster or crisis, economic vulnerability, major life events)
- Presence of violence
- Psychological problems in caregiver
- Psychological problems in care receiver
- Substance abuse
- Unpredictable illness course

Impaired Parenting (00056)
(1978, 1998)

Domain 7: Role Relationships
Class 1: Caregiving Roles

Definition   Inability of the primary caretaker to create, maintain, or regain an environment that promotes the optimum growth and development of the child

Defining Characteristics

Infant or Child

- Behavioral disorders
- Failure to thrive
- Frequent accidents
- Frequent illness
- Incidence of abuse
- Incidence of trauma (e.g., physical and psychological)
- Lack of attachment
- Lack of separation anxiety
- Poor academic performance
- Poor cognitive development
- Poor social competence
- Runaway

Parental

- Abandonment
- Child abuse
- Child neglect
- Frequently punitive
- Hostility to child
- Inadequate attachment
- Inadequate child health maintenance
- Inappropriate caretaking skills
- Inappropriate child care arrangements
- Inappropriate stimulation (e.g., visual, tactile, auditory)
- Inconsistent behavior management
- Inconsistent care
- Inflexibility in meeting needs of child
- Little cuddling
- Maternal–child interaction deficit
- Negative statements about child
- Paternal–child interaction deficit
- Rejection of child
- Reports frustration
- Reports inability to control child
- Reports role inadequacy
- Statements of inability to meet child's needs
- Unsafe home environment

Related Factors

Infant or Child

- Altered perceptual abilities
- Attention deficit hyperactivity disorder
- Developmental delay
- Difficult temperament
- Handicapping condition
- Illness
- Multiple births

- Not desired gender
- Premature birth
- Separation from parent

- Temperamental conflicts with parental expectations

Knowledge

- Deficient knowledge about child development
- Deficient knowledge about child health maintenance
- Deficient knowledge about parenting skills
- Inability to respond to infant cues

- Lack of cognitive readiness for parenthood
- Lack of education
- Limited cognitive functioning
- Poor communication skills
- Preference for physical punishment
- Unrealistic expectations

Physiological

- Physical illness

Psychological

- Closely spaced pregnancies
- Depression
- Difficult birthing process
- Disability
- Disturbed sleep pattern
- High number of pregnancies

- History of mental illness
- History of substance abuse
- Lack of prenatal care
- Sleep deprivation
- Young parental age

Social

- Change in family unit
- Chronic low self-esteem
- Economically disadvantaged
- Father of child not involved
- Financial difficulties
- History of being abused
- History of being abusive
- Inability to put child's needs before own
- Inadequate child care arrangements
- Job problems
- Lack of family cohesiveness
- Lack of parental role model
- Lack of resources
- Lack of social support networks
- Lack of transportation
- Lack of valuing of parenthood

- Legal difficulties
- Maladaptive coping strategies
- Marital conflict
- Mother of child not involved
- Poor home environment
- Poor parental role model
- Poor problem-solving skills
- Presence of stress (e.g., financial, legal, recent crisis, cultural move)
- Relocations
- Role strain
- Single parent
- Situational low self-esteem
- Social isolation
- Unemployment
- Unplanned pregnancy
- Unwanted pregnancy

Readiness for Enhanced Parenting (00164)
(2002, LOE 2.1)

Domain 7: Role Relationships
Class 1: Caregiving Roles

Definition A pattern of providing an environment for children or other dependent person(s) that is sufficient to nurture growth and development, and can be strengthened

Defining Characteristics

- Children report satisfaction with home environment
- Emotional support of children
- Emotional support of other dependent person(s)
- Evidence of attachment
- Exhibits realistic expectations of children
- Exhibits realistic expectations of other dependent person(s)
- Expresses willingness to enhance parenting
- Needs of children are met (e.g., physical and emotional)
- Needs of other dependent person(s) is/are met (e.g., physical and emotional)
- Other dependent person(s) express(es) satisfaction with home environment

Risk for Impaired Parenting (00057)
(1978, 1998)

Domain 7: Role Relationships
Class 1: Caregiving Roles

Definition At risk for inability of the primary caretaker to create, maintain, or regain an environment that promotes the optimum growth and development of the child

Risk Factors

Infant or Child

- Altered perceptual abilities
- Attention deficit hyperactivity disorder
- Developmental delay
- Difficult temperament
- Handicapping condition
- Illness
- Multiple births
- Not gender desired
- Premature birth
- Prolonged separation from parent
- Temperamental conflicts with parental expectation

Knowledge

- Deficient knowledge about child development
- Deficient knowledge about child health maintenance
- Deficient knowledge about parenting skills
- Inability to respond to infant cues
- Lack of cognitive readiness for parenthood
- Low cognitive functioning
- Low educational level
- Poor communication skills
- Preference for physical punishment
- Unrealistic expectations of child

Physiological

- Physical illness

Psychological

- Closely spaced pregnancies
- Depression
- Difficult birthing process
- Disability
- High number of pregnancies
- History of mental illness
- History of substance abuse
- Sleep deprivation
- Sleep disruption
- Young parental age

Social

- Change in family unit
- Chronic low self-esteem
- Economically disadvantaged
- Father of child not involved
- Financial difficulties
- History of being abused
- History of being abusive
- Inadequate child care arrangements
- Job problems
- Lack of access to resources
- Lack of family cohesiveness
- Lack of parental role model
- Lack of prenatal care
- Lack of resources
- Lack of social support network
- Lack of transportation
- Lack of valuing of parenthood
- Late prenatal care

- Legal difficulties
- Maladaptive coping strategies
- Marital conflict
- Mother of child not involved
- Parent–child separation
- Poor home environment
- Poor parental role model
- Poor problem-solving skills
- Relocation
- Role strain
- Single parent
- Situational low self-esteem
- Social isolation
- Stress
- Unemployment
- Unplanned pregnancy
- Unwanted pregnancy

Risk for Impaired Attachment* (00058)
(1994, 2008, LOE 2.1)

Domain 7: Role Relationships
Class 2: Family Relationships

Definition At risk for disruption of the interactive process between parent/significant other and child that fosters the development of a protective and nurturing reciprocal relationship

Risk Factors

- Anxiety associated with the parent role
- Disorganized infant behavior
- Ill child who is unable effectively to initiate parental contact
- Inability of parent(s) to meet personal needs
- Lack of privacy
- Parental conflict resulting from disorganized infant behavior
- Parent–child separation
- Physical barriers
- Premature infant
- Substance abuse

*This diagnosis formerly held the label *Risk for Impaired Parent/Child Attachment.*

Dysfunctional Family Processes* (00063)
(1994, 2008, LOE 2.1)

Domain 7: Role/Relationships
Class 2: Family Relationships

Definition Psychosocial, spiritual, and physiological functions of the family unit are chronically disorganized, which leads to conflict, denial of problems, resistance to change, ineffective problem-solving, and a series of self-perpetuating crises

Defining Characteristics

Behavioral

- Agitation
- Blaming
- Broken promises
- Chaos
- Complicated grieving
- Conflict avoidance
- Contradictory communication
- Controlling communication
- Criticizing
- Deficient knowledge about substance abuse
- Denial of problems
- Dependency
- Difficulty having fun
- Difficulty with intimate relationships
- Difficulty with life cycle transitions
- Diminished physical contact
- Disturbances in academic performance in children
- Disturbances in concentration
- Enabling maintenance of substance use pattern (e.g., alcohol)
- Escalating conflict
- Failure to accomplish developmental tasks
- Family special occasions are substance-use centered
- Harsh self-judgment
- Immaturity
- Impaired communication
- Inability to accept a wide range of feelings
- Inability to accept help
- Inability to adapt to change
- Inability to deal constructively with traumatic experiences
- Inability to express a wide range of feelings
- Inability to meet the emotional needs of its members
- Inability to meet the security needs of its members
- Inability to meet the spiritual needs of its members
- Inability to receive help appropriately
- Inadequate understanding of substance abuse
- Inappropriate expression of anger
- Ineffective problem-solving skills
- Lack of reliability
- Lying
- Manipulation
- Nicotine addiction
- Orientation toward tension relief rather than achievement of goals
- Paradoxical communication
- Power struggles
- Rationalization
- Refusal to get help
- Seeking affirmation
- Seeking approval
- Self-blaming
- Social isolation

*This diagnosis formerly held the label *Dysfunctional Family Processes: Alcoholism.*

- Stress-related physical illnesses
- Substance abuse
- Verbal abuse of children

- Verbal abuse of parent
- Verbal abuse of spouse

Feelings

- Abandonment
- Anger
- Anxiety
- Being different from other people
- Being unloved
- Chronic low self-esteem
- Confuses love and pity
- Confusion
- Depression
- Dissatisfaction
- Distress
- Embarrassment
- Emotional control by others
- Emotional isolation
- Failure
- Fear
- Frustration
- Guilt
- Hopelessness
- Hostility

- Hurt
- Insecurity
- Lack of identity
- Lingering resentment
- Loneliness
- Loss
- Mistrust
- Moodiness
- Powerlessness
- Rejection
- Reports feeling misunderstood
- Repressed emotions
- Responsibility for substance abuser's behavior
- Suppressed rage
- Shame
- Tension
- Unhappiness
- Vulnerability
- Worthlessness

Roles and Relationships

- Altered role function
- Chronic family problems
- Closed communication systems
- Deterioration in family relationships
- Disrupted family rituals
- Disrupted family roles
- Disturbed family dynamics
- Economic problems
- Family denial
- Family does not demonstrate respect for autonomy of its members
- Family does not demonstrate respect for individuality of its members
- Inconsistent parenting

- Ineffective spouse communication
- Intimacy dysfunction
- Lack of cohesiveness
- Lack of skills necessary for relationships
- Low perception of parental support
- Marital problems
- Neglected obligations
- Pattern of rejection
- Reduced ability of family members to relate to each other for mutual growth and maturation
- Triangulating family relationships

Related Factors

- Addictive personality
- Biochemical influences
- Family history of resistance to treatment
- Family history of substance abuse
- Genetic predisposition to substance abuse
- Inadequate coping skills
- Lack of problem-solving skills
- Substance abuse

Interrupted Family Processes (00060)
(1982, 1998)

Domain 7: Role Relationships
Class 2: Family Relationships

Definition Change in family relationships and/or functioning

Defining Characteristics

- Changes in assigned tasks
- Changes in availability for affective responsiveness
- Changes in availability for emotional support
- Changes in communication patterns
- Changes in effectiveness in completing assigned tasks
- Changes in expressions of conflict with community resources
- Changes in expressions of conflict within family
- Changes in expressions of isolation from community resources
- Changes in mutual support
- Changes in participation in decision-making
- Changes in participation in problem-solving
- Changes in satisfaction with family
- Changes in somatic complaints
- Communication pattern changes
- Intimacy changes
- Pattern changes
- Power alliance changes
- Ritual changes
- Stress-reduction behavior changes

Related Factors

- Developmental crises
- Developmental transition
- Interaction with community
- Modification in family finances
- Modification in family social status
- Power shift of family members
- Shift in family roles
- Shift in health status of a family member
- Situation transition
- Situational crises

Readiness for Enhanced
Family Processes (00159)
(2002, LOE 2.1)

Domain 7: Role Relationships
Class 2: Family Relationships

Definition   A pattern of family functioning that is sufficient to support the well-being of family members and can be strengthened

Defining Characteristics

- Activities support the growth of family members
- Activities support the safety of family members
- Balance exists between autonomy and cohesiveness
- Boundaries of family members are maintained
- Communication is adequate
- Energy level of family supports activities of daily living
- Expresses willingness to enhance family dynamics
- Family adapts to change
- Family functioning meets needs of family members
- Family resilience is evident
- Family roles are appropriate for developmental stages
- Family roles are flexible for developmental stages
- Family tasks are accomplished
- Interdependent with community
- Relationships are generally positive
- Respect for family members is evident

Ineffective Relationship (00223)
(2010, LOE 2.1)

Domain 7: Role Relationships
Class 3: Role Performance

Definition A pattern of mutual partnership that is insufficient to provide for each other's needs

Defining Characteristics

- Does not identify partner as a key person
- Does not meet developmental goals appropriate for family life-cycle stage
- Inability to communicate in a satisfying manner between partners
- No demonstration of mutual respect between partners
- No demonstration of mutual support in daily activities between partners
- No demonstration of understanding of partner's insufficient (physical, social, psychological) functioning
- No demonstration of well-balanced autonomy between partners
- No demonstration of well-balanced collaboration between partners
- Reports dissatisfaction with complementary relation between partners
- Reports dissatisfaction with fulfilling emotional needs between partners
- Reports dissatisfaction with fulfilling physical needs between partners
- Reports dissatisfaction with sharing of ideas between partners
- Reports dissatisfaction with sharing of information between partners

Related Factors

- Cognitive changes in one partner
- Developmental crises
- History of domestic violence
- Incarceration of one partner
- Poor communication skills
- Stressful life events
- Substance abuse
- Unrealistic expectations

References

Aoki, Y., Kato, N., & Hirasawa, M. (eds). (2002). *Josangaku Taikei 5 Boshi no Shinri Shakaigaku* [*Midwifery System*. Vol. 5: *Psychosociology for Mother and Child*]. Tokyo: Japanese Nursing Association Publishing.

Chandola, T., Marmot, M., & Siegrist, J. (2007). Failed reciprocity in close social relationships and health: Findings from the Whitehall II study. *Journal of Psychosomatic Research, 63*(4), 403–411.

Kanbara, F. (1991). *Gendai no Kekkon to Fufu Kankei* [*Today's marriage and marital relationship*]. Tokyo: Baifukan.

Kawano, M. (1999). *Sexuality no Kango* [*Nursing for sexuality*]. Tokyo: Medical Friend.

Mochizuki, T. (1996). *Kazoku Shyakai-gaku Nyumon* [*Introduction to family sociology*]. Tokyo: Baifukan.

Muramoto, J., & Mori, A. (eds). (2007). *Bosei Kango-gaku Joron* [*Introduction to maternal nursing* (2nd ed.)]. Tokyo: Ishiyaku.

Murry, V., Harrell, A., Brody, G., Chen, Y., Simons, R., Black, A., Cutrona, C., & Gibbons, F. (2008). Long-term effects of stressors on relationship well-being and parenting among rural African American women. *Family Relations, 57*(2), 117–127.

Nojima, S., & Suzuki, K. (eds). (2005). *Kazoku Kango-gaku* [*Family nursing*]. Tokyo: Kenpansha.

Roy, C. (1984). *Introduction to nursing: Adaptation model* (2nd ed.). Upper Saddle River, NJ: Prentice-Hall.

Starratt, V., Goetz, A., Shackelford, T., McKibbin, W., & Stewart-Williams, S. (2008). Men's partner-directed insults and sexual coercion in intimate relationships. *Journal of Family Violence, 23*(5), 315–323.

Strawbridge, W., Wallhagen, M., & Shema, S. (2010). Spousal interrelations in self-reports of cognition in the context of marital problems. *Gerontology, 57*(2), 148–152.

Domain 7: Role Relationships
Class 3: Role Performance

Definition A pattern of mutual partnership that is sufficient to provide for each other's needs and can be strengthened

Defining Characteristics

- Demonstrates mutual respect between partners
- Demonstrates mutual support in daily activities between partners
- Demonstrates understanding of partner's insufficient (physical, social, psychological) function
- Demonstrates well-balanced autonomy between partners
- Demonstrates well-balanced collaboration between partners
- Identifies each other as a key person
- Meets developmental goals appropriate for family life-cycle stage
- Reports desire to enhance communication between partners
- Reports satisfaction with complementary relationship between partners
- Reports satisfaction with fulfilling emotional needs by one's partner
- Reports satisfaction with fulfilling physical needs by one's partner
- Reports satisfaction with sharing of ideas between partners
- Reports satisfaction with sharing of information between partners

References

Aoki, Y., Kato, N., & Hirasawa, M. (eds). (2002). *Josangaku Taikei 5 Boshi no Shinri Shakaigaku* [*Midwifery System*. Vol. 5: *Psychosociology for Mother and Child*]. Tokyo: Japanese Nursing Association Publishing.
Kanbara, F. (1991). *Gendai no Kekkon to Fufu Kankei* [*Today's marriage and marital relationship*]. Tokyo: Baifukan.
Kawano, M. (1999). *Sexuality no Kango* [*Nursing for sexuality*]. Tokyo: Medical Friend.
Mochizuki, T. (1996). *Kazoku Shyakai-gaku Nyumon* [*Introduction to family sociology*]. Tokyo: Baifukan.
Muramoto, J., & Mori, A. (eds). (2007). *Bosei Kango-gaku Joron* [*Introduction to maternal nursing* (2nd ed.)]. Tokyo: Ishiyaku.
Nojima, S., & Suzuki, K. (eds). (2005). *Kazoku Kango-gaku* [*Family nursing*]. Tokyo: Kenpansha.
Roy, C. (1984). *Introduction to nursing: Adaptation model* (2nd ed.). Upper Saddle River, NJ: Prentice-Hall.

Risk for Ineffective Relationship (00229)
(2010, LOE 2.1)

Domain 7: Role Relationships
Class 3: Role Performance

Definition Risk for a pattern of mutual partnership that is insufficient to provide for each other's needs

Risk Factors

- Cognitive changes in one partner
- Developmental crises
- History of domestic violence
- Incarceration of one partner
- Poor communication skills
- Stressful life events
- Substance abuse
- Unrealistic expectations

References

Aoki, Y., Kato, N., & Hirasawa, M. (eds). (2002). *Josangaku Taikei 5 Boshi no Shinri Shakaigaku* [*Midwifery System*. Vol. 5: *Psychosociology for Mother and Child*]. Tokyo: Japanese Nursing Association Publishing.

Chandola, T., Marmot, M., & Siegrist, J. (2007). Failed reciprocity in close social relationships and health: Findings from the Whitehall II study. *Journal of Psychosomatic Research, 63*(4), 403–411.

Kanbara, F. (1991). *Gendai no Kekkon to Fufu Kankei* [*Today's marriage and marital relationship*]. Tokyo: Baifukan.

Kawano, M. (1999). *Sexuality no Kango* [*Nursing for sexuality*]. Tokyo: Medical Friend.

Mochizuki, T. (1996). *Kazoku Shyakai-gaku Nyumon* [*Introduction to family sociology*]. Tokyo: Baifukan.

Muramoto, J., & Mori, A. (eds). (2007). *Bosei Kango-gaku Joron* [*Introduction to maternal nursing* (2nd ed.)]. Tokyo: Ishiyaku.

Murry, V., Harrell, A., Brody, G., Chen, Y., Simons, R., Black, A., Cutrona, C., & Gibbons, F. (2008). Long-term effects of stressors on relationship well-being and parenting among rural African American women. *Family Relations, 57*(2), 117–127.

Nojima, S., & Suzuki, K. (eds). (2005). *Kazoku Kango-gaku* [*Family nursing*]. Tokyo: Kenpansha.

Roy, C. (1984). *Introduction to nursing: Adaptation model* (2nd ed.). Upper Saddle River, NJ: Prentice-Hall.

Starratt, V., Goetz, A., Shackelford, T., McKibbin, W., & Stewart-Williams, S. (2008). Men's partner-directed insults and sexual coercion in intimate relationships. *Journal of Family Violence, 23*(5), 315–323.

Strawbridge, W., Wallhagen, M., & Shema, S. (2010). Spousal interrelations in self-reports of cognition in the context of marital problems. *Gerontology, 57*(2), 148–152.

7. Role Relationships

Parental Role Conflict (00064)
(1988)

Domain 7: Role Relationships
Class 3: Role Performance

Definition   Parental experience of role confusion and conflict in response to crisis

Defining Characteristics

- Anxiety
- Demonstrates disruption in caretaking routines
- Fear
- Reluctant to participate in usual caretaking activities
- Reports concern about changes in parental role
- Reports concern about family (e.g., functioning, communication, health)
- Reports concern about perceived loss of control over decisions relating to child
- Reports feelings of frustration
- Reports feelings of guilt
- Reports feeling of inadequacy to provide for child's needs (e.g., physical, emotional)

Related Factors

- Change in marital status
- Home care of a child with special needs
- Interruptions of family life due to home care regimen (e.g., treatments, caregivers, lack of respite)
- Intimidation by invasive modalities (e.g., intubation)
- Intimidation by restrictive modalities (e.g., isolation)
- Parent–child separation due to chronic illness
- Specialized care center

Ineffective Role Performance (00055)
(1978, 1996, 1998)

Domain 7: Role Relationships
Class 3: Role Performance

Definition Patterns of behavior and self-expression that do not match the environmental context, norms, and expectations

Defining Characteristics

- Altered role perceptions
- Anxiety
- Change in capacity to resume role
- Change in other's perception of role
- Change in self-perception of role
- Change in usual patterns of responsibility
- Deficient knowledge
- Depression
- Discrimination
- Domestic violence
- Harassment
- Inadequate adaptation to change
- Inadequate confidence
- Inadequate external support for role enactment
- Inadequate motivation
- Inadequate opportunities for role enactment
- Inadequate self-management
- Inadequate skills
- Inappropriate developmental expectations
- Ineffective coping
- Ineffective role performance
- Pessimism
- Powerlessness
- Role ambivalence
- Role conflict
- Role confusion
- Role denial
- Role dissatisfaction
- Role overload
- Role strain
- System conflict
- Uncertainty

Related Factors

Knowledge

- Inadequate role model
- Inadequate role preparation (e.g., role transition, skill rehearsal, validation)
- Lack of education
- Lack of role model
- Unrealistic role expectations

Physiological

- Body image alteration
- Chronic low self-esteem
- Cognitive deficits
- Depression
- Fatigue
- Mental illness
- Neurological defects
- Pain
- Physical illness
- Situational low self-esteem
- Substance abuse

Social

- Conflict
- Developmental level
- Domestic violence
- Economically disadvantaged
- Inadequate role socialization
- Inadequate support system
- Inappropriate linkage with the healthcare system
- Job schedule demands
- Lack of resources
- Lack of rewards
- Stress
- Young age

Impaired Social Interaction (00052)
(1986)

Domain 7: Role Relationships
Class 3: Role Performance

Definition   Insufficient or excessive quantity or ineffective quality of social exchange

Defining Characteristics

- Discomfort in social situations
- Dysfunctional interaction with others
- Family reports changes in interaction (e.g., style, pattern)
- Inability to communicate a satisfying sense of social engagement (e.g., belonging, caring, interest, shared history)
- Inability to receive a satisfying sense of social engagement (e.g., belonging, caring, interest, shared history)
- Use of unsuccessful social interaction behaviors

Related Factors

- Absence of significant others
- Communication barriers
- Deficit about ways to enhance mutuality (e.g., knowledge, skills)
- Disturbed thought processes
- Environmental barriers
- Limited physical mobility
- Self-concept disturbance
- Sociocultural dissonance
- Therapeutic isolation

Domain 8
Sexuality

NANDA International Nursing Diagnoses: Definitions & Classification 2012–2014, First Edition.
Edited by T. Heather Herdman.
© 2012 NANDA International. Published 2012 by Blackwell Publishing Ltd.

Sexual Dysfunction (00059)
(1980, 2006, LOE 2.1)

Domain 8: Sexuality
Class 2: Sexual Function

Definition The state in which an individual experiences a change in sexual function during the sexual response phases of desire, excitation, and/or orgasm, which is viewed as unsatisfying, unrewarding, or inadequate

Defining Characteristics

- Actual limitations imposed by disease
- Actual limitations imposed by therapy
- Alterations in achieving perceived sex role
- Alterations in achieving sexual satisfaction
- Change of interest in others
- Change of interest in self
- Inability to achieve desired satisfaction
- Perceived alteration in sexual excitation
- Perceived deficiency of sexual desire
- Perceived limitations imposed by disease
- Perceived limitations imposed by therapy
- Seeking confirmation of desirability
- Verbalization of problem

Related Factors

- Absent role models
- Altered body function (e.g., pregnancy, recent childbirth, drugs, surgery, anomalies, disease process, trauma, radiation)
- Altered body structure (e.g., pregnancy, recent childbirth, surgery, anomalies, disease process, trauma, radiation)
- Biopsychosocial alteration of sexuality
- Deficient knowledge
- Ineffectual role models
- Lack of privacy
- Lack of significant other
- Misinformation
- Physical abuse
- Psychosocial abuse (e.g., harmful relationships)
- Values conflict
- Vulnerability

References

Cavalcanti, R., & Cavalcanti, M. (1996). *Tratamento clinico das inadequacies sexuals* (2nd ed.). São Paulo: Roca.

Fehring, R.J. (1994). The Fehring model. In R.M. Carrol-Johnson, & M. Paquete (eds), *Classification of nursing diagnoses: Proceedings of the Tenth Conference*. Philadelphia: J.B. Lippincott, pp. 55–62.

Hogan, R.M. (1985). *Human sexuality: A nursing perspective*. New York: Appleton-Century-Crofts.

Hoskins, L.M. (1989). Clinical validation, methodologies for nursing diagnoses research. In R.M. Carrol-Johnson, & M. Paquete (eds), *Classification of nursing diagnoses: Proceedings of the eighth conference of North American Nursing Diagnosis Association*. Philadelphia: Lippincott, pp. 126–131.

Kaplan, H.S. (1977). *A nova terapia do sexo: Tratamento dinâmico das disfuncões sexuals*. Rio de Janeiro: Nova Fronteira.

Kaplan, H.S. (1983). *O desejo sexual – e novos conceitos etécnicas da terapia do sexo*. Rio de Janeiro: Nova Fronteira.

8. Sexuality

Ineffective Sexuality Pattern (00065)
(1986, 2006, LOE 2.1)

Domain 8: Sexuality
Class 2: Sexual Function

Definition
Expressions of concern regarding own sexuality

Defining Characteristics

- Alteration in achieving perceived sex role
- Alteration in relationship with significant other
- Reports changes in sexual activities
- Reports changes in sexual behaviors
- Reports difficulties with sexual activities
- Reports difficulties with sexual behaviors
- Reports limitations in sexual activities
- Reports limitations in sexual behaviors
- Values conflict

Related Factors

- Absent role model
- Conflicts with sexual orientation
- Conflicts with variant preferences
- Deficient knowledge about alternative responses to health-related transitions, altered body function or structure, illness, or medical treatment
- Fear of acquiring a sexually transmitted infection
- Fear of pregnancy
- Impaired relationship with a significant other
- Ineffective role model
- Lack of privacy
- Lack of significant other
- Skill deficit about alternative responses to health-related transitions, altered body function or structure, illness, or medical treatment

References

Cavalcanti, R., & Cavalcanti, M. (1996). *Tratamento clinico das inadequacies sexuals* (2nd ed.). São Paulo: Roca.

Fehring, R.J. (1994). The Fehring model. In R.M. Carrol-Johnson, & M. Paquete (eds), *Classification of nursing diagnoses: Proceedings of the Tenth Conference*. Philadelphia: J.B. Lippincott, pp. 55–62.

Hogan, R.M. (1985). *Human sexuality: A nursing perspective*. New York: Appleton-Century-Crofts.

Hoskins, L.M. (1989). Clinical validation, methodologies for nursing diagnoses research. In R.M. Carrol-Johnson, & M. Paquete (eds), *Classification of nursing diagnoses: Proceedings of the eighth conference of North American Nursing Diagnosis Association*. Philadelphia: Lippincott, pp. 126–131.

Kaplan, H.S. (1977). *A nova terapia do sexo: Tratamento dinâmico das disfuncões sexuals*. Rio de Janeiro: Nova Fronteira.

Kaplan, H.S. (1983). *O desejo sexual – e novos conceitos etécnicas da terapia do sexo*. Rio de Janeiro: Nova Fronteira.

8. Sexuality

Ineffective Childbearing Process (00221)
(2010, LOE 2.1)

Domain 8: Sexuality
Class 3: Reproduction

Definition Pregnancy and childbirth process and care of the newborn* that does not match the environmental context, norms, and expectations

Defining Characteristics

During Pregnancy

- Does not access support systems appropriately
- Does not report appropriate physical preparations
- Does not report appropriate prenatal lifestyle (e.g., nutrition, elimination, sleep, bodily movement, exercise, personal hygiene)
- Does not report availability of support systems
- Does not report managing unpleasant symptoms in pregnancy
- Does not report realistic birth plan
- Does not seek necessary knowledge (e.g., of labor and delivery, newborn care)
- Failure to prepare necessary newborn care items
- Inconsistent prenatal health visits
- Lack of prenatal visits
- Lack of respect for unborn baby

During Labor and Delivery

- Does not access support systems appropriately
- Does not demonstrate attachment behavior to the newborn baby
- Does not report availability of support systems
- Does not report lifestyle (e.g., diet, elimination, sleep, bodily movement, personal hygiene) that is appropriate for the stage of labor
- Does not respond appropriately to onset of labor
- Lacks proactivity during labor and delivery

After Birth*

- Does not access support systems appropriately
- Does not demonstrate appropriate baby feeding techniques
- Does not demonstrate appropriate breast care
- Does not demonstrate attachment behavior to the baby

---

*The original Japanese term for "childbearing" (*shussan ikuji koudou*), which encompasses both childbirth and rearing of the neonate. It is one of the main concepts of Japanese midwifery.

- Does not demonstrate basic baby care techniques
- Does not provide safe environment for the baby
- Does not report appropriate postpartum lifestyle (e.g., diet, elimination, sleep, bodily movement, exercise, personal hygiene)
- Does not report availability of support systems

Related Factors

- Deficient knowledge (e.g., of labor and delivery, newborn care)
- Domestic violence
- Inconsistent prenatal health visits
- Lack of appropriate role models for parenthood
- Lack of cognitive readiness for parenthood
- Lack of maternal confidence
- Lack of prenatal health visits
- Lack of a realistic birth plan
- Lack of sufficient support systems
- Maternal powerlessness
- Maternal psychological distress
- Suboptimal maternal nutrition
- Substance abuse
- Unplanned pregnancy
- Unsafe environment
- Unwanted pregnancy

References

Aoki, Y. (ed.) (1998). *Bosei Hoken wo meguru Shidou Kyouiku Soudan 2* [*Coaching, education, and counseling in maternal health*, Vol. 2]. Tokyo: Life Science Co.

Aoki, Y., Kato, N., & Hirasawa, M. (eds) (2002). *Josangaku Taikei 5 Boshi no Shinri Shakaigaku* [*Midwifery System*. Vol. 5: *Psychosociology for mother and child*]. Tokyo: Japanese Nursing Association Publishing .

Aoki, Y., Kato, N., & Hirasawa, M. (eds) (2003). *Josangaku Taikei 8 Josan Shindan Gijyutsu-gaku 2* [*Midwifery System*. Vol. 8: *Maternity diagnoses and techniques* 2]. Tokyo: Japanese Nursing Association Publishing .

Callister, L.C., Holt, S.T., & Kuhre, M. (2010). Giving birth: The voices of Australian women. *Journal of Perinatal and Neonatal Nursing*, 24(2), 128–136.

Darvill, R., Skirton, H., & Farrand, P. (2008). Psychological factors that impact on women's experiences of first-time motherhood: A qualitative study of the transition. *Midwifery*, 26(3), 357–366.

Furber, C., Garrod, D., Maloney, E., Lovell, K., & McGowan, L. (2009). A qualitative study of mild to moderate psychological distress during pregnancy. *International Journal of Nursing Studies*, 46(5), 669–677.

Japan Society for Maternity Diagnoses (ed.). (2004). *Maternity Shindan guidebook* [*Guidebook of maternity diagnoses*]. Tokyo: Igakushoin.

Kabeyama, K. (ed.). (2006). *Rinsho Josanfu Hikkei: Seimei to Bunka wo Fumaeta Shigen* [*Essentials of clinical midwifery: Caring based on life and culture* (2nd ed.)]. Tokyo: Igakushoin.

Okayama National Hospital (ed.) (2000). *Akachan ni Yasashii Byouin no Bonyuu Ikuji Shidou* [*Breast-feeding and newborn-care teaching manuals from a baby-friendly hospital*]. Tokyo: Medica Publishing.

Savage, C. (2009). A proposed framework related to the care of addicted mothers. *Journal of Addictions Nursing*, 20(3), 158–160.

Sharps, P., Laughon, K., & Giangrande, S. (2007). Intimate partner violence and the childbearing year: Maternal and infant health consequences. *Trauma Violence Abuse*, 8(2), 105–116.

Taketani, Y. , & Kabeyama, S. (eds). (2007). *Josangaku Kouza 6* [*Midwifery Course*, Vol. 6]. Tokyo: Igakushoin.

8. Sexuality

Readiness for Enhanced Childbearing Process* (00208)
(2008, LOE 2.1)

Domain 8: Sexuality
Class 3: Reproduction

Definition A pattern of preparing for and maintaining a healthy pregnancy, childbirth process, and care of the newborn that is sufficient for ensuring well-being and can be strengthened

Defining Characteristics

During Pregnancy

- Attends regular prenatal health visits
- Demonstrates respect for unborn baby
- Prepares necessary newborn care items
- Reports appropriate physical preparations
- Reports appropriate prenatal lifestyle (e.g., nutrition, elimination, sleep, bodily movement, exercise, personal hygiene)
- Reports availability of support systems
- Reports realistic birth plan
- Reports managing unpleasant symptoms in pregnancy
- Seeks necessary knowledge (e.g., of labor and delivery, newborn care)

During Labor and Delivery

- Demonstrates attachment behavior to the newborn baby
- Is proactive during labor and delivery
- Reports lifestyle (e.g., diet, elimination, sleep, bodily movement, personal hygiene) that is appropriate for the stage of labor
- Responds appropriately to onset of labor
- Uses relaxation techniques appropriate for the stage of labor
- Utilizes support systems appropriately

After Birth*

- Demonstrates appropriate baby-feeding techniques
- Demonstrates appropriate breast care
- Demonstrates attachment behavior to the baby
- Demonstrates basic baby care techniques

*The original Japanese term for "childbearing" (*shussan ikuji koudou*), which encompasses both childbirth and rearing of the neonate. It is one of the main concepts of Japanese midwifery.

- Provides safe environment for the baby
- Reports appropriate postpartum lifestyle (e.g. diet, elimination, sleep, bodily movement, exercise, personal hygiene)
- Utilizes support system appropriately

References

Aoki, Y. (ed.). (1998). *Bosei Hoken wo meguru Shidou Kyouiku Soudan 2* [*Coaching, education, and counseling in maternal health,* Vol. 2]. Tokyo: Life Science Co.

Aoki, Y., Kato, N., & Hirasawa, M. (eds.). (2002). *Josangaku Taikei 5 Boshi no Shinri Shakaigaku* [*Midwifery System.* Vol. 5: *Psychosociology for mother and child*]. Tokyo: Japanese Nursing Association Publishing.

Aoki, Y., Kato, N., & Hirasawa, M. (eds.). (2003). *Josangaku Taikei 8 Josan Shindan Gijyutsu-gaku 2* [*Midwifery System.* Vol. 8: *Maternity diagnoses and techniques* 2]. Tokyo: Japanese Nursing Association Publishing .

Japan Society for Maternity Diagnoses (ed.). (2004). *Maternity Shindan guidebook* [*Guidebook of maternity diagnoses*]. Tokyo: Igakushoin.

Kabeyama, K. (ed.). (2006). *Rinsho Josanfu Hikkei: Seimei to Bunka wo Fumaeta Shigen* [*Essentials of clinical midwifery: Caring based on life and culture* (2nd ed.)]. Tokyo: Igakushoin.

Okayama National Hospital (ed.). (2000). *Akachan ni Yasashii Byouin no Bonyuu Ikuji Shidou* [*Breast-feeding and newborn-care teaching manuals from a baby-friendly hospital*]. Tokyo: Medica Publishing.

Taketani, Y. , & Kabeyama, S. (eds). (2007). *Josangaku Kouza 6* [*Midwifery Course*, Vol. 6]. Tokyo: Igakushoin.

Risk for Ineffective Childbearing Process (00227)

(2010, LOE 2.1)

Domain 8: Sexuality
Class 3: Reproduction

Definition Risk for a pregnancy and childbirth process and care of the newborn* that does not match the environmental context, norms, and expectations

Risk Factors

- Deficient knowledge (e.g., of labor and delivery, newborn care)
- Domestic violence
- Inconsistent prenatal health visits
- Lack of appropriate role models for parenthood
- Lack of cognitive readiness for parenthood
- Lack of maternal confidence
- Lack of prenatal health visits
- Lack of a realistic birth plan
- Lack of sufficient support systems
- Maternal powerlessness
- Maternal psychological distress
- Suboptimal maternal nutrition
- Substance abuse
- Unplanned pregnancy
- Unwanted pregnancy

References

Aoki, Y. (ed.). (1998). *Bosei Hoken wo meguru Shidou Kyouiku Soudan 2* [*Coaching, education, and counseling in maternal health*, Vol. 2]. Tokyo: Life Science Co.

Aoki, Y., Kato, N., & Hirasawa, M. (eds). (2002). *Josangaku Taikei 5 Boshi no Shinri Shakaigaku* [*Midwifery System*. Vol. 5: *Psychosociology for mother and child*]. Tokyo: Japanese Nursing Association Publishing.

Aoki, Y., Kato, N., & Hirasawa, M. (eds). (2003). *Josangaku Taikei 8 Josan Shindan Gijyutsu-gaku 2* [*Midwifery System*. Vol. 8: *Maternity diagnoses and techniques* 2]. Tokyo: Japanese Nursing Association Publishing.

Callister, L.C., Holt, S.T., & Kuhre, M. (2010). Giving birth: The voices of Australian women. *Journal of Perinatal and Neonatal Nursing*, 24(2), 128–136.

Darvill, R., Skirton, H., & Farrand, P. (2008). Psychological factors that impact on women's experiences of first-time motherhood: A qualitative study of the transition. *Midwifery*, 26(3), 357–366.

Furber, C., Garrod, D., Maloney, E., Lovell, K., & McGowan, L. (2009). A qualitative study of mild to moderate psychological distress during pregnancy. *International Journal of Nursing Studies*, 46(5), 669–677.

Japan Society for Maternity Diagnoses (ed.). (2004). *Maternity Shindan guidebook* [*Guidebook of maternity diagnoses*]. Tokyo: Igakushoin.

Kabeyama, K. (ed.). (2006). *Rinsho Josanfu Hikkei: Seimei to Bunka wo Fumaeta Shigen* [*Essentials of clinical midwifery: Caring based on life and culture* (2nd ed.)]. Tokyo: Igakushoin.

Okayama National Hospital (ed.). (2000). *Akachan ni Yasashii Byouin no Bonyuu Ikuji Shidou* [*Breast-feeding and newborn-care teaching manuals from a baby-friendly hospital*]. Tokyo: Medica Publishing.

Savage, C. (2009). A proposed framework related to the care of addicted mothers. *Journal of Addictions Nursing*, 20(3), 158–160.

Sharps, P., Laughon, K., & Giangrande, S. (2007). Intimate partner violence and the childbearing year: Maternal and infant health consequences. *Trauma Violence Abuse*, 8(2), 105–116.

Taketani, Y., & Kabeyama, S. (eds). (2007). *Josangaku Kouza 6* [*Midwifery Course*, Vol. 6]. Tokyo: Igakushoin.

*The original Japanese term for "childbearing" (*shussan ikuji koudou*), which encompasses both childbirth and rearing of the neonate. It is one of the main concepts of Japanese midwifery.

Risk for Disturbed Maternal–Fetal Dyad (00209)
(2008, LOE 2.1)

Domain 8: Sexuality
Class 3: Reproduction

Definition At risk for disruption of the symbiotic maternal–fetal dyad as a result of comorbid or pregnancy-related conditions

Risk Factors

- Complications of pregnancy (e.g., premature rupture of membranes, placenta previa or abruption, late prenatal care, multiple gestation)
- Compromised oxygen transport (e.g., anemia, cardiac disease, asthma, hypertension, seizures, premature labor, hemorrhage)
- Impaired glucose metabolism (e.g., diabetes, steroid use)
- Physical abuse
- Substance abuse (e.g., tobacco, alcohol, drugs)
- Treatment-related side effects (e.g., pharmaceutical agents, surgery)

References

Berg, M. (2005). Pregnancy and diabetes: How women handle the challenges. *Journal of Perinatal Education, 14*(3), 23–32.

Curran, C.A. (2003). Intrapartum emergencies. *Journal of Obstetric, Gynecologic, and Neonatal Nursing, 32*(6), 802–813.

Higgins, L.P., & Hawkins, J.W. (2005). Screening for abuse during pregnancy: Implementing a multisite program. *American Journal of Maternal/Child Nursing, 30*(2), 109–114.

Lange, S.S., & Jenner, M. (2004). Myocardial infarction in the obstetric patient. *Critical Care Nursing Clinics of North America: Obstetric and Neonatal Intensive Care, 16*(2), 211–219.

McCarter-Spaulding, D.E. (2005). Medications in pregnancy and lactation. *American Journal of Maternal/Child Nursing, 30*(1), 10–17.

Poole, J.H. (2004). Multiorgan dysfunction in the perinatal patient. *Critical Care Nursing Clinics of North America: Obstetric and Neonatal Intensive Care, 16*(2), 193–204.

Rudisill, P.T. (2004). Amniotic fluid embolism. *Critical Care Nursing Clinics of North America: Obstetric and Neonatal Intensive Care, 16*(2), 221–225.

Shannon, M., King, T.L., & Kennedy, H.P. (2007). Allostasis: A theoretical framework for understanding and evaluating perinatal health outcomes. *Journal of Obstetric, Gynecologic, and Neonatal Nursing, 36*(2), 125–134.

Simpson, K.R. (2004). Monitoring the preterm fetus during labor. *American Journal of Maternal/Child Nursing, 29*(6), 380–388.

Stark, C.J., & Stepans, M.B.F. (2004). A comparison of blood pressure in term, low birth weight infants of smoking and nonsmoking mothers. *Journal of Perinatal Education, 13*(4), 17–26.

Stringer, M., Miesnik, S. R., Brown, L., Martz, A.H., & Macones, G. (2004). Nursing care of the patient with preterm premature rupture of membranes. *American Journal of Maternal/Child Nursing, 29*(3), 144–150.

Torgersen, K.L., & Curran, C.A. (2006). A systematic approach to the physiologic adaptations of pregnancy. *Critical Care Nursing Quarterly, 29*(1), 2–19.

Wolfe, B.E. (2005). Reproductive health in women with eating disorders. *Journal of Obstetric, Gynecologic, and Neonatal Nursing, 34*(2), 255–263.

8. Sexuality

Domain 9
Coping/Stress Tolerance

NANDA International Nursing Diagnoses: Definitions & Classification 2012–2014, First Edition.
Edited by T. Heather Herdman.
© 2012 NANDA International. Published 2012 by Blackwell Publishing Ltd.

Post-Trauma Syndrome (00141)
(1986, 1998, 2010)

Domain 9: Coping/Stress Tolerance
Class 1: Post-Trauma Responses

Definition Sustained maladaptive response to a traumatic, overwhelming event

Defining Characteristics

- Aggression
- Alienation
- Altered mood states
- Anger
- Anxiety
- Avoidance
- Compulsive behavior
- Denial
- Depression
- Detachment
- Difficulty concentrating
- Enuresis (in children)
- Exaggerated startle response
- Fear
- Flashbacks
- Gastric irritability
- Grieving
- Guilt
- Headaches
- Hopelessness
- Horror
- Hypervigilance
- Intrusive dreams
- Intrusive thoughts
- Irritability
- Neurosensory irritability
- Nightmares
- Palpitations
- Panic attacks
- Psychogenic amnesia
- Rage
- Reports feeling numb
- Repression
- Shame
- Substance abuse

Related Factors

- Being held prisoner of war
- Criminal victimization
- Disasters
- Epidemics
- Events outside the range of usual human experience
- Physical abuse
- Psychological abuse
- Serious accidents (e.g., industrial, motor vehicle)
- Serious injury to loved ones
- Serious injury to self
- Serious threat to loved ones
- Serious threat to self
- Sudden destruction of one's community
- Sudden destruction of one's home
- Torture
- Tragic occurrence involving multiple deaths
- War
- Witnessing mutilation
- Witnessing violent death

Risk for Post-Trauma Syndrome (00145)
(1998)

Domain 9: Coping/Stress Tolerance
Class 1: Post-Trauma Responses

Definition   At risk for sustained maladaptive response to a traumatic, overwhelming event

Risk Factors

- Diminished ego strength
- Displacement from home
- Duration of the event
- Exaggerated sense of responsibility
- Inadequate social support
- Occupation (e.g., police, fire, rescue, corrections, emergency room staff, mental health worker)
- Perception of event
- Survivor's role in the event
- Unsupportive environment

Rape-Trauma Syndrome (00142)

(1980, 1998)

Domain 9: Coping/Stress Tolerance
Class 1: Post-Trauma Responses

Definition Sustained maladaptive response to a forced, violent sexual penetration against the victim's will and consent

Defining Characteristics

- Aggression
- Agitation
- Anger
- Anxiety
- Change in relationships
- Chronic self-esteem
- Confusion
- Denial
- Dependence
- Depression
- Disorganization
- Dissociative disorders
- Disturbed sleep pattern
- Embarrassment
- Fear
- Guilt
- Helplessness
- Humiliation
- Hyperalertness
- Impaired decision-making
- Mood swings
- Muscle spasms
- Muscle tension
- Nightmares
- Paranoia
- Phobias
- Physical trauma
- Powerlessness
- Revenge
- Self-blame
- Sexual dysfunction
- Shame
- Shock
- Substance abuse
- Suicide attempts
- Vulnerability

Related Factors

- Rape

Relocation Stress Syndrome (00114)
(1992, 2000)

Domain 9: Coping/Stress Tolerance
Class 1: Post-Trauma Responses

Definition   Physiological and/or psychosocial disturbance following transfer from one environment to another

Defining Characteristics

- Alienation
- Aloneness
- Anger
- Anxiety (e.g., separation)
- Chronic low self-esteem
- Concern over relocation
- Dependency
- Depression
- Fear
- Frustration
- Increased illness
- Increased physical symptoms
- Increased verbalization of needs
- Insecurity
- Loneliness
- Loss of identity
- Loss of self-worth
- Pessimism
- Reports unwillingness to move
- Situational low self-esteem
- Sleep pattern disturbance
- Withdrawal
- Worry

Related Factors

- Decreased health status
- Impaired psychosocial health
- Isolation
- Lack of adequate support system
- Lack of predeparture counseling
- Language barrier
- Losses
- Move from one environment to another
- Passive coping
- Reports feelings of powerlessness
- Unpredictability of experience

Risk for Relocation Stress Syndrome (00149)
(2000)

Domain 9: Coping/Stress Tolerance
Class 1: Post-Trauma Responses

Definition At risk for physiological and/or psychosocial disturbance following transfer from one environment to another

Risk Factors

- Decreased health status
- Lack of adequate support system
- Lack of predeparture counseling
- Losses
- Moderate-to-high degree of environmental change
- Moderate mental competence
- Move from one environment to another
- Passive coping
- Reports powerlessness
- Unpredictability of experiences

Ineffective Activity Planning (00199)
(2008, LOE 2.2)

Domain 9: Coping/Stress Tolerance
Class 2: Coping Responses

Definition Inability to prepare for a set of actions fixed in time and under certain conditions

Defining Characteristics

- Failure pattern of behavior
- History of procrastination
- Lack of plan
- Lack of resources
- Lack of sequential organization
- Reports excessive anxieties about a task to be undertaken
- Reports fear toward a task to be undertaken
- Reports worries about a task to be undertaken
- Unmet goals for chosen activity

Related Factors

- Compromised ability to process information
- Defensive flight behavior when faced with proposed solution
- Hedonism
- Lack of family support
- Lack of friend support
- Unrealistic perception of events
- Unrealistic perception of personal competence

References

American Psychiatric Association (2004). *Mini DSM IV-TR*. Paris: Masson.

Auger, L. (1980). *S'aider soi-même d'avantage*. Québec: Les éditions de l'homme.

Auger, L. (1992). *Prendre soin de soi. Guide pratique de micro-thérapie*. Montreal: CIM.

Auger, L. (2001). *Savoir vivre*. Quebec: Les éditions Un monde différent ltée.

Auger, L. (2006). *Vivre avec sa tête ou avec son cœur*. Quebec: Centre la Pensée Réaliste, republication par Pierre Bovo.

Barth, B.M. (1985). Jérôme Bruner et l'innovation pédagogique. *Communication et Langages*, 66, 45–58.

Beck, A.T., Rush, A.J., Shaw, B.F., & Emery, G. (1979). *Cognitive therapy of depression*. New York: Guilford Press.

Corbière, M., Laisné, F., & Mercier, C. (2001). Élaboration du questionnaire: obstacles à l'insertion au travail et sentiment d'efficacité pour les surmonter. Manuscrit inédit, Centre de recherche Femand-Seguin, Unité 218, Hôpital Louis-H. Montreal: Lafontaine.

Debray, Q., Kindynis, S., Leclère, M., & Seigneurie, A. (2005). *Protocoles de traitement des personnalités pathologiques. Approche cognitivo-comportementale*: Paris: Masson.

Ellis, A. (1962). *Reason and emotion in psychotherapy*. New York: Secausus, Lyle Stuart.

Ellis, A., & Harper, R. (1992). *L'approche émotivo-rationnelle. Une nouvelle façon de vivre*. Québec: Les éditions de l'homme.

Filion, F. (1989). *J'améliore mes plans d'action*. Quebec: CAER Ed.

Greenberg, D. & Padesky, C. (2004). *Dépression et anxiété: comprendre et surmonter par l'approche cognitive*. Quebec: Décarie Éditeur.

Ladouceur, R., Marchand, A., & Boivert, J.-M. (1999). *Les troubles anxieux. Approche cognitive et comporte-mentale*. Gaétan Morin & Paris: Masson.

Lalonde, P., Aubut, J., & Grunberg, F. (eds) (2001). *Psychiatrie clinique. Une approche bio-psyco-sociale*. Quebec: Tome II.

Lecomte, T., & Leclerc, C. (2004). *Manuel de réadaptation psychiatrique*. Quebec: Presses de l'Université du Québec.

Monastès, J.L., & Boyer, C. (2006). *Les thérapies comportementales et cognitives. Se libérer des troubles psy*. Milan: Les essentiels Milan.

Morin, C., Briand, C., & Lalonde, P. (1999). De la symptomatologie à la résolution de problèmes: approche intégrée pour les personnes atteintes de schizophrénie. In: *Santé Mentale au Québec. Dossier schizophrénie, délires et thérapie cognitive*, Vol XXIV, No. 1, p. 277.

Riberio, K.L. (1999). The labyrinth of community mental health: In search of meaningful occupation. *Psychiatric Rehabilitation Journal*, 23(2), 143–153.

Seyle, H. (1959). *The stress of life*. New York: McGraw-Hill.

Townsend, M.C. (2004). *Soins infirmiers. Psychiatrie et santé mentale*. Quebec: ERPI.

Wilson, R., & Branch, R. (2004). *Les thérapies comportementales et cognitives pour les nuls*. Paris: First.

Risk for Ineffective Activity Planning (00226)

(2010, LOE 2.1)

Domain 9: Coping/Stress Tolerance
Class 2: Coping Responses

Definition At risk for an inability to prepare for a set of actions fixed in time and under certain conditions

Risk Factors

- Compromised ability to process information
- Defensive flight behavior when faced with proposed solution
- Hedonism
- History of procrastination
- Ineffective support systems
- Insufficient support systems
- Unrealistic perception of events
- Unrealistic perception of personal competence

References

American Psychiatric Association (2004). *Mini DSM IV-TR*. Paris: Masson.

Auger, L. (1980). *S'aider soi-même d'avantage*. Québec: Les éditions de l'homme.

Auger, L. (1992). *Prendre soin de soi. Guide pratique de micro-thérapie*. Montreal: CIM.

Auger, L. (2001). *Savoir vivre*. Quebec: Les éditions Un monde différent ltée.

Auger, L. (2006). *Vivre avec sa tête ou avec son cœur*. Quebec: Centre la Pensée Réaliste, republication par Pierre Bovo.

Barth, B.M. (1985). Jérôme Bruner et l'innovation pédagogique. *Communication et Langages*, 66, 45–58.

Beck, A.T., Rush, A.J., Shaw, B.F., & Emery, G. (1979). *Cognitive therapy of depression*. New York: Guilford Press.

Corbière, M., Laisné, F., & Mercier, C. (2001). *Élaboration du questionnaire: obstacles à l'insertion au travail et sentiment d'efficacité pour les surmonter*. Manuscrit inédit, Centre de recherche Femand-Seguin, Unité 218, Hôpital Louis-H. Montreal: Lafontaine.

Debray, Q., Kindynis, S., Leclère, M., & Seigneurie, A. (2005). *Protocoles de traitement des personnalités pathologiques. Approche cognitivo-comportementale*: Paris: Masson.

Ellis, A. (1962). *Reason and emotion in psychotherapy*. New York: Secausus, Lyle Stuart.

Ellis, A., & Harper, R. (1992). *L'approche émotivo-rationnelle. Une nouvelle façon de vivre*. Québec: Les éditions de l'homme.

Filion, F. (1989). *J'améliore mes plans d'action*. Quebec: CAER Ed.

Greenberg, D. & Padesky, C. (2004). *Dépression et anxiété: comprendre et surmonter par l'approche cognitive*. Quebec: Décarie Éditeur.

Ladouceur, R., Marchand, A., & Boivert, J.-M. (1999). *Les troubles anxieux. Approche cognitive et comporte-mentale*. Gaétan Morin & Paris: Masson.

Lalonde, P., Aubut, J., & Grunberg, F. (eds). (2001). *Psychiatrie clinique. Une approche bio-psyco-sociale*. Quebec: Tome II.

Lecomte, T., & Leclerc, C. (2004). *Manuel de réadaptation psychiatrique*. Quebec: Presses de l'Université du Québec.

Monastès, J.L., & Boyer, C. (2006). *Les thérapies comportementales et cognitives. Se libérer des troubles psy*. Milan: Les essentiels Milan.

Morin, C., Briand, C., & Lalonde, P. (1999). De la symptomatologie à la résolution de problèmes: approche intégrée pour les personnes atteintes de schizophrénie. In: *Santé Mentale au Québec. Dossier schizophrénie, délires et thérapie cognitive*, Vol XXIV, No. 1, p. 277.

Riberio, K.L. (1999). The labyrinth of community mental health: In search of meaningful occupation. *Psychiatric Rehabilitation Journal*, 23(2), 143–153.

Seyle, H. (1959). *The stress of life*. New York: McGraw-Hill.

Townsend, M.C. (2004). *Soins infirmiers. Psychiatrie et santé mentale*. Quebec: ERPI.

Wilson, R., & Branch, R. (2004). *Les thérapies comportementales et cognitives pour les nulls*. Paris: First.

9. Coping/Stress Tolerance

Anxiety (00146)
(1973, 1982, 1998)

Domain 9: Coping/Stress Tolerance
Class 2: Coping Responses

Definition Vague uneasy feeling of discomfort or dread accompanied by an autonomic response (the source often nonspecific or unknown to the individual); a feeling of apprehension caused by anticipation of danger. It is an alerting signal that warns of impending danger and enables the individual to take measures to deal with threat

Defining Characteristics

Behavioral

- Diminished productivity
- Extraneous movement
- Fidgeting
- Glancing about
- Insomnia
- Poor eye contact
- Reports concerns due to change in life events
- Restlessness
- Scanning
- Vigilance

Affective

- Anguish
- Apprehensive
- Distressed
- Fear
- Feelings of inadequacy
- Focus on self
- Increased wariness
- Irritability
- Jittery
- Overexcited
- Painful increased helplessness
- Persistent increased helplessness
- Rattled
- Regretful
- Uncertainty
- Worried

Physiological

- Facial tension
- Hand tremors
- Increased perspiration
- Increased tension
- Shakiness
- Trembling
- Voice quivering

Sympathetic

- Anorexia
- Cardiovascular excitation
- Diarrhea
- Dry mouth
- Facial flushing
- Heart pounding
- Increased blood pressure
- Increased pulse

- Increased reflexes
- Increased respiration
- Pupil dilation
- Respiratory difficulties

- Superficial vasoconstriction
- Twitching
- Weakness

Parasympathetic

- Abdominal pain
- Decreased blood pressure
- Decreased pulse
- Diarrhea
- Faintness
- Fatigue

- Nausea
- Sleep disturbance
- Tingling in extremities
- Urinary frequency
- Urinary hesitancy
- Urinary urgency

Cognitive

- Awareness of physiological symptoms
- Blocking of thought
- Confusion
- Decreased perceptual field
- Difficulty concentrating
- Diminished ability to learn

- Diminished ability to problem-solve
- Fear of unspecified consequences
- Forgetfulness
- Impaired attention
- Preoccupation
- Rumination
- Tendency to blame others

Related Factors

- Change in:
  - Economic status
  - Environment
  - Health status
  - Interaction patterns
  - Role function
  - Role status
- Exposure to toxins
- Familial association
- Heredity
- Interpersonal contagion
- Interpersonal transmission
- Maturational crises
- Situational crises
- Stress

- Substance abuse
- Threat of death
- Threat to:
  - Economic status
  - Environment
  - Health status
  - Interaction patterns
  - Role function
  - Role status
  - Self-concept
- Unconscious conflict about essential goals of life
- Unconscious conflict about essential values
- Unmet needs

Class 2: Coping Responses 345

9. Coping/Stress Tolerance

Defensive Coping (00071)

(1988, 2008, LOE 2.1)

Domain 9: Coping/Stress Tolerance
Class 2: Coping Responses

Definition Repeated projection of falsely positive self-evaluation based on a self-protective pattern that defends against underlying perceived threats to positive self-regard

Defining Characteristics

- Denial of obvious problems
- Denial of obvious weaknesses
- Difficulty establishing relationships
- Difficulty in perception of reality testing
- Difficulty maintaining relationships
- Grandiosity
- Hostile laughter
- Hypersensitivity to criticism
- Hypersensitivity to slight

- Lack of follow-through in therapy
- Lack of follow-through in treatment
- Lack of participation in therapy
- Lack of participation in treatment
- Projection of blame
- Projection of responsibility
- Rationalization of failures
- Reality distortion
- Ridicule of others
- Superior attitude toward others

Related Factors

- Conflict between self-perception and value system
- Deficient support system
- Fear of failure
- Fear of humiliation
- Fear of repercussions

- Lack of resilience
- Low level of confidence in others
- Low level of self-confidence
- Uncertainty
- Unrealistic expectations of self

References

Balder, L., & Denour, A.K. (1984). Couples' reactions and adjustment to mastectomy. *International Journal of Psychiatry in Medicine, 14*(3), 265–276.

Bartek, S.E., Krebs, D.L., & Taylor, M.C. (1993). Coping, defending, and the relations between moral judgment and moral behavior in prostitutes and other female juvenile delinquents. *Journal of Abnormal Psychology, 102*(1), 66–73.

Bean, G., Cooper, S., Alpert, R., & Kipnis, D. (1980). Coping mechanisms of cancer patients: A study of 33 patients receiving chemotherapy. *CA: A Cancer Journal For Clinicians, 30*(5), 257–259.

Brown, J.D., & Dutton, K.A. (1995). The thrill of victory, the complexity of defeat: Self-esteem and people's emotional reactions to success and failure. *Journal of Personality and Social Psychology, 68*(4), 712–722.

Cassileth, B.R., Lusk, E.J., Strouse, T.B., Miller, D.S., Brown, L.L., & Cross, P.A. (1985). Psychological analysis of cancer patients and their next of kin. *Cancer, 55*(1), 72–76.

Coelho, G.V., Hamburg, D.A., & Adams, J.E. (1974). *Coping and adaptation*. New York: Basic Books.

Coopersmith, S. (1967). *Antecedents of self-esteem*. San Francisco, CA: Freeman, Cooper.

Creswell, C., & Chalder, T. (2001). Defensive coping styles in chronic fatigue syndrome. *Journal Of Psychosomatic Research, 51*(4), 607–610.

Cysouw-Guitouni, A. (2001). L'avenir et la sauvegarde des valeurs. *Psychologie Préventive*, *37*, 18–23.

Dalle Grave, R., Calugi, S., Molinari, E. et al.; QUOVADIS Study Group (2005). Weight loss expectations in obese patients and treatment attrition: An observational multicenter study. *Obesity Research*, *13*(11), 1961–1969.

George, J.M., Scott, D.S., Turner, S.P., & Gregg, J.M. (1980). The effects of psychological factors of physical trauma on recovery from oral surgery. *Journal of Behavioral Medicine*, *3*(3), 291–310.

Guitouni, M. (2002). Le choix d'une génération: Démisionner ou résister. *Psychologie Préventive*, *38*, 25–29.

Jaramillo-Vélez, D.E., Ospina-Muñoz, D.E., Cabarcas-Iglesias, G., & Humphreys, J. (2005). Resiliencia, espiritualidad, aflicción y tácticas de resolución de conflictos en mujeres Maltratadas [Resilience, spirituality, distress and tactics for battered women's conflict resolution]. *Revista de Salud Pública*, *7*(3), 281–292.

Kools, S. (1999). Self-protection in adolescents in foster care. *Journal of Child and Adolescent Psychiatric Nursing*, *12*(4), 139–152.

Lazarus, R.S. (1966). *Psychological stress and the coping process*. New York: McGraw-Hill.

Lindstrom, T.C. (1989). Defence mechanisms and some notes on their relevance for the caring professions. *Scandinavian Journal of Caring Sciences*, *3*(3), 99–104.

McFarland, G.K., and McFarlane, E.A. (1995). *Traité de diagnostic infirmier* (adaptation of S. Truchon & D. Fleury). St-Laurent: ERPI.

Meredith, P.J., Strong, J., & Feeney, J.A. (2006) The relationship of adult attachment to emotion, catastrophizing, control, threshold and tolerance, in experimentally-induced pain. *Pain*, *120*(1–2), 44–52.

Morris, C.A. (1985). Self-concept as altered by the diagnosis of cancer. *Nursing Clinics of North America*, *20*(4), 611–630.

Noy, S. (2004). Minimizing casualties in biological and chemical threats (war and terrorism): The importance of information to the public in a prevention program. *Prehospital and Disaster Medicine*, *19*(1), 29–36.

Perez-Sales, P., & Vazquez Valverde, C. (2003). [Support psychotherapy in traumatic situations]. *Revista de enfermería*, *26*(12), 44–52.

Taubes, I. (2002). Tout commence par une confiance primitive dans la vie: entretien avec Boris Cyulnik. *Psychologies*, March, 90–94.

Taubes, I. (2005). Je fuis les responsabilités. *Psychologies*, Mar, 88–89.

Tod, A.M., & Lacey, A. (2004). Overweight and obesity: Helping clients to take action. *British Journal of Community Nursing*, *9*(2), 59–66.

Tromp, D.M., Brouha, X.D., De Leeuw, J.R., Hordijk, G.J., & Winnubst, J.A. (2004). Psychological factors and patient delay in patients with head and neck cancer. *European Journal of Cancer*, *40*(10), 1509–1516.

Worder, J.W., & Sobel, J. (1978). Ego strength and psychosocial adaptation to cancer. *Psychosomatic Medicine*, *40*(8), 585–592.

Yehuda, R., McFarlane, A.C., & Shalev, A.Y. (1998). Predicting the development of posttraumatic stress disorder from the acute response to a traumatic event. *Biological Psychiatry*, *44*(2), 1305–1313.

Ineffective Coping (00069)
(1978, 1998)

Domain 9: Coping/Stress Tolerance
Class 2: Coping Responses

Definition Inability to form a valid appraisal of the stressors, inadequate choices of practiced responses, and/or inability to use available resources

Defining Characteristics

- Change in usual communication patterns
- Decreased use of social support
- Destructive behavior toward others
- Destructive behavior toward self
- Difficulty organizing information
- Fatigue
- High illness rate
- Inability to attend to information
- Inability to meet basic needs
- Inability to meet role expectations
- Inadequate problem-solving
- Lack of goal-directed behavior
- Lack of resolution of problem
- Poor concentration
- Reports inability to ask for help
- Reports inability to cope
- Risk-taking
- Sleep pattern disturbance
- Substance abuse
- Use of forms of coping that impede adaptive behavior

Related Factors

- Disturbance in pattern of appraisal of threat
- Disturbance in pattern of tension release
- Gender differences in coping strategies
- High degree of threat
- Inability to conserve adaptive energies
- Inadequate level of confidence in ability to cope
- Inadequate level of perception of control
- Inadequate opportunity to prepare for stressor
- Inadequate resources available
- Inadequate social support created by characteristics of relationships
- Maturational crisis
- Situational crisis
- Uncertainty

Readiness for Enhanced Coping (00158)

(2002, LOE 2.1)

Domain 9: Coping/Stress Tolerance
Class 2: Coping Responses

Definition A pattern of cognitive and behavioral efforts to manage demands that is sufficient for well-being and can be strengthened

Defining Characteristics

- Acknowledges power
- Aware of possible environmental changes
- Defines stressors as manageable
- Seeks knowledge of new strategies
- Seeks social support
- Uses a broad range of emotion-oriented strategies
- Uses a broad range of problem-oriented strategies
- Uses spiritual resources

Ineffective Community Coping (00077)
(1994, 1998)

Domain 9: Coping/Stress Tolerance
Class 2: Coping Responses

Definition Pattern of community activities for adaptation and problem-solving that is unsatisfactory for meeting the demands or needs of the community

Defining Characteristics

- Community does not meet its own expectations
- Deficits in community participation
- Excessive community conflicts
- High illness rates
- Increased social problems (e.g., homicides, vandalism, arson, terrorism, robbery, infanticide, abuse, divorce, unemployment, poverty, militancy, mental illness)
- Reports of community powerlessness
- Reports of community vulnerability
- Stressors perceived as excessive

Related Factors

- Deficits in community social support resources
- Deficits in community social support services
- Inadequate resources for problem-solving
- Ineffective community systems (e.g., lack of emergency medical system, transportation system, disaster planning systems)
- Man-made disasters
- Natural disasters
- Nonexistent community systems

Readiness for Enhanced Community Coping (00076)

(1994)

Domain 9: Coping/Stress Tolerance
Class 2: Coping Responses

Definition A pattern of community activities for adaptation and problem-solving that is sufficient for meeting the demands or needs of the community for the management of current and future problems/stressors and can be strengthened

Defining Characteristics

- Active planning by community for predicted stressors
- Active problem-solving by community when faced with issues
- Agreement that community is responsible for stress management
- Positive communication among community members
- Positive communication between community/aggregates and larger community
- Programs available for recreation
- Programs available for relaxation
- Resources sufficient for managing stressors

Compromised Family Coping (00074)
(1980, 1996)

Domain 9: Coping/Stress Tolerance
Class 2: Coping Responses

Definition An usually supportive primary person (family member, significant other, or close friend) provides insufficient, ineffective, or compromised support, comfort, assistance, or encouragement that may be needed by the client to manage or master adaptive tasks related to his or her health challenge

Defining Characteristics

Objective

- Significant person attempts assistive behaviors with unsatisfactory results
- Significant person attempts supportive behaviors with unsatisfactory results
- Significant person displays protective behavior disproportionate to client's abilities
- Significant person displays protective behavior disproportionate to client's need for autonomy
- Significant person enters into limited personal communication with client
- Significant person withdraws from client

Subjective

- Client reports a complaint about significant person's response to health problem
- Client reports a concern about significant person's response to health problem
- Significant person reports an inadequate knowledge base, which interferes with effective supportive behaviors
- Significant person reports an inadequate understanding, which interferes with effective supportive behaviors
- Significant person reports preoccupation with personal reaction (e.g., fear, anticipatory grief, guilt, anxiety) to client's need

Related Factors

- Coexisting situations affecting the significant person
- Developmental crises that the significant person may be facing
- Exhaustion of supportive capacity of significant people
- Inadequate information available to a primary person
- Inadequate understanding of information by a primary person
- Incorrect information obtained by a primary person

- Incorrect understanding of information by a primary person
- Lack of reciprocal support
- Little support provided by client, in turn, for primary person
- Prolonged disease that exhausts supportive capacity of significant people
- Situational crises that the significant person may be facing
- Temporary family disorganization
- Temporary family role changes
- Temporary preoccupation by a significant person

Disabled Family Coping (00073)

(1980, 1996, 2008, LOE 2.1)

Domain 9: Coping/Stress Tolerance
Class 2: Coping Responses

Definition Behavior of primary person (family member, significant other, or close friend) that disables his or her capacities and the client's capacities to effectively address tasks essential to either person's adaptation to the health challenge

Defining Characteristics

- Abandonment
- Aggression
- Agitation
- Carrying on usual routines without regard for client's needs
- Client's development of dependence
- Depression
- Desertion
- Disregarding client's needs
- Distortion of reality regarding client's health problem
- Family behaviors that are detrimental to well-being
- Hostility
- Impaired individualization
- Impaired restructuring of a meaningful life for self
- Intolerance
- Neglectful care of client in regard to basic human needs
- Neglectful care of client in regard to illness treatment
- Neglectful relationships with other family members
- Prolonged overconcern for client
- Psychosomaticism
- Rejection
- Taking on illness signs of client

Related Factors

- Arbitrary handling of family's resistance to treatment
- Dissonant coping styles for dealing with adaptive tasks by the significant person and client
- Dissonant coping styles among significant people
- Highly ambivalent family relationships
- Significant person with chronically unexpressed feelings (e.g., guilt, anxiety, hostility, despair)

Readiness for Enhanced Family Coping (00075)
(1980)

Domain 9: Coping/Stress Tolerance
Class 2: Coping Responses

Definition A pattern of management of adaptive tasks by primary person (family member, significant other, or close friend) involved with the client's health challenge that is sufficient for health and growth, in regard to self and in relation to the client, and can be strengthened

Defining Characteristics

- Chooses experiences that optimize wellness
- Individual expresses interest in making contact with others who have experienced a similar situation
- Significant person attempts to describe growth impact of crisis
- Significant person moves in direction of enriching lifestyle
- Significant person moves in direction of health promotion

Death Anxiety (00147)
(1998, 2006, LOE 2.1)

Domain 9: Coping/Stress Tolerance
Class 2: Coping Responses

Definition Vague uneasy feeling of discomfort or dread generated by perceptions of a real or imagined threat to one's existence

Defining Characteristics

- Reports concerns of overworking the caregiver
- Reports deep sadness
- Reports fear of developing terminal illness
- Reports fear of loss of mental abilities when dying
- Reports fear of pain related to dying
- Reports fear of premature death
- Reports fear of prolonged dying
- Reports fear of suffering related to dying
- Reports fear of the process of dying
- Reports feeling powerless over dying
- Reports negative thoughts related to death and dying
- Reports worry about the impact of one's own death on significant others

Related Factors

- Anticipating adverse consequences of general anesthesia
- Anticipating impact of death on others
- Anticipating pain
- Anticipating suffering
- Confronting the reality of terminal disease
- Discussions on the topic of death
- Experiencing dying process
- Near-death experience
- Nonacceptance of own mortality
- Observations related to death
- Perceived proximity of death
- Uncertainty about an encounter with a higher power
- Uncertainty about the existence of a higher power
- Uncertainty about life after death
- Uncertainty of prognosis

References

Abdel-Khalek, A.M., & Tomàs-Sàbado, J. (2005). Anxiety and death anxiety in Egyptian and Spanish nursing students. *Death Studies, 29*(2), 157–169.

Aday, R.H. (1984–85). Belief in afterlife and death anxiety: Correlates and comparisons. *Omega: Journal of Death and Dying, 15*(1), 67–75.

Adelbratt, S., & Strang, P. (2000). Death anxiety in brain tumour patients and their spouses. *Palliative Medicine, 14*(6), 499–507.

Alvarado, J.A., Templer, D.I., Bresler, C., & Thomas-Dobson, S. (1995). The relationship of religious variables to death depression and death anxiety. *Journal of Clinical Psychology, 51*(2), 202–204.

Amenta, M.M. (1984). Death anxiety purpose in life and duration of service in hospice volunteers. *Psychological Reports, 54,* 979–984.

Angst, J., Angst, F., & Stassen, H.H. (1999). Suicide risk in patients with major depressive disorder. *Journal of Clinical Psychiatry, 60*(Suppl. 2), 57–62; discussion 75–76, 113–116.

Bay, E., & Algase, D.L. (1999). Fear and anxiety: A simultaneous concept analysis. *Nursing Diagnosis, 10*(3), 103–111.

Beck, C.T. (1997). Nursing students' experiences caring for dying patients. *Journal of Nursing Education, 36*(9), 408–415.

Bene, B., & Foxall, M.J. (1991). Death anxiety and job stress in hospice and medical-surgical nurses. *Hospice Journal, 7*(3), 25–41.

Bolt, M. (1977). Religious orientation and death fears. *Review of Religious Research, 19*(1), 73–76.

Braunstein, J.W. (2004). An investigation of irrational beliefs and death anxiety as a function of HIV status. *Journal of Rational-Emotive and Cognitive-Behavior Therapy, 22*, 21–38.

Brockopp, D.Y,. King, D.B., & Hamilton, J.E. (1991). The dying patient: A comparative study of nurse caregiver characteristics. *Death Studies, 15*(3), 245–248.

Chiappetta, W., Floyd, H.H., & McSeveney, D.R. (1977). Sex differences in coping with death anxiety. *Psychological Reports, 39*(3), 945–946.

Clements, R. (1998). Intrinsic religious motivation and attitudes toward death among the elderly. *Current Psychology, 17*(2–3), 237–248.

Cully, J.A., La Voie, D., & Gfeller, J.D. (2001). Reminiscence, personality, and psychological functioning in older adults. *Gerontologist, 41*(1), 89–95.

Hunt, B., & Rosenthal, D.A. (2000). Rehabilitation counselors' experiences with client death anxiety. *Journal of Rehabilitation, 66*(4), 44–50.

Kastenbaum, R. (1992). *The psychology of death.* New York: Guilford Press.

Kuuppelomaky, M. (2000). Cancer patients', family members' and professional helpers' conceptions and beliefs concerning death. *European Journal of Oncology Nursing, 4*(1), 39–47.

Matalon, T.H. (2000). The relationship among children's conceptualisation of death, parental communication about death, and parental death anxiety. *Dissertation Abstracts International Section A: Humanities & Social Sciences, 61*, (2-A), 510–511. Retrieved from http://fordham.bepress.com/dissertations/AAI99609501.

Mok, E., Lee, W.M., & Wong, F.K. (2002). The issue of death and dying: employing problem-based learning in nursing education. *Nurse Education Today, 22*(4), 319–329.

Nelson, L.D., & Cantrell, C.H. (1980). Religiosity and death anxiety: A multi-dimensional analysis. *Review of Religious Research, 21*(2), 148–157.

Rasmussen, C.A., & Brems, C. (1996). The relationship of death anxiety with age psychosocial maturity. *Journal of Psychology, 130*(2), 141–144.

Rasmussen, C.H., & Johnson, M.E. (1994). Spirituality and religiosity: Relative relationships to death anxiety. *Omega: Journal of Death and Dying, 29*(4), 313–318.

Robbins, R.A. (1992). Death competency: A study of hospice volunteers. *Death Studies, 16*(6), 557–569.

Rosenhein, E., & Muchnick, B. (1984–85). Death concerns in differential levels of consciousness as functions of defence strategy and religious belief. *Omega: Journal of Death and Dying, 15*(1), 15–24.

Sanders, J.F., Poole, T.E., & Rivero, W.T. (1980). Death anxiety among the elderly. *Psychological Reports, 46*, 53–54.

Sherman, D.W. (1996). Nurses' willingness to care for AIDS patients and spirituality, social support, and death anxiety. *Image: Journal of Nursing Scholarship, 28*(3), 205–213.

Stoller, E.P. (1980–81). The impact of death-related fears on attitudes of nurses in hospital work setting. *Omega: Journal of Death and Dying, 11*, 85–96.

Straub, S.H., & Roberts, J.M. (2001). Fear of death in widows: Effects of age at widowhood and suddenness of death. *Omega: Journal of Death and Dying, 43*(1), 25–41.

Sulmasy, D.P., & McIlvane, J.M. (2002). Patients' ratings of quality and satisfaction with care at the end of life. *Archive of Internal Medicine, 162*(18), 2098–2104.

Whitley, G.G. (1994). Expert validation and differentiation of the nursing diagnosis anxiety and fear. *Nursing Diagnosis, 5*(4), 143–150.

Whitley, G.G. & Tousman, S.A. (1996). A multivariate approach for validation of anxiety and fear. *Nursing Diagnosis, 7*(3), 116–124.

Ineffective Denial (00072)
(1988, 2006, LOE 2.1)

Domain 9: Coping/Stress Tolerance
Class 2: Coping Responses

Definition Conscious or unconscious attempt to disavow the knowledge or meaning of an event to reduce anxiety and/or fear, leading to the detriment of health

Defining Characteristics

- Delays seeking healthcare attention
- Displaces fear of impact of the condition
- Displaces source of symptoms to other organs
- Displays inappropriate affect
- Does not admit fear of death
- Does not admit fear of invalidism
- Does not perceive personal relevance of danger
- Does not perceive personal relevance of symptoms
- Makes dismissive comments when speaking of distressing events
- Makes dismissive gestures when speaking of distressing events
- Minimizes symptoms
- Refuses healthcare attention
- Unable to admit impact of disease on life pattern
- Uses self-treatment

Related Factors

- Anxiety
- Fear of death
- Fear of loss of autonomy
- Fear of separation
- Lack of competency in using effective coping mechanisms
- Lack of control of life situation
- Lack of emotional support from others
- Overwhelming stress
- Threat of inadequacy in dealing with strong emotions
- Threat of unpleasant reality

References

Bartle, S.H. (1980). Denial of cardiac warnings. *Psychosomatics, 12*(1), 74–77.

Bennet, D.H., & Holmes, D.S. (1975). Influence of denial (situation redefinition) and projection on anxiety associated with threat to self-esteem. *Journal of Personality and Social Psychology, 32*(5), 915–921.

Byrne, B. (2000). Relationships between anxiety, fear, self-esteem, and coping strategies in adolescence. *Adolescence, 35*(137), 201–215.

Davey, G.C., Burgess, I., & Rashes, R. (1995). Coping strategies and phobias: The relationship between fears, phobias and methods of coping with stressors. *British Journal of Clinical Psychology, 34*(Pt 3), 423–434.

Fryer, S., Waller, G., & Kroese, B.S. (1997). Stress, coping, and disturbed eating attitudes in teenage girls. *International Journal of Eating Disorders, 22*(4), 427–436.

Gammon, J. (1998). Analysis of the stressful effects of hospitalisation and source isolation coping and psychological constructs. *International Journal of Nursing Practice, 4*(2), 84–96.

Gottschalk, L.A., Fronczek, J., Abel, L., Buchsbaum, M.S., & Fallon, J.H. (2001). The cerebral neurobiology of anxiety, anxiety displacement, and anxiety denial. *Psychotherapy and Psychosomatics, 70*(1), 17–24.

Greenberg, J., Solomon, S., Pyszczynski, T. et al. (1992). Why do people need self-esteem? Converging evidence that self-esteem serves an anxiety-buffering function. *Journal of Personality and Social Psychology, 63*(6), 913–922.

Heilbrun, A.B., & Pepe, V. (1985). Awareness of cognitive defences and stress management. *British Journal of Medical Psychology, 58*(Pt 1), 9–17.

Hobfoll, S.E., & Walfisch, S. (1984). Coping with a threat to life: A longitudinal study of self-concept, social support, and psychological distress. *American Journal of Community Psychology, 12*(1), 87–100.

Hovey, J.D., & Magana, C.G. (2002). Exploring the mental health of Mexican migrant farm workers in Midwest: Psychosocial predictors of psychological distress and suggestions for prevention and treatment. *Journal of Psychology, 136*(5), 493–513.

Kennedy, P., Duff, J., Evans, M., & Beedie, A. (2003). Coping effectiveness training reduces depression and anxiety following traumatic spinal cord injuries. *British Journal of Clinical Psychology, 42*(Pt 1), 41–52.

Kollbrunner, J., Zbaren, P., & Quack, K. (2001). Quality of life stress in patients with large tumors of the mouth. Dealing with the illness: Coping, anxiety and depressive symptoms. *HNO, 49*(12), 998–1007.

Leserman, J., Perkins, D.O., & Evans, D.L. (1992). Coping with the threat of AIDS: The role of social support. *American Journal of Psychiatry, 149*(11), 1514–1520.

Mogg, K., Mathews, A., Bird, C., & Macgregor-Morris, R. (1990). Effects of stress and anxiety on the processing of threat stimuli. *Journal of Personality and Social Psychology, 59*(6), 1230–1237.

Monat, A., & Lazarus, R.S. (1991). *Stress and Coping: An anthology* (3rd ed.). New York: Columbia University Press.

Muller, L., & Spitz, E. (2003). [Multidimensional assessment of coping: validation of the Brief COPE among French population]. *Encephale, 29*(6), 507–518.

Sandstrom, M.J., & Cramer, P. (2003). Defense mechanisms and psychological adjustment in childhood. *Journal of Nervous and Mental Disease, 191*(8), 487–495.

Schimel, J., Greenberg, J., & Martens, A. (2003). Evidence that projection of a feared trait can serve a defensive function. *Personality and Social Psychology Bulletin, 29*(8), 969–979.

Skinner, N., & Brewer, N. (2002). The dynamics of threat and challenge appraisals prior to stressful achievement events. *Journal of Personality and Social Psychology, 83*(3), 678–692.

Westman, A.S. (1992). Existential anxiety as related to conceptualization of self and of death, denial of death, and religiosity. *Psychological Reports, 71*(3 Pt 2), 1064–1066.

9. Coping/Stress Tolerance

Adult Failure to Thrive (00101)
(1998)

Domain 9: Coping/Stress Tolerance
Class 2: Coping Responses

Definition Progressive functional deterioration of a physical and cognitive nature. The individual's ability to live with multisystem diseases, cope with ensuing problems, and manage his or her care is remarkably diminished

Defining Characteristics

- Altered mood state
- Anorexia
- Apathy
- Cognitive decline
  - Decreased perception
  - Demonstrated difficulty responding to environmental stimuli
  - Demonstrated difficulty with concentration
  - Demonstrated difficulty with decision-making
  - Demonstrated difficulty with judgment
  - Demonstrated difficulty with memory
  - Demonstrated difficulty with reasoning
- Consumption of minimal to no food at most meals (e.g., consumes <75% of normal requirements)
- Decreased participation in activities of daily living
- Decreased social skills
- Frequent exacerbations of chronic health problems
- Inadequate nutritional intake
- Neglect of financial responsibilities
- Neglect of home environment
- Physical decline (e.g., fatigue, dehydration, incontinence of bowel and bladder)
- Reports desire for death
- Reports loss of interest in pleasurable outlets
- Self-care deficit
- Social withdrawal
- Unintentional weight loss (e.g., 5% in 1 month, 10% in 6 months)

Related Factors

- Depression

Fear (00148)
(1980, 1996, 2000)

Domain 9: Coping/Stress Tolerance
Class 2: Coping Responses

Definition Response to perceived threat that is consciously recognized as a danger

Defining Characteristics

- Reports alarm
- Reports apprehension
- Reports being scared
- Reports decreased self-assurance
- Reports dread

- Reports excitement
- Reports increased tension
- Reports jitteriness
- Reports panic
- Reports terror

Cognitive

- Diminished learning ability
- Diminished problem-solving ability
- Diminished productivity

- Identifies object of fear
- Stimulus believed to be a threat

Behaviors

- Attack behaviors
- Avoidance behaviors
- Impulsiveness

- Increased alertness
- Narrowed focus on the source of the fear

Physiological

- Anorexia
- Diarrhea
- Dry mouth
- Dyspnea
- Fatigue
- Increased perspiration
- Increased pulse

- Increased respiratory rate
- Increased systolic blood pressure
- Muscle tightness
- Nausea
- Pallor
- Pupil dilation
- Vomiting

Related Factors

- Innate origin (e.g., sudden noise, height, pain, loss of physical support)
- Innate releasers (neurotransmitters)

- Language barrier
- Learned response (e.g., conditioning, modeling from or identification with others)

9. Coping/Stress Tolerance

- Phobic stimulus
- Sensory impairment
- Separation from support system in potentially stressful situation
- (e.g., hospitalization, hospital procedures)
- Unfamiliarity with environmental experience(s)

Domain 9: Coping/Stress Tolerance
Class 2: Coping Responses

Definition A normal complex process that includes emotional, physical, spiritual, social, and intellectual responses and behaviors by which individuals, families, and communities incorporate an actual, anticipated, or perceived loss into their daily lives

Defining Characteristics

- Alteration in activity level
- Alterations in dream patterns
- Alterations in immune function
- Alterations in neuroendocrine function
- Anger
- Blame
- Despair
- Detachment
- Disorganization
- Disturbed sleep pattern
- Experiencing relief
- Maintaining the connection to the deceased
- Making meaning of the loss
- Pain
- Panic behavior
- Personal growth
- Psychological distress
- Suffering

Related Factors

- Anticipatory loss of significant object (e.g., possession, job, status, home, parts and processes of body)
- Anticipatory loss of a significant other
- Death of a significant other
- Loss of significant object (e.g., possession, job, status, home, parts and processes of body)

References

Center for the Advancement of Health (2004a). Report on bereavement and grief research. Outcomes of bereavement. *Death Studies*, 28(1), 520–542.

Center for the Advancement of Health (2004b). Report on bereavement and grief research. Themes in research on bereavement and grief. *Death Studies*, 28(6), 498–505.

Christ, G., Bonnano, G., Malkinson, R., & Rubin, S. (2003). Bereavement experiences after the death of a child. In M. Field, & R. Berhman, (eds), *When children die: Improving palliative and end-of-life care for children and their families*. Washington, DC: National Academy Press, pp. 553–579.

Davis, C., & Nolen-Hocksema, S. (2001). Loss and meaning: How do people make sense of loss? *American Behavioral Scientist*, 44(5), 726–741.

Gamino, L., Sewell, K., & Easterling, L. (2000). Scott and White Grief Study – Phase 2: Toward an adaptive model of grief. *Death Studies*, 24(7), 633–660.

Gamino, L., Hogan, N., & Sewell, K. (2002). Feeling the absence: A content analysis from the Scott and White grief study. *Death Studies*, 26(10), 793–813.

9. Coping/Stress Tolerance

Hall, M., & Irwin, M. (2001). Physiological indices of functioning in bereavement. In M. Stroebe, R. Hannson, W. Stroebe, & H. Schut (eds), *Handbook of bereavement research: Consequences, coping and care*. Washington DC: American Psychological Association, pp. 473–493.

Hansson, R., & Stroebe, M. (2003). Grief, older adulthood. In T. Gullotta, & M. Bloom (eds.), *Encyclopedia of primary prevention and health promotion*. New York: Plenum Press, pp. 515–521.

Hogan, N., Worden, J.W., & Schmidt, L. (2004). An empirical study of the proposed complicated grief disorder criteria. *OMEGA – Journal of Death and Dying*, 48(3), 263–277.

Jacobs, S. (1999). *Traumatic grief: Diagnosis, treatment, and prevention*. Caselton, NY: Brunner/Mazel.

Matthews, L., & Marwit, S. (2004). Complicated grief and the trend toward cognitive-behavioral therapy. *Death Studies*, 28(9), 849–863.

Ogrodniczuk, J., Piper, W., Joyce, A. et al. (2003). Differentiating symptoms of complicated grief and depression among psychiatric outpatients. *Canadian Journal of Psychiatry*, 48(2), 87–93.

Ott, C. (2003). The impact of complicated grief on mental and physical health at various points in the bereavement process. *Death Studies*, 27(3), 249–272.

Prigerson, H., & Jacobs, S. (2001). Traumatic grief as a distinct disorder: A rationale, consensus criteria, and a preliminary empirical test. In M. Stroebe, R. Hannson, W. Stroebe, & H. Schut (eds), *Handbook of bereavement research: Consequences, coping and care*. Washington, DC: American Psychological Association, pp. 613–646.

Domain 9: Coping/Stress Tolerance
Class 2: Coping Responses

Definition A disorder that occurs after the death of a significant other, in which the experience of distress accompanying bereavement fails to follow normative expectations and manifests in functional impairment

Defining Characteristics

- Decreased functioning in life roles
- Decreased sense of well-being
- Depression
- Experiencing somatic symptoms of the deceased
- Fatigue
- Grief avoidance
- Longing for the deceased
- Low levels of intimacy
- Persistent emotional distress
- Preoccupation with thoughts of the deceased
- Reports anxiety
- Reports distressful feelings about the deceased
- Reports feeling dazed
- Reports feeling empty
- Reports feeling in shock
- Reports feeling stunned
- Reports feelings of anger
- Reports feelings of detachment from others
- Reports feelings of disbelief
- Reports feelings of mistrust
- Reports lack of acceptance of the death
- Reports persistent painful memories
- Reports self-blame
- Rumination
- Searching for the deceased
- Self-blame
- Separation distress
- Traumatic distress
- Yearning

Related Factors

- Death of a significant other
- Emotional instability
- Lack of social support

References

Center for the Advancement of Health (2004a). Report on bereavement and grief research. Outcomes of bereavement. *Death Studies*, 28(1), 520–542.

Center for the Advancement of Health (2004b). Report on bereavement and grief research. Themes in research on bereavement and grief. *Death Studies*, 28(6), 498–505.

Christ, G., Bonnano, G., Malkinson, R., & Rubin, S. (2003). Bereavement experiences after the death of a child. In M. Field, & R. Berhman, (eds), *When children die: Improving palliative and end-of-life care for children and their families*. Washington, DC: National Academy Press, pp. 553–579.

Davis, C., & Nolen-Hocksema, S. (2001). Loss and meaning: How do people make sense of loss? *American Behavioral Scientist*, 44(5), 726–741.

9. Coping/Stress Tolerance

Gamino, L., Sewell, K., & Easterling, L. (2000). Scott and White Grief Study – Phase 2: Toward an adaptive model of grief. *Death Studies, 24*(7), 633–660.

Gamino, L., Hogan, N., & Sewell, K. (2002). Feeling the absence: A content analysis from the Scott and White grief study. *Death Studies, 26*(10), 793–813.

Hall, M., & Irwin, M. (2001). Physiological indices of functioning in bereavement. In M. Stroebe, R. Hannson, W. Stroebe, & H. Schut (eds), *Handbook of bereavement research: Consequences, coping and care.* Washington DC: American Psychological Association, pp. 473–493.

Hansson, R., & Stroebe, M. (2003). Grief, older adulthood. In T. Gullotta, & M. Bloom (eds), *Encyclopedia of primary prevention and health promotion.* New York: Plenum Press, pp. 515–521.

Hogan, N., Worden, J.W., & Schmidt, L. (2004). An empirical study of the proposed complicated grief disorder criteria. *OMEGA – Journal of Death and Dying, 48*(3), 263–277.

Jacobs, S. (1999). *Traumatic grief: Diagnosis, treatment, and prevention.* Caselton, NY: Brunner/Mazel.

Matthews, L., & Marwit, S. (2004). Complicated grief and the trend toward cognitive-behavioral therapy. *Death Studies, 28*(9), 849–863.

Ogrodniczuk, J., Piper, W., Joyce, A. et al. (2003). Differentiating symptoms of complicated grief and depression among psychiatric outpatients. *Canadian Journal of Psychiatry, 48*(2), 87–93.

Ott, C. (2003). The impact of complicated grief on mental and physical health at various points in the bereavement process. *Death Studies, 27*(3), 249–272.

Prigerson, H., & Jacobs, S. (2001). Traumatic grief as a distinct disorder: A rationale, consensus criteria, and a preliminary empirical test. In M. Stroebe, R. Hannson, W. Stroebe, & H. Schut (eds), *Handbook of bereavement research: Consequences, coping and care.* Washington, DC: American Psychological Association, pp. 613–646.

Risk for Complicated Grieving (00172)

(2004, 2006, LOE 2.1)

Domain 9: Coping/Stress Tolerance
Class 2: Coping Responses

Definition At risk for a disorder that occurs after the death of a significant other, in which the experience of distress accompanying bereavement fails to follow normative expectations and manifests in functional impairment

Risk Factors

- Death of a significant other
- Emotional instability
- Lack of social support

References

Center for the Advancement of Health (2004a). Report on bereavement and grief research. Outcomes of bereavement. *Death Studies*, *28*(1), 520–542.

Center for the Advancement of Health (2004b). Report on bereavement and grief research. Themes in research on bereavement and grief. *Death Studies*, *28*(6), 498–505.

Christ, G., Bonnano, G., Malkinson, R., & Rubin, S. (2003). Bereavement experiences after the death of a child. In M. Field, & R. Berhman, (eds), *When children die: Improving palliative and end-of-life care for children and their families*. Washington, DC: National Academy Press, pp. 553–579.

Davis, C., & Nolen-Hocksema, S. (2001). Loss and meaning: How do people make sense of loss? *American Behavioral Scientist*, *44*(5), 726–741.

Gamino, L., Sewell, K., & Easterling, L. (2000). Scott and White Grief Study – Phase 2: Toward an adaptive model of grief. *Death Studies*, *24*(7), 633–660.

Gamino, L., Hogan, N., & Sewell, K. (2002). Feeling the absence: A content analysis from the Scott and White grief study. *Death Studies*, *26*(10), 793–813.

Hall, M., & Irwin, M. (2001). Physiological indices of functioning in bereavement. In M. Stroebe, R. Hannson, W. Stroebe, & H. Schut (eds), *Handbook of bereavement research: Consequences, coping and care*. Washington DC: American Psychological Association, pp. 473–493.

Hansson, R., & Stroebe, M. (2003). Grief, older adulthood. In T. Gullotta, & M. Bloom (eds.), *Encyclopedia of primary prevention and health promotion*. New York: Plenum Press, pp. 515–521.

Hogan, N., Worden, J.W., & Schmidt, L. (2004). An empirical study of the proposed complicated grief disorder criteria. *OMEGA – Journal of Death and Dying*, *48*(3), 263–277.

Jacobs, S. (1999). *Traumatic grief: Diagnosis, treatment, and prevention*. Caselton, NY: Brunner/Mazel.

Matthews, L., & Marwit, S. (2004). Complicated grief and the trend toward cognitive-behavioral therapy. *Death Studies*, *28*(9), 849–863.

Ogrodniczuk, J., Piper, W., Joyce, A. et al. (2003). Differentiating symptoms of complicated grief and depression among psychiatric outpatients. *Canadian Journal of Psychiatry*, *48*(2), 87–93.

Ott, C. (2003). The impact of complicated grief on mental and physical health at various points in the bereavement process. *Death Studies*, *27*(3), 249–272.

Prigerson, H., & Jacobs, S. (2001). Traumatic grief as a distinct disorder: A rationale, consensus criteria, and a preliminary empirical test. In M. Stroebe, R. Hannson, W. Stroebe, & H. Schut (eds), *Handbook of bereavement research: Consequences, coping and care*. Washington, DC: American Psychological Association, pp. 613–646.

Readiness for Enhanced Power (00187)*
(2006, LOE 2.1)

Domain 9: Coping/Stress Tolerance
Class 2: Coping Responses

Definition A pattern of participating knowingly in change that is sufficient for well-being and can be strengthened

Defining Characteristics

- Expresses readiness to enhance awareness of possible changes to be made
- Expresses readiness to enhance freedom to perform actions for change
- Expresses readiness to enhance identification of choices that can be made for change
- Expresses readiness to enhance involvement in creating change
- Expresses readiness to enhance knowledge for participation in change
- Expresses readiness to enhance participation in choices for daily living
- Expresses readiness to enhance participation in choices for health
- Expresses readiness to enhance power

References

Anderson, R.M., & Funnell, M.M. (2005). Patient empowerment: Reflections on the challenge of fostering the adoption of a new paradigm. *Patient Education and Counseling*, 57(2), 153–157.

Barrett, E.A.M. (1990). A measure of power as knowing participation in change. In O. Strickland, & C. Waltz (eds), *Measurement of nursing outcomes*, Vol. 4. *Measuring client self-care and coping skills*. New York: Springer, pp. 159–180.

Caroselli, C., & Barrett, E.A.M. (1998). A review of the power as knowing participation in change literature. *Nursing Science Quarterly*, 11(1), 9–16.

Cowling, W.R. (2004). Pattern, participation, praxis, and power in unitary appreciative inquiry. *Nursing Science Quarterly*, 27, 202–14.

Funnell, M.M. (2004). Patient empowerment. *Critical Care Nursing Quarterly*, 27(3), 201–204.

Guinn, M.J. (2004). A daughter's journey promoting geriatric self-care: Promoting positive health care interactions. *Geriatric Nursing*, 25(5), 267–271.

Harkness, J. (2005). Patient involvement: A vital principle for patient-centered health care. *World Hospitals and Health Services*, 41(2), 12–16, 40–43.

Hashimoto, H., & Fukuhara, S. (2003). The influence of locus of control on preferences for information and decision making. *Patient Education and Counseling*, 55(2), 236–240.

Jeng, C., Yang, S., Chang, P., & Tsao, L. (2004). Menopausal women: Perceiving continuous power through the experience of regular exercise. *Journal of Clinical Nursing*, 13(4), 447–454.

Mok, E. (2001). Empowerment of cancer patients: From a Chinese perspective. *Nursing Ethics*, 8(1), 69–76.

Pender, N.J., Murdaugh, C.L., & Parsons, M.A. (2006). *Health promotion in nursing practice* (5th ed.). Stamford, CT: Appleton & Lange.

*Note: even though power (a response) and empowerment (an intervention approach) are different concepts, the literature related to both concepts supports the defining characteristics of this diagnosis.

Pibernik-Okanovic, M., Prasek, M., Poljicanin-Filipovic, T., Pavlic-Renar, I., & Metelko, Z. (2003). Effects of an empowerment-based psychosocial intervention on quality of life and metabolic control in type 2 diabetic patients. *Patient Education and Counseling, 52*(2), 193–199.

Shearer, N.B.C., & Reed, P.G. (2004). Empowerment: reformulation of a non-Rogerian concept. *Nursing Science Quarterly, 17*(3), 253–259.

Wright, B.W. (2004). Trust and power in adults: An investigation using Rogers' science of unitary human beings. *Nursing Science Quarterly, 17*(2), 139–146.

Powerlessness (00125)
(1982, 2010, LOE 2.1)

Domain 9: Coping/Stress Tolerance
Class 2: Coping Responses

Definition The lived experience of lack of control over a situation, including a perception that one's actions do not significantly affect an outcome

Defining Characteristics

- Dependence on others
- Depression over physical deterioration
- Nonparticipation in care
- Reports alienation
- Reports doubt regarding role performance
- Reports frustration over inability to perform previous activities
- Reports lack of control
- Reports shame

Related Factors

- Illness-related regimen
- Institutional environment
- Unsatisfying interpersonal interactions

References

Andershed, B., & Harstäde, C. (2007). Next of kin's feelings of guilt and shame in end-of-life care. *Contemporary Nurse: A Journal for the Australian Nursing Profession, 27*(1), 61–72.

Colyer, H. (1996). Women's experience of living with cancer. *Journal of Advanced Nursing, 23*(3), 496–501.

Davidhizar, R. (1994). Powerlessness of caregivers in home care. *Journal of Clinical Nursing, 3*(3), 155–158.

Efraimsson, E., Rasmussen, B., Gilje, F., & Sandman, P. (2003). Expressions of power and powerlessness in discharge planning: A case study of an older woman on her way home. *Journal of Clinical Nursing, 12*(5), 707–716.

Fisker, T., & Strandmark, M. (2007). Experiences of surviving spouse of terminally ill spouse: A phenomenological study of an altruistic perspective. *Scandinavian Journal of Caring Sciences, 21*(2), 274–281.

Gibson, J., & Kenrick, M. (1998). Pain and powerlessness: the experience of living with peripheral vascular disease. *Journal of Advanced Nursing, 27*(4), 737–745.

Hägglund, D., & Ahlström, G. (2007). The meaning of women's experience of living with long-term urinary incontinence is powerlessness. *Journal of Clinical Nursing, 16*(10), 1946–1954.

Hansson, L., & Björkman, T. (2005). Empowerment in people with a mental illness: Reliability and validity of the Swedish version of an empowerment scale. *Scandinavian Journal of Caring Sciences, 19*(1), 32–38.

Kain, V. (2007). Moral distress and providing care to dying babies in neonatal nursing. *International Journal of Palliative Nursing, 13*(5), 243–248.

Koch, T., & Webb, C. (1996). The biomedical construction of ageing: Implications for nursing care of older people. *Journal of Advanced Nursing, 23*(5), 954–959.

Nystrom, A., & Segesten, K. (1994). On sources of powerlessness in nursing home life. *Journal of Advanced Nursing, 19*(1), 124–133.

Papadatou, D., & Bellali, T. (2002). Greek nurse and physician grief as a result of caring for children dying of cancer. *Pediatric Nursing, 28*(4), 345.

Rydahl-Hansen, S. (2005). Hospitalized patients experienced suffering in life with incurable cancer. *Scandinavian Journal of Caring Sciences*, *19*(3), 213–222.

Strandmark, M. (2004). Ill health is powerlessness: A phenomenological study about worthlessness, limitations and suffering. *Scandinavian Journal of Caring Sciences*, *18*(2), 135–144.

Thomas, S., & Gonzalez-Prendes, A. (2009). Powerlessness, anger, and stress in African American women: Implications for physical and emotional health. *Health Care for Women International*, *30*(1–2), 93–113.

Van Den Tillaart, S., Kurtz, D., & Cash, P. (2009). Powerlessness, marginalized identity, and silencing of health concerns: Voiced realities of women living with a mental health diagnosis. *International Journal of Mental Health Nursing*, *18*(3), 153–163.

Walding, M. (1991). Pain, anxiety and powerlessness. *Journal of Advanced Nursing*, *16*(4), 388–397.

Risk for Powerlessness (00152)
(2000, 2010, LOE 2.1)

Domain 9: Coping/Stress Tolerance
Class 2: Coping Responses

Definition At risk for the lived experience of lack of control over a situation, including a perception that one's actions do not significantly affect an outcome.

Risk Factors

- Anxiety
- Caregiving
- Chronic low self-esteem
- Deficient knowledge
- Economically disadvantaged
- Illness
- Ineffective coping patterns
- Lack of social support
- Pain
- Progressive debilitating disease
- Situational low self-esteem
- Social marginalization
- Stigmatized condition
- Stigmatized disease
- Unpredictable course of illness

References

Andershed, B., & Harstäde, C. (2007). Next of kin's feelings of guilt and shame in end-of-life care. *Contemporary Nurse: A Journal for the Australian Nursing Profession, 27*(1), 61–72.

Colyer, H. (1996). Women's experience of living with cancer. *Journal of Advanced Nursing, 23*(3), 496–501.

Davidhizar, R. (1994). Powerlessness of caregivers in home care. *Journal of Clinical Nursing, 3*(3), 155–158.

Efraimsson, E., Rasmussen, B., Gilje, F., & Sandman, P. (2003). Expressions of power and powerlessness in discharge planning: A case study of an older woman on her way home. *Journal of Clinical Nursing, 12*(5), 707–716.

Fisker, T., & Strandmark, M. (2007). Experiences of surviving spouse of terminally ill spouse: A phenomenological study of an altruistic perspective. *Scandinavian Journal of Caring Sciences, 21*(2), 274– 281.

Gibson, J., & Kenrick, M. (1998). Pain and powerlessness: the experience of living with peripheral vascular disease. *Journal of Advanced Nursing, 27*(4), 737–745.

Hägglund, D., & Ahlström, G. (2007). The meaning of women's experience of living with long-term urinary incontinence is powerlessness. *Journal of Clinical Nursing, 16*(10), 1946–1954.

Hansson, L., & Björkman, T. (2005). Empowerment in people with a mental illness: Reliability and validity of the Swedish version of an empowerment scale. *Scandinavian Journal of Caring Sciences, 19*(1), 32–38.

Kain, V. (2007). Moral distress and providing care to dying babies in neonatal nursing. *International Journal of Palliative Nursing, 13*(5), 243–248.

Koch, T., & Webb, C. (1996). The biomedical construction of ageing: Implications for nursing care of older people. *Journal of Advanced Nursing, 23*(5), 954–959.

Nystrom, A., & Segesten, K. (1994). On sources of powerlessness in nursing home life. *Journal of Advanced Nursing, 19*(1), 124–133.

Papadatou, D., & Bellali, T. (2002). Greek nurse and physician grief as a result of caring for children dying of cancer. *Pediatric Nursing, 28*(4), 345.

Rydahl-Hansen, S. (2005). Hospitalized patients experienced suffering in life with incurable cancer. *Scandinavian Journal of Caring Sciences, 19*(3), 213–222.

Strandmark, M. (2004). Ill health is powerlessness: A phenomenological study about worthlessness, limitations and suffering. *Scandinavian Journal of Caring Sciences, 18*(2), 135–144.

Thomas, S., & Gonzalez-Prendes, A. (2009). Powerlessness, anger, and stress in African American women: Implications for physical and emotional health. *Health Care for Women International, 30*(1–2), 93–113.

Van Den Tillaart, S., Kurtz, D., & Cash, P. (2009). Powerlessness, marginalized identity, and silencing of health concerns: Voiced realities of women living with a mental health diagnosis. *International Journal of Mental Health Nursing, 18*(3), 153–163.

Walding, M. (1991). Pain, anxiety and powerlessness. *Journal of Advanced Nursing, 16*(4), 388–397.

Impaired Individual Resilience (00210)

(2008, LOE 2.1)

Domain 9: Coping/Stress Tolerance
Class 2: Coping Responses

Definition Decreased ability to sustain a pattern of positive responses to an adverse situation or crisis

Defining Characteristics

- Decreased interest in academic activities
- Decreased interest in vocational activities
- Depression
- Guilt
- Isolation
- Lower perceived health status
- Low self-esteem
- Renewed elevation of distress
- Shame
- Social isolation
- Using maladaptive coping skills (i.e., drug use, violence, etc.)

Related Factors

- Demographics that increase chance of maladjustment
- Gender
- Inconsistent parenting
- Large family size
- Low intelligence
- Low maternal education
- Minority status
- Neighborhood violence
- Parental mental illness
- Poor impulse control
- Poverty
- Psychological disorders
- Substance abuse
- Violence
- Vulnerability factors which encompass indices that exacerbate the negative effects of the risk condition

References

Armstrong, M., Birnie-Lefcovitch, S., & Ungar, M (2005) Pathways between social support family well-being, quality of parenting and child resilience: What we know. *Journal of Child and Family Studies*, 14(2), 269–281.

Bonanno, G.A. (2005). Clarifying and extending the construct of adult resilience. *American Psychologist*, 60, 265–267.

Brown, J.H. & Brown, D. (2005). Why "at risk" is at risk. *American School Board Journal*, 192(11): 44–46.

Crosnoe, R., & Elder, G. (2004). Family dynamics, supportive relationships, and educational resilience during adolescence. *Journal of Family Issues*, 25(5), 571–602.

Kaylor, G., & Otis, M. (2003). The effect of childhood maltreatment on adult criminality: A Tobit regression analysis. *Child Maltreatment*, 8(2), 129–137.

Luthar, S.S., & Cicchetti, D. (2000). The construct of resilience: Implications for interventions and social policies. *Developmental Psychopathology*, 12(4), 857–885.

Richardson, G.E. (2002). The metatheory of resilience and resiliency. *Journal of Clinical Psychology, 58*(3), 307–321.

Rutter, M., & Sroufe, A. (2000). Developmental psychopathology: Concepts and challenges. *Developmental Psychopathology, 12*(3), 265–296.

Taylor, J. (2000). Sisters of the yam: African American women's healing and self-recovery from intimate male partner violence. *Issues in Mental Health Nursing, 21*(5), 515–531.

9. Coping/Stress Tolerance

Domain 9: Coping/Stress Tolerance
Class 2: Coping Responses

Definition
A pattern of positive responses to an adverse situation or crisis that is sufficient for optimizing human potential and can be strengthened

Defining Characteristics

- Access to resources
- Demonstrates positive outlook
- Effective use of conflict management strategies
- Enhances personal coping skills
- Expressed desire to enhance resilience
- Identifies available resources
- Identifies support systems
- Increases positive relationships with others
- Involvement in activities
- Makes progress toward goals
- Presence of a crisis
- Reports enhanced sense of control
- Reports self-esteem
- Safe environment is maintained
- Sets goals
- Takes responsibilities for actions
- Use of effective communication skills

References

Bolger, K., & Patterson, C. (2003). Sequelae of child maltreatment: Vulnerability and resilience. In S. Luthar (eds), *Resilience and vulnerability: Adaptation in the context of childhood adversities*. Cambridge: Cambridge University Press, pp. 156–181.

Bolger, K., Patterson, C., & Kupersmidt, J. (1998). Peer relationships and self-esteem among children who have been maltreated. *Child Development*, 69(4), 1171–1197.

Bonanno, G.A. (2005). Clarifying and extending the construct of adult resilience. *American Psychologist*, 60, 265–267.

Brown, J.H., & Brown, D. (2005). Why 'at risk' is at risk. *American School Board Journal*, 192(11), 44–46.

Crosnoe, R., & Elder, G. (2004). Family dynamics, supportive relationships, and educational resilience during adolescence. *Journal of Family Issues*, 25(5), 571–602.

Evans, G.W., & Kantrowitz, E. (2002). Socioeconomic status and health: The potential role of environmental risk exposure. *Annual Review of Public Health*, 23(1), 303–331.

Fergus, S., & Zimmerman, M. (2005). Adolescent resilience: A framework for understanding healthy development in the face of risk. *Annual Review of Public Health*, 26, 399–419.

Haskett, M., & Willoughby, M. (2007). Paths to child social adjustment: Parenting quality and children's processing of social information. *Child: Care, Health and Development*, 33(1), 67–77.

Kelley, T.M. (2005). Natural resilience and innate mental health. *American Psychologist*, 60(3), 265.

Kim, J., & Cicchetti, D. (2003). Social self-efficacy and behavior problems in maltreated children. *Journal of Clinical Child and Adolescent Psychology*, 32(1), 106–117.

Luthar, S.S., & Cicchetti, D. (2000). The construct of resilience: Implications for interventions and social policies. *Developmental Psychopathology*, 12(4), 857–885.

Luthar, S., Cicchetti, D., & Becker, B. (2000). The construct of resilience: A critical evaluation and guidelines for future work. *Child Development*, 71(3), 543–562.

Manly, J.T., Kim, J.E., Rogosch, F.A., & Cicchetti, D. (2001). Dimensions of child maltreatment and children's adjustment: Contributions of developmental timing and subtype. *Developmental Psychopathology*, 13(4), 759–782.

9. Coping/Stress Tolerance

Masten, A.S. (2001). Ordinary magic: Resilience processes in development. *American Psychologist, 56*(3), 227–238.

Masten, A.S. (2004). Regulatory processes, risk and resilience in adolescent development. *Annals of the New York Academy of Science, 1021*(1), 310–319.

Masten, A., & Powell, J. (2003). A resilience framework for research policy and practice. In S. Luthar (ed.), *Resilience and vulnerability: Adaptation in the context of childhood adversities.* Cambridge: Cambridge University Press, pp. 1–25.

Masten, A., Burt, K., Roisman, G., Obradovic, J., Long, J., & Tellegen, A. (2004). Resources and resilience in the transition to adulthood: Continuity and change. *Development and Psychopathology, 16*(4), 1071–1094.

Richardson, G.E. (2002). The metatheory of resilience and resiliency. *Journal of Clinical Psychology, 58*(3), 307–321.

Rutter, M. (1987). Psychosocial resilience and protective mechanism. *American Journal of Orthopsychiatry, 57*(3), 316–331.

Rutter, M., & O'Conner, T. (2004). Are there biological programming effects of psychological development? Findings from a study of Romanian adoptees. *Developmental Psychology, 40*(1), 81–94.

Rutter, M., & Sroufe, A. (2000). Developmental psychopathology: Concepts and challenges. *Developmental Psychopathology, 12*(3), 265–296.

Sinclair, V.G., & Wallston, K.A. (2004). The development and psychometric evaluation of the brief resilient coping scale. *Assessment, 11*(1), 94–101.

Tusaie, K., & Dyer, J. (2004). Resilience: A historical review of the construct. *Holistic Nursing Practice, 18*(1), 3–8.

Werner, E.E. (1996a). Protective factors and individual resilience. In S. Meisels, & J. Shonkoff (eds), *Handbook of early childhood interventions.* New York: Cambridge University Press, pp. 115–133.

Werner, E.E. (1996b). Vulnerable but invincible. *European Child and Adolescent Psychiatry, 5*(1), 47–51.

Risk for Compromised Resilience (00211)
(2008, LOE 2.1)

Domain 9: Coping/Stress Tolerance
Class 2: Coping Responses

Definition At risk for decreased ability to sustain a pattern of positive responses to an adverse situation or crisis

Risk factors

- Chronicity of existing crises
- Multiple coexisting adverse situations

- Presence of an additional new crisis (e.g., unplanned pregnancy, death of a spouse, loss of job, illness, loss of housing, death of family member)

References

Armstrong, M., Birnie-Lefcovitch, S., & Ungar, M. (2005) Pathways between social support family well-being, quality of parenting and child resilience: What we know. *Journal of Child and Family Studies*, *14*(2), 269–281.

Black, C., & Ford-Gilboe, M. (2004). Adolescent mothers: Resilience, family health, work and health promoting practices. *Journal of Advanced Nursing*, *48*(4), 351–360.

Bonanno, G.A. (2005). Clarifying and extending the construct of adult resilience. *American Psychologist*, *60*, 265–267.

Brown, J.H., & Brown, D. (2005). Why "at risk" is at risk. *American School Board Journal*, *192*(11), 44–46.

Evans, G.W., & Kantrowitz, E. (2002). Socioeconomic status and health: The potential role of environmental risk exposure. *Annual Review of Public Health*, *23*(1), 303–331.

Fergus, S., & Zimmerman, M. (2005). Adolescent resilience: A framework for understanding healthy development in the face of risk. *Annual Review of Public Health*, *26*, 399–419.

Gorman, C., Dale, S. S., Grossman, W., Klarreich, K., McDowell, J., & Whitaker, L. (2005). The importance of resilience. *Time*, *165*(3), A52–A55.

Greef, A., & Ritman, I. (2005). Individual characteristics associated with resilience in single-parent families. *Psychological Reports*, *96*(1), 36–42.

Kelley, T.M. (2005). Natural resilience and innate mental health. *American Psychologist*, *60*(3), 265.

Luthar, S.S., & Cicchetti, D. (2000). The construct of resilience: Implications for interventions and social policies. *Developmental Psychopathology*, *12*(4), 857–885.

Manly, J.T., Kim, J.E., Rogosch, F.A., & Cicchetti, D. (2001). Dimensions of child maltreatment and children's adjustment: Contributions of developmental timing and subtype. *Developmental Psychopathology*, *13*(4), 759–782.

Martin, A.J., & Marsh, H.W. (2006). Academic resilience and its psychological and educational correlates: A construct validity approach. *Psychology in the Schools*, *43*(3), 267–281.

Masten, A.S. (2001). Ordinary magic: Resilience processes in development. *American Psychologist*, *56*(3), 227–238.

Rogers, S., Muir, K., & Evenson, C.R. (2003). Signs of resilience: assets that support deaf adults' success in bridging the deaf and hearing worlds. *American Annals of the Deaf*, *148*(3), 222–232.

Sinclair, V.G., & Wallston, K.A. (2004). The development and psychometric evaluation of the brief resilient coping scale. *Assessment*, *11*(1), 94–101.

Taylor, J. (2000). Sisters of the yam: African American women's healing and self-recovery from intimate male partner violence. *Issues in Mental Health Nursing*, *21*(5), 515–531.

Werner, E.E. (1996a). Protective factors and individual resilience. In S. Meisels, & J. Shonkoff (eds), *Handbook of early childhood interventions*. New York: Cambridge University Press, pp. 115–133.

Werner, E.E. (1996b). Vulnerable but invincible. *European Child and Adolescent Psychiatry*, *5*(1), 47–51.

Chronic Sorrow (00137)

(1998)

Domain 9: Coping/Stress Tolerance
Class 2: Coping Responses

Definition Cyclical, recurring, and potentially progressive pattern of pervasive sadness experienced (by a parent, caregiver, individual with chronic illness or disability) in response to continual loss, throughout the trajectory of an illness or disability

Defining Characteristics

- Reports feelings of sadness (e.g., periodic, recurrent)
- Reports feelings that interfere with ability to reach highest level of personal well-being
- Reports feelings that interfere with ability to reach highest level of social well-being
- Reports negative feelings (e.g., anger, being misunderstood, confusion, depression, disappointment, emptiness, fear, frustration, guilt, self-blame, helplessness, hopelessness, loneliness, low self-esteem, recurring loss, being overwhelmed)

Related Factors

- Crises in management of the disability
- Crises in management of the illness
- Crises related to developmental stages
- Death of a loved one
- Experiences chronic disability (e.g., physical or mental)
- Experiences chronic illness (e.g., physical or mental)
- Missed opportunities
- Missed milestones
- Unending caregiving

9. Coping/Stress Tolerance

Domain 9: Coping/Stress Tolerance
Class 2: Coping Responses

Definition Excessive amounts and types of demands that require action

Defining Characteristics

- Demonstrates increased feelings of anger
- Demonstrates increased feelings of impatience
- Reports a feeling of pressure
- Reports a feeling of tension
- Reports difficulty in functioning
- Reports excessive situational stress (e.g., rates stress level as 7 or above on a 10-point scale)
- Reports increased feelings of anger
- Reports increased feelings of impatience
- Reports negative impact from stress (e.g., physical symptoms, psychological distress, feeling of being sick or of going to get sick)
- Reports problems with decision-making

Related Factors

- Inadequate resources (e.g., financial, social, education/knowledge level)
- Intense stressors (e.g., family violence, chronic illness, terminal illness)
- Multiple coexisting stressors (e.g., environmental threats/demands, physical threats/demands, social threats/demands)
- Repeated stressors (e.g., family violence, chronic illness, terminal illness)

References

Al-Hassan, M., & Sagr, L. (2002). Stress and stressors of myocardial infarction patients in the early period after discharge. *Journal of Advanced Nursing, 40*(2), 181–188.

Bay, E., Hagerty, B., Williams, R.A., & Kirsch, N. (2005). Chronic stress, salivary cortisol response, interpersonal relatedness, and depression among community-dwelling survivors of traumatic brain injury. *Journal of Neuroscience Nursing, 37*(1), 4–14.

Boardman, J.D. (2004). Stress and physical health: The role of neighborhoods as mediating and moderating mechanisms. *Social Science and Medicine, 58*(12), 2473–2483.

Booth, K., Beaver, K., Kitchener, H., O'Neill, J., & Farrell, C. (2005). Women's experiences of information, psychological distress and worry after treatment for gynecological cancer. *Patient Education and Counseling, 56*(2), 225–232.

Carlson-Catalano, J. (1998). Nursing diagnoses and interventions for postacute phase battered women. *Nursing Diagnoses, 9*(3), 101–110.

Choenarom, C., Williams, R.A., & Hagerty, B.M. (2005). The role of sense of belonging and social support on stress and depression in individuals with depression. *Archives in Psychiatric Nursing, 19*(1), 18–29.

Cropley, M., & Steptoe, A. (2005). Social support, life events and physical symptoms: A prospective study of chronic and recent life stress in men and women. *Psychological Medicine, 33*(2),299–306.

Davidson, M., Penney, E.D., Muller, B., & Grey, M. (2004). Stressors and self care challenges faced by adolescents living with type 1 diabetes. *Applied Nursing Research, 17*(1), 72–80.

Diong, S.M., Bishop, G.D., Enkelmann, H.C. et al. (2005). Anger, stress, coping, social support and health, Modelling the relationships. *Psychology and Health, 20*(4), 467–495.

Drew, D., Goodenough, B., Maurice, L., Foreman, T., & Willis, L. (2005). Parental grieving after a child dies from cancer: Is stress from stem cell transplant a factor? *International Journal of Palliative Nursing, 11*(6), 266–273.

Eby, K.K. (2004). Exploring the stressors of low-income women with abusive partners: Understanding their needs and developing effective community responses. *Journal of Family Violence, 19*(6), 221–232.

Golden-Kreutz, D.M., Thorton, L.M., Wells-Di Gregoria, S. et al. (2005). Traumatic stress, perceived global stress, and life events: Prospectively predicting quality of life in breast cancer patients. *Health Psychology, 24*(3), 288–296.

Hannigan, B., Edwards, D., & Burnard, P. (2004). Stress and stress management in clinical psychology: Findings from a systematic review. *Journal of Mental Health, 13*(3), 235–245.

Harwood, L., Locking-Cusolito, H., Spittal, J., Wilson, B., & White, S. (2005). Preparing for hemodialysis: Patients' stressors and responses. *Nephrology Nursing Journal, 32*(3), 295–303.

Holmes. T.H., & Rahe, R.H. (1967). The Social Readjustment Rating Scale. *Journal of Psychometric Research, 11*(2), 213–218.

Hung, C.-H. (2005), Measuring postpartum stress. *Journal of Advanced Nursing, 50*(4), 417–424.

Ilgen, M.A., & Hutchinson, K.E. (2005). A history of major depressive disorder and the response to stress. *Journal of Affective Disorders, 86*(2–3), 143–150.

Janz, N.K., Dodge, J.A., Janevic, M.R., Lin, X., Donaldson, A.E., & Clark, N.M. (2004). Understanding and reducing stress and psychological distress in older women with heart disease. *Journal of Women and Aging, 16*(3/4), 19–38.

Kanner, A.D., Coyne, J.C., Schaefer, C., & Lazarus, R.S. (1981). Comparison of two measures of stress measurement: Daily hassles and uplifts versus major life events. *Journal of Behavioral Medicine, 4*(1), 1–37.

Keil, R.M.K. (2004). Coping and stress: A conceptual analysis. *Journal of Advanced Nursing, 45*(5), 659–665.

Krause, N. (2004). Stressors arising in highly valued roles, meaning in life, and the physical health status of older adults. *Journal of Gerontology: Social Sciences, 59*(5), S287–S297.

Lazarus, R.S., & Folkman, S. (1984). *Stress, appraisal, and coping.* New York: Springer.

Lim, L.S., Williams, D.E., & Hagan, P.T. (2005). Validation of a five-point self rated stress score. *American Journal of Health Promotion, 19*(6), 438–441.

Lloyd, C., Smith, J., & Weinger, K. (2005). Stress and diabetes: A review of the links. *Diabetes Spectrum, 18*(2), 121–127.

Lunney, M., & Myszak, C. (1997). Abstract: Stress overload: A new diagnosis. In M.J. Rantz, & P. LeMone (eds), *Classification of nursing diagnoses: Proceedings of the twelfth conference, North American Nursing Diagnosis Association.* Glendale, CA: CINAHL Information Systems, pp. 190–191.

Lustky, M.K., Widman, L., Paschane, A., & Ecker, E. (2004). Stress, quality of life and physical activity in women with varying degrees of premenstrual symptomatology. *Women and Health, 39*(3), 35–44.

McNulty, P.A.F. (2005). Reported stressors and health care needs of active duty Navy personnel during three phases of deployment in support of the war in Iraq. *Military Medicine, 170*(6), 530–535.

Maller, M.H., Almeida, D.M., & Neupert, S.D. (2005). Women's daily physical health symptoms and stressful experiences across adulthood. *Psychology and Health, 20*(3), 389–403.

Mariano, C. (1993). Case study: The method. In P.L. Munhall, & C.O. Oiler (eds), *Nursing research: A qualitative perspective* (2nd ed.). New York: National League for Nursing, pp. 311–337.

Miles, M.B., & Huberman, A.M. (1984). *Qualitative data analysis: A sourcebook of new methods.* Newbury Park, CA: Sage.

Motzer, S.A., & Hertig, V. (2004). Stress, stress response and health. *Nursing Clinics of North America, 39*(1), 1–17.

Neilsen, N.R., Zhang, Z.F., Kristensen, T.S., Netterstrm, B., Schnohr, P., & Grebaek, M. (2005). Self reported stress and risk of breast cancer: Prospective cohort study. *British Medical Journal, 331*(7516), 548–550.

Pender, N.J., Murtaugh, C.L., & Parsons, M.A. (2006). *Health promotion in nursing practice* (5th ed.). Upper Saddle River, NJ: Prentice Hall.

Power, T.G. (2004). Stress and coping in childhood: The parents' role. *Parenting: Science and Practice, 4*(4), 271–317.

9. Coping/Stress Tolerance

Ridner, S.H. (2004). Psychological distress: Concept analysis. *Journal of Advanced Nursing, 45*(5), 536–545.

Robinson, K.L., McBeth, J., & McFarlane, G.J. (2004). Psychological distress and premature mortality in the general population: A prospective study. *Annals of Epidemiology, 14*(7), 467–472.

Ryan, M. (2001). Biases that influence the diagnostic process. In M. Lunney (ed.), *Critical thinking and nursing diagnoses: Case studies and analyses*. Philadelphia: NANDA, pp. 8, 156–158.

Ryan-Wenger, N.A., Sharrer, V.W., & Campbell, K.K. (2005). Changes in children's stressors over the past 30 years. *Pediatric Nursing, 31*(4), 282–291.

Sarid, O., Anson, O., Yaari, A., & Margalith, M. (2004). Academic stress, immunological reaction, and academic performance among students of nursing and physiotherapy. *Research in Nursing and Health, 27*(5), 370–377.

Scollan-Koliopoulos, M. (2005). Managing stress response to control hypertension in type 2 diabetes. *Nurse Practitioner, 30*(2), 46–49.

Selye, H. (1956). *The stress of life*. New York: McGraw Hill.

Selye, H. (1974*). Stress without distress*. Philadelphia: JB Lippincott.

Selye, H. (1976). Further thoughts on "stress without distress." *Medical Times, 104*(11), 124–132.

Sepa, A., Wahlberg, J., Vaarsala, O., Frodi, A., & Ludvigsson, J. (2005). Psychological stress may induce diabetes-related autoimmunity in infancy. *Diabetes Care, 28*(2), 290–295.

So, H.M., & Chan, D.S.K. (2004). Perceptions of stressors by patients and nurses of critical care units in Hong Kong. *International Journal of Nursing Studies, 41*(1), 77–84.

Sternberg, E. (2001). *The balance within: The science of connecting health and emotions*. New York: WH Freeman.

Stewart, K.E., Cianfrani, L.R., & Walker, J.F. (2005). Stress, social support and housing are related to health status among HIV-positive persons in the Deep South of the United States. *AIDS Care, 17*(3), 350–358.

Taxis, J.C., Rew, L., Jackson, K., & Kouzekanani, K. (2004). Protective resources and perceptions of stress in a multi-ethnic sample of school-age children. *Pediatric Nursing, 30*(6), 477–482, 487.

Vondras, D.D., Powless, M.R., Olson, A.K., Wheeler, D., & Snudden, A.L. (2005). Differential effects of everyday stress on the episodic memory test performances of young, mid-life, and older adults. *Aging and Mental Health, 9*(1), 60–70.

9. Coping/Stress Tolerance

Autonomic Dysreflexia (00009)
(1988)

Domain 9: Coping/Stress Tolerance
Class 3: Neurobehavioral Stress

Definition
Life-threatening, uninhibited sympathetic response of the nervous system to a noxious stimulus after a spinal cord injury at T7 or above

Defining Characteristics

- Blurred vision
- Bradycardia
- Chest pain
- Chilling
- Conjunctival congestion
- Diaphoresis (above the injury)
- Headache (a diffuse pain in different portions of the head and not confined to any nerve distribution area)
- Horner's syndrome
- Metallic taste in mouth
- Nasal congestion
- Pallor (below the injury)
- Paresthesia
- Paroxysmal hypertension
- Pilomotor reflex
- Red splotches on skin (above the injury)
- Tachycardia

Related Factors

- Bladder distension
- Bowel distension
- Deficient caregiver knowledge
- Deficient patient knowledge
- Skin irritation

Risk for Autonomic Dysreflexia (00010)
(1998, 2000)

Domain 9: Coping/Stress Tolerance
Class 3: Neurobehavioral Stress

Definition At risk for life-threatening, uninhibited response of the sympathetic nervous system, postspinal shock, in an individual with spinal cord injury or lesion at T6 or above (has been demonstrated in patients with injuries at T7 and T8)

Risk Factors

An injury at T6 or above or a lesion at T6 or above AND at least one of the following noxious stimuli.

Cardiopulmonary Stimuli

- Deep vein thrombosis
- Pulmonary emboli

Gastrointestinal Stimuli

- Bowel distension
- Constipation
- Difficult passage of feces
- Digital stimulation
- Enemas
- Esophageal reflux
- Fecal impaction
- Gallstones
- Gastric ulcers
- Gastrointestinal system pathology
- Hemorrhoids
- Suppositories

Musculoskeletal–Integumentary Stimuli

- Cutaneous stimulation (e.g., pressure ulcer, ingrown toenail, dressings, burns, rash)
- Fractures
- Heterotopic bone
- Pressure over bony prominences
- Pressure over genitalia
- Range-of-motion exercises
- Spasm
- Sunburns
- Wounds

Neurological Stimuli

- Irritating stimuli below level of injury
- Painful stimuli below level of injury

Regulatory Stimuli

- Extreme environmental temperatures
- Temperature fluctuations

Reproductive Stimuli

- Ejaculation
- Labor and delivery
- Menstruation

- Ovarian cyst
- Pregnancy
- Sexual intercourse

Situational Stimuli

- Constrictive clothing (e.g., straps, stockings, shoes)
- Narcotic/opiate withdrawal
- Positioning

- Reactions to pharmaceutical agents (e.g., decongestants, sympathomimetics, vasoconstrictors)
- Surgical procedure

Urological Stimuli

- Bladder distension
- Bladder spasm
- Calculi
- Catheterization
- Cystitis
- Detrusor sphincter dyssynergia

- Epididymitis
- Instrumentation
- Surgery
- Urethritis
- Urinary tract infection

9. Coping/Stress Tolerance

Disorganized Infant Behavior (00116)
(1994, 1998)

Domain 9: Coping/Stress Tolerance
Class 3: Neurobehavioral Stress

Definition Disintegrated physiological and neurobehavioral responses of infant to the environment

Defining Characteristics

Attention–Interaction System

- Abnormal response to sensory stimuli (e.g., difficult to soothe, unable to sustain alert status)

Motor System

- Altered primitive reflexes
- Changes to motor tone
- Finger splaying
- Fisting
- Hands to face
- Hyperextension of extremities
- Jittery
- Startles
- Tremors
- Twitches
- Uncoordinated movement

Physiological

- Arrhythmias
- Bradycardia
- Desaturation
- Feeding intolerances
- Skin color changes
- Tachycardia
- Time-out signals (e.g., gaze, grasp, hiccough, cough, sneeze, sigh, slack jaw, open mouth, tongue thrust)

Regulatory Problems

- Inability to inhibit startle
- Irritability

State–Organization System

- Active–awake (fussy, worried gaze)
- Diffuse sleep
- Irritable crying
- Quiet–awake (staring, gaze aversion)
- State–oscillation

Related Factors

Caregiver

- Cue misreading
- Deficient knowledge regarding behavioral cues
- Environmental stimulation contribution

Environmental

- Lack of containment within environment
- Physical environment inappropriateness
- Sensory deprivation
- Sensory inappropriateness
- Sensory overstimulation

Individual

- Illness
- Immature neurological system
- Low postconceptual age
- Prematurity

Postnatal

- Feeding intolerance
- Invasive procedures
- Malnutrition
- Motor problems
- Oral problems
- Pain

Prenatal

- Congenital disorders
- Genetic disorders
- Teratogenic exposure

Readiness for Enhanced Organized Infant Behavior (00117)

(1994)

Domain 9: Coping/Stress Tolerance
Class 3: Neurobehavioral Stress

Definition A pattern of modulation of the physiological and behavioral systems of functioning (i.e., autonomic, motor, state–organization, self-regulatory, and attentional–interactional systems) in an infant that is sufficient for well-being and can be strengthened

Defining Characteristics

- Definite sleep–wake states
- Response to stimuli (e.g., visual, auditory)
- Stable physiological measures
- Use of some self-regulatory behaviors

Risk for Disorganized Infant Behavior (00115)
(1994)

Domain 9: Coping/Stress Tolerance
Class 3: Neurobehavioral Stress

Definition At risk for alteration in integrating and modulation of the physiological and behavioral systems of functioning (i.e., autonomic, motor, state–organization, self-regulatory, and attentional–interactional systems)

Risk Factors

- Environmental overstimulation
- Invasive procedures
- Lack of containment within environment
- Motor problems
- Oral problems
- Pain
- Painful procedures
- Prematurity

Decreased Intracranial Adaptive Capacity (00049)
(1994)

Domain 9: Coping/Stress Tolerance
Class 3: Neurobehavioral Stress

Definition Intracranial fluid dynamic mechanisms that normally compensate for increases in intracranial volumes are compromised, resulting in repeated disproportionate increases in intracranial pressure (ICP) in response to a variety of noxious and non-noxious stimuli

Defining Characteristics

- Baseline ICP ≥10 mmHg
- Disproportionate increase in ICP following stimulus
- Elevated P2 ICP waveform
- Repeated increases of >10 mmHg for more than 5 minutes following any of a variety of external stimuli
- Volume–pressure response test variation (volume:pressure ratio 2, pressure–volume index <10)
- Wide-amplitude ICP waveform

Related Factors

- Brain injuries
- Decreased cerebral perfusion ≤50–60 mmHg
- Sustained increase in ICP of 10–15 mmHg
- Systemic hypotension with intracranial hypertension

Domain 10
Life Principles

NANDA International Nursing Diagnoses: Definitions & Classification 2012–2014, First Edition.
Edited by T. Heather Herdman.
© 2012 NANDA International. Published 2012 by Blackwell Publishing Ltd.

Readiness for Enhanced Hope (00185)

(2006, LOE 2.1)

Domain 10: Life Principles
Class 1: Values

Definition A pattern of expectations and desires for mobilizing energy on one's own behalf that is sufficient for well-being and can be strengthened

Defining Characteristics

- Expresses desire to enhance ability to set achievable goals
- Expresses desire to enhance belief in possibilities
- Expresses desire to enhance congruency of expectations with desires
- Expresses desire to enhance hope
- Expresses desire to enhance interconnectedness with others
- Expresses desire to enhance problem-solving to meet goals
- Expresses desire to enhance sense of meaning to life
- Expresses desire to enhance spirituality

References

Benzein, E.G. (2005). The level of and relation between hope, hopelessness and fatigue in patients and family members in palliative care. *Palliative Medicine, 19*(3), 234–240.

Benzein, E., & Saveman, B.-L. (1998). One step towards the understanding of hope: A concept analysis. *International Journal of Nursing Studies, 35*(6), 322–329.

Davis, B. (2005). Mediators of the relationship between hope and well-being in older adults. *Clinical Nursing Research, 14*(3), 253–272.

10. Life Principles

Readiness for Enhanced Spiritual Well-Being (00068)
(1994, 2002, LOE 2.1)

Domain 10: Life Principles
Class 2: Beliefs

Definition A pattern of experiencing and integrating meaning and purpose in life through connectedness with self, others, art, music, literature, nature, and/or a power greater than oneself that is sufficient for well-being and can be strengthened

Defining Characteristics

Connections to Self

- Expresses desire for enhanced acceptance
- Expresses desire for enhanced coping
- Expresses desire for enhanced courage
- Expresses desire for enhanced hope
- Expresses desire for enhanced joy
- Expresses desire for enhanced love
- Expresses desire for enhanced meaning in life
- Expresses desire for enhanced purpose in life
- Expresses desire for enhanced satisfying philosophy of life
- Expresses desire for enhanced self-forgiveness
- Expresses desire for enhanced serenity (e.g., peace)
- Expresses desire for enhanced surrender
- Meditation

Connections with Others

- Provides service to others
- Requests forgiveness of others
- Requests interactions with significant others
- Requests interactions with spiritual leaders

Connections with Art, Music, Literature, Nature

- Displays creative energy (e.g., writing, poetry, singing)
- Listens to music
- Reads spiritual literature
- Spends time outdoors

Connections with Power Greater Than Self

- Expresses awe
- Expresses reverence
- Participates in religious activities
- Prays
- Reports mystical experiences

Readiness for Enhanced Decision-Making (00184)

(2006, LOE 2.1)

Domain 10: Life Principles
Class 3: Value/Belief/Action Congruence

Definition A pattern of choosing a course of action that is sufficient for meeting short- and long-term health-related goals and can be strengthened

Defining Characteristics

- Expresses desire to enhance congruency of decisions with goals
- Expresses desire to enhance congruency of decisions with personal values
- Expresses desire to enhance congruency of decisions with sociocultural goals
- Expresses desire to enhance congruency of decisions with sociocultural values
- Expresses desire to enhance decision-making
- Expresses desire to enhance risk–benefit analysis of decisions
- Expresses desire to enhance understanding of choices for decision-making
- Expresses desire to enhance understanding of the meaning of choices
- Expresses desire to enhance use of reliable evidence for decisions

References

Evans, R., Elwyn, G., & Edwards, A. (2004). Making interactive decision support for patients a reality. *Informatics in Primary Care, 12*(2), 109–113.

Harkness, J. (2005). Patient involvement: A vital principle for patient-centered health care. *World Hospitals and Health Services: The Official Journal of the International Hospital Federation, 41*(2), 12–16.

O'Connor, A.M., Drake, E.R., Wells, G.A., Tugwell, P., Laupacis, A., & Elmslie, T. (2003). A survey of the decision-making need of Canadians faced with complex health decisions. *Health Expectations, 6*(2), 97–109.

O'Connor, A.M., Tugwell, P., Wells, G.A. et al. (1998). A decision aid for women considering hormone therapy after menopause: Decision support framework and evaluation. *Patient Education and Counseling, 33*(3), 267–279.

Paterson, B.L., Russell, C., & Thorne, S. (2001). Critical analysis of everyday self-care decision making in chronic illness. *Journal of Advanced Nursing, 35*(3), 335–341.

Pender, N.J., Murdaugh, C.L., & Parsons, M.A. (2006). *Health promotion in nursing practice* (5th edn). Upper Saddle River, NJ: Pearson Prentice-Hall.

Roelands, M., Van Oost, P., Stevens, V., Depoorter, A., & Buysse, A. (2004). Clinical practice guidelines to improve shared decision-making about assistive device use in home care: A pilot interventions study. *Patient Education and Counseling, 55*(2), 252–64.

Ross, M.M., Carswell, A., Hing, M., Hollingworth, G., & Dalziel, W.B. (2001). Seniors decision making about pain management. *Journal of Advanced Nursing, 35*(3), 442–451.

Rothert, M.L., Holmes-Rovner, M., Rovner, D. et al. (1997). An educational intervention as decision support for menopausal women. *Research in Nursing and Health, 20,* 377–387.

Tunis, S.R. (2005). Perspective: A clinical research strategy to support shared decision making. *Health Affairs, 24*(1), 180–184.

10. Life Principles

Decisional Conflict (00083)
(1988, 2006, LOE 2.1)

Domain 10: Life Principles
Class 3: Value/Belief/Action Congruence

Definition Uncertainty about course of action to be taken when choice among competing actions involves risk, loss, or challenge to values and beliefs

Defining Characteristics

- Delayed decision-making
- Physical signs of distress (e.g., increased heart rate, restlessness)
- Physical signs of tension
- Questioning moral principles while attempting a decision
- Questioning moral rules while attempting a decision
- Questioning moral values while attempting a decision
- Questioning personal beliefs while attempting a decision
- Questioning personal values while attempting a decision
- Self-focusing
- Vacillation among alternative choices
- Verbalizes feeling of distress while attempting a decision
- Verbalizes uncertainty about choices
- Verbalizes undesired consequences of alternative actions being considered

Related Factors

- Divergent sources of information
- Interference with decision-making
- Lack of experience with decision-making
- Lack of relevant information
- Moral obligations require not performing action
- Moral obligations require performing action
- Moral principles support mutually inconsistent courses of action
- Moral rules support mutually inconsistent courses of action
- Moral values support mutually inconsistent courses of action
- Multiple sources of information
- Perceived threat to value system
- Support system deficit
- Unclear personal beliefs
- Unclear personal values

References

Audi, R. (1999). *The Cambridge dictionary of philosophy* (2nd ed.). New York: Cambridge University Press.
Beauchamp, T.L., & Childress, J.F. (2001). *Principles of biomedical ethics* (5th ed.). New York: Oxford University Press.
Canadian Nurses' Association (2002). *Code of ethics for registered nurses*. Ottawa, ON: Canadian Nurses' Association.
Fletcher, J.C., Lombardo, P.A., Marshall, M.F., & Miller, F.G. (1995). *Introduction to clinical ethics* (2nd ed.). Hagerston, MD: University Publishing.
Jameton, A. (1984). *Nursing practice: The ethical issues*. Englewood Cliffs, NJ: Prentice-Hall.

Kopala, B., & Burkhart, L. (2005). Ethical dilemma and moral distress: Proposed new NANDA diagnoses. *International Journal of Nursing Terminologies and Classifications, 16*(1), 3–13.

Redman, B.K., & Fry, S.T. (1998). Ethical conflicts reported by certified registered rehabilitation nurses. *Rehabilitation Nursing, 23*(4), 179–184.

Webster, G.C., & Baylis, F. (2000). *Moral residue.* In S.B. Rubin, & L. Zoloth (eds), *Margin of error. The ethics of mistakes in the practice of medicine.* Hagerstown, MD: University Publishing.

10. Life Principles

Moral Distress (00175)
(2006, LOE 2.1)

Domain 10: Life Principles
Class 3: Values/Belief/Action Congruence

Definition Response to the inability to carry out one's chosen ethical/moral decision/action

Defining Characteristics

- Expresses anguish (e.g., powerlessness, guilt, frustration, anxiety, self-doubt, fear) over difficulty acting on one's moral choice

Related Factors

- Conflict among decision-makers
- Conflicting information guiding ethical decision-making
- Conflicting information guiding moral decision-making
- Cultural conflicts
- End-of-life decisions
- Loss of autonomy
- Physical distance of decision-maker
- Time constraints for decision-making
- Treatment decisions

References

Audi, R. (1999). *The Cambridge dictionary of philosophy* (2nd ed.). New York: Cambridge University Press.

Beauchamp, T.L., & Childress, J.F. (2001). *Principles of biomedical ethics* (5th ed.). New York: Oxford University Press.

Berger, M.C., Seversen, A., & Chvatal, R. (1991). Ethical issues in nursing. *Western Journal of Nursing Research*, 13(4), 514–521.

Burkhardt, M.A., & Nathaniel, A.K. (2002). *Ethics and Issues in Contemporary Nursing*. Albany, NY: Delmar.

Canadian Nurses' Association (2002). *Code of ethics for registered nurses*. Ottawa, ON: Canadian Nurses' Association.

Corley, M.C., Elswick, R.K., Gorman, M., & Clor, T. (2001). Development and evaluation of a moral distress scale. *Journal of Advanced Nursing*, 33(2), 250–256.

Ferrell, B.R., & Rivera, L.M. (1995). Ethical decision making in oncology. *Cancer Practice*, 3(2), 94–99.

Fry, S.T., & Duffy, M.E. (2001). The development and psychometric evaluation of the ethical issues scale. *Image: Journal of Nursing Scholarship*, 33(3), 273–277.

Gwin, R.R., & Richters, J.E. (1998). Selected ethical issues in cancer care. In J. Itano, & K. Taoka (eds), *Core curriculum for oncology nurses* (3rd ed.). Philadelphia, PA: WB Saunders, pp. 741–745.

Jameton, A. (1984). *Nursing practice: The ethical issues*. Englewood Cliffs, NJ: Prentice-Hall.

Jameton, A. (1993). Dilemmas of moral distress: Moral responsibility and nursing practice. *AWHONN's Clinical Issues in Perinatal and Women's Health Nursing*, 4(4), 542–551.

Kopala, B., & Burkhart, L. (2005). Ethical dilemma and moral distress: Proposed new NANDA diagnoses. *International Journal of Nursing Terminologies and Classifications*, 16(1), 3–13.

McGee, G., Spanogle, J.P., Caplan, A.L., & Asch, D.A. (2001). A national study of ethics committees. *American Journal of Bioethics*, 1(4), 60–64.

Moore, M.L. (2000). Ethical issues for nurses providing perinatal care in community settings. *Journal of Perinatal and Neonatal Nursing*, 14(2), 25–35.

Omery, A., Henneman, E., Billet, B., Luna-Raines, M., & Brown-Saltzman, K. (1995). Ethical issues in hospital-based nursing practice. *Journal of Cardiovascular Nursing, 9*(3), 43–53.

Pinch, W.J. & Spielman, M.L. (1993). Parental perceptions of ethical issues post-NICU discharge. *Western Journal of Nursing Research, 15*(4), 422–437.

Redman, B.K., & Fry, S.T. (1998a). Ethical conflicts reported by certified registered rehabilitation nurses. *Rehabilitation Nursing, 23*(4), 179–184.

Redman, B.K., & , Fry, S.T. (1998b). Ethical conflicts reported by registered nurse/certified diabetes educators: a replication. *Journal of Advanced Nursing, 28*(6), 1320–1325.

Rodney, P., & Starzomsky, R. (1993). Constraints on the moral agency of nurses. *Canadian Nurse, 89*(9), 23–26.

Scanlon, C. (1994). Survey yields significant results. *American Nurses Association Center for Ethics and Human Rights Communique, 3*(3), 1–3.

Tiedje, L.B. (2000). Moral distress in perinatal nursing. *Journal of Perinatal and Neonatal Nursing, 14*(2), 36–43.

Volbrecht, R.M. (2002). *Nursing ethics: Communities in dialogue.* Upper Saddle River, NJ: Prentice Hall.

Webster, G.C., & Baylis, F. (2000). Moral residue. In S.B. Rubin, & L. Zoloth (eds), *Margin of error: The ethics of mistakes in the practice of medicine.* Hagerstown, MD: University Publishing.

Wilkinson, J.M. (1987/88). Moral distress in nursing practice: Experience and effect. *Nursing Forum, 23*(1), 16–28.

10. Life Principles

Noncompliance (00079)
(1973, 1996, 1998)

Domain 10: Life Principles
Class 3: Value/Belief/Action Congruence

Definition Behavior of person and/or caregiver that fails to coincide with a health-promoting or therapeutic plan agreed on by the person (and/or family and/or community) and healthcare professional. In the presence of an agreed upon, health–promoting, or therapeutic plan, the person's or caregiver's behavior is fully or partially nonadherent and may lead to clinically ineffective or partially ineffective outcomes

Defining Characteristics

- Behavior indicative of failure to adhere
- Evidence of development of complications
- Evidence of exacerbation of symptoms
- Failure to keep appointments
- Failure to progress
- Objective tests provide evidence of failure to adhere (e.g., physiological measures, detection of physiological markers)

Related Factors

Health System

- Access to care
- Communication skills of the provider
- Convenience of care
- Credibility of provider
- Difficulty in client–provider relationship
- Individual health coverage
- Provider continuity
- Provider regular follow-up
- Provider reimbursement
- Satisfaction with care
- Teaching skills of the provider

Healthcare Plan

- Complexity
- Cost
- Duration
- Financial flexibility of plan
- Intensity

Individual

- Cultural influences
- Deficient knowledge related to the regimen behavior
- Developmental abilities
- Health beliefs
- Individual's value system

- Motivational forces
- Personal abilities
- Significant others

- Skill relevant to the regimen behavior
- Spiritual values

Network

- Involvement of members in health plan
- Perceived beliefs of significant others

- Social value regarding plan

10. Life Principles

Impaired Religiosity (00169)
(2004, LOE 2.1)

Domain 10: Life Principles
Class 3: Value/Belief/Action Congruence

Definition Impaired ability to exercise reliance on beliefs and/or participate in rituals of a particular faith tradition

Defining Characteristics

- Difficulty adhering to prescribed religious beliefs
- Difficulty adhering to prescribed religious rituals (e.g., religious ceremonies, dietary regulations, clothing, prayer, worship/religious services, private religious behaviors/reading religious materials/media, holiday observances, meetings with religious leaders)
- Questions religious belief patterns
- Questions religious customs
- Reports a need to reconnect with previous belief patterns
- Reports a need to reconnect with previous customs
- Reports emotional distress because of separation from faith community

Related Factors

Developmental and Situational

- Aging
- End-stage life crises
- Life transitions

Physical

- Illness
- Pain

Psychological

- Anxiety
- Fear of death
- Ineffective coping
- Ineffective support
- Lack of security
- Personal crisis
- Use of religion to manipulate

Sociocultural

- Cultural barriers to practicing religion
- Environmental barriers to practicing religion
- Lack of social integration
- Lack of sociocultural interaction

Spiritual

- Spiritual crises
- Suffering

References

Bellingham, R., Cohen, B., Jones, T., Spaniol, L. (1989). Connectedness: Some skills for spiritual health. *American Journal of Health Promotion, 4*(1), 18–24.

Bergan, A., & McConatha, J.T. (2000). Religiosity and life satisfaction. *Activities, Adaptation and Aging, 24*(3), 23–34.

Besthorn, F.H. (2001). Transpersonal psychology and deep ecological philosophy: Exploring linkages and applications for social work. *Social Thought, 20*(1/2), 23–44.

Burkhardt, M.A. (1989). Spirituality: An analysis of the concept. *Holistic Nursing Practice, 3*(3), 69–77.

Burkhardt, M.A. (1994). Environmental connections and reawakened spirit. In E.A. Schuster, & C.L. Brown (eds), *Exploring our environmental connections*. New York: National League for Nursing, pp. 287–306.

Burkhart, L., & Solari-Twadell, P.A. (2001). Spirituality and religiousness: Differentiating the diagnosis through a review of the nursing literature. *Nursing Diagnosis: International Journal of Nursing Language and Classification, 12*(2), 45–54.

Carroll, M.M. (2001). Conceptual models of spirituality. *Social Thought, 20*(1/2), 5–21.

Carson, V.B., Winkelstein, M., Soeken, K., & Bruinins, M. (1986). The effect of didactic teaching on spiritual attitudes. *Image: Journal of Nursing Scholarship, 18*(4), 161–164.

Charnes, L.S., & Moore, P.S. (1992). Meeting patients' spiritual needs. The Jewish perspective. *Holistic Nursing Practice, 6*(3), 64–72.

Chatters, L.M., Taylor, R.J., & Lincoln, K.D. (2001). Advances in the measurement of religiosity among older African Americans: Implications for health and mental health researchers. *Journal of Mental Health and Aging, 7*(1), 181–200.

Dudley, J.R., Smith, C., & Millison, M.B. (1995). Unfinished business: Assessing the spiritual needs of hospice clients. *American Journal of Hospice and Palliative Care, 12*(2), 30–37.

Durienz, B., Luyten, P., Snauwaert, B., & Hutsebaut, D. (2002). The importance of religiosity and values in predicting political attitudes: Evidence for the continuing importance of religiosity in Flanders (Belgium). *Mental Health, Religion, and Culture, 5*(1), 35–54.

El Haase, J., Britt, T., Copward, D.D., Leidy, N.K., & Penn, P.E. (1992). Simultaneous concept analysis of spiritual perspective, hope, acceptance, and self-transcendence. *Image, 24*(2), 141–147.

Fahlberg, L., Wolfer, J., & Fahlberg, L.A. (1992). Personal crisis: Growth or pathology? *Health Promotion, 7*(1), 45–52.

Fehring, R.J., Brennan, P.F., & Keller, M.L. (1987). Psychological and spiritual well-being in college students. *Research in Nursing and Health, 10*, 391–398.

Freeman, D.R. (2001). The relationship between spiritual development and ethnicity in violent men. *Social Thought, 20*(1/2), 95–107.

Fry, P.S. (2000). Religious involvement, spirituality and personal meaning for life: Existential predictors of psychological wellbeing in community-residing and institutional care elders. *Aging and Mental Health, 4*(4), 375–387.

Hover-Kramer, D. (1989). Creating a context for self-healing: The transpersonal perspective. *Holistic Nursing Practice, 3*(3), 27–34.

Labun, E. (1988). Spiritual care: An element in nursing care planning. *Journal of Advanced Nursing, 13*(3), 314–320.

Maltby, J., & Day, L. (2002). Religious experience, religious orientation and schizotypy. *Mental Health, Religion and Culture, 5*(2), 163–174.

Mansen, T.J. (1993). The spiritual dimension of individuals: Conceptual development. *Nursing Diagnosis, 4*(4), 140–147.

Mayer, J. (1992). Wholly responsible for a part, or partly responsible for a whole? The concept of spiritual care in nursing. *Second Opinion, 17*(3), 26–55.

Mickley, J.R., Soeken, K., & Belcher, A. (1992) Spiritual well-being, religiousness and hope among women with breast cancer. *Image: Journal of Nursing Scholarship, 24*(4), 267–336.

Moberg, D.O. (1984). Subjective measures of spiritual well-being. *Review of Religious Research, 25*(4), 351–364.

10. Life Principles

Nagai-Jacobson, M.G., & Burkhardt, M.A. (1989). Spirituality: Cornerstone of holistic nursing practice. *Holistic Nursing Practice, 3*(3), 18–26.

Narayanasamy, A. (1996). Spiritual care of chronically ill patients. *British Journal of Nursing, 5*(7), 411–416.

Pullen, L., Modrcin-Talbott, M.A., West, W.R., & Muenchen, R. (1999). Spiritual high vs high on spirits: Is religiosity related to adolescent alcohol and drug abuse? *Journal of Psychiatric and Mental Health Nursing, 6,* 3–8.

Reed, P. (1987). Spirituality and well-being in terminally ill hospitalized adults. *Research in Nursing and Health, 15,* 349–357.

Reed, P.G. (1991). Preferences for spiritually related nursing interventions among terminally ill and on terminally ill hospitalized adults and well adults. *Applied Nursing Research, 4*(3), 122–128.

Reed, P.G. (1992). An emerging paradigm for the investigation of spirituality in nursing. *Research in Nursing and Health, 15,* 349–357.

Siddle, R., Haddock, G., Tarrier, N., & Faragher, E.B. (2002). The validation of a religiosity measure for individuals with schizophrenia. *Mental Health, Religion and Culture, 5*(3), 267–284.

Stolley, J.M., Buckwalter, K.C., & Koenig, H.G. (1999). Prayer and religious coping for caregivers of persons with Alzheimer's disease and related disorders. *American Journal of Alzheimer's Disease, 14*(3), 181–191.

Thomas, S.A. (1989). Spirituality: An essential dimension in the treatment of hypertension. *Holistic Nursing Practice, 3*(3), 47–55.

Watson, J. (1994). A frog, a rock, a ritual: Myth, mystery, and metaphors for an ecocaring cosmology in a universe that is turning over. In E.A. Schuster, & C.L. Brown (eds.), *Exploring our environmental connections.* New York: National League for Nursing, pp. 17–39.

Whitfield, W. (2002). Research in religion and mental health: Naming of parts – some reflections. *International Journal of Psychiatric Nursing Research, 8*(1), 891–896.

Readiness for Enhanced Religiosity (00171)

(2004, LOE 2.1)

Domain 10: Life Principles
Class 3: Value/Belief/Action Congruence

Definition A pattern of reliance on religious beliefs and/or participation in rituals of a particular faith tradition that is sufficient for well-being and can be strengthened

Defining Characteristics

- Expresses desire to strengthen belief patterns that have provided religion in the past
- Expresses desire to strengthen religious belief patterns that have provided comfort in the past
- Expresses desire to strengthen religious customs that have provided comfort in the past
- Questions belief patterns that are harmful
- Questions customs that are harmful
- Rejects belief patterns that are harmful
- Rejects customs that are harmful
- Requests assistance to expand religious options
- Requests assistance to increase participation in prescribed religious beliefs (e.g., religious ceremonies, dietary regulations/rituals, clothing, prayer, worship/religious services, private religious behaviors, reading religious materials/media, holiday observances)
- Requests forgiveness
- Requests meeting with religious leaders/facilitators
- Requests reconciliation
- Requests religious experiences
- Requests religious materials

References

Bellingham, R., Cohen, B., Jones, T., Spaniol, L. (1989). Connectedness: Some skills for spiritual health. *American Journal of Health Promotion, 4*(1), 18–24.

Bergan, A., & McConatha, J.T. (2000). Religiosity and life satisfaction. *Activities, Adaptation and Aging, 24*(3), 23–34.

Besthorn, F.H. (2001). Transpersonal psychology and deep ecological philosophy: Exploring linkages and applications for social work. *Social Thought, 20*(1/2), 23–44.

Burkhardt, M.A. (1989). Spirituality: An analysis of the concept. *Holistic Nursing Practice, 3*(3), 69–77.

Burkhardt, M.A. (1994). Environmental connections and reawakened spirit. In E.A. Schuster, & C.L. Brown (eds), *Exploring our environmental connections*. New York: National League for Nursing, pp. 287–306.

Burkhart, L., & Solari-Twadell, P.A. (2001). Spirituality and religiousness: Differentiating the diagnosis through a review of the nursing literature. *Nursing Diagnosis: International Journal of Nursing Language and Classification, 12*(2), 45–54.

Carroll, M.M. (2001). Conceptual models of spirituality. *Social Thought, 20*(1/2), 5–21.

Carson, V.B., Winkelstein, M., Soeken, K., & Bruinins, M. (1986). The effect of didactic teaching on spiritual attitudes. *Image: Journal of Nursing Scholarship, 18*(4), 161–164.

Charnes, L.S., & Moore, P.S. (1992). Meeting patients' spiritual needs. The Jewish perspective. *Holistic Nursing Practice, 6*(3), 64–72.

Chatters, L.M., Taylor, R.J., & Lincoln, K.D. (2001). Advances in the measurement of religiosity among older African Americans: Implications for health and mental health researchers. *Journal of Mental Health and Aging, 7*(1), 181–200.

Dudley, J.R., Smith, C., & Millison, M.B. (1995). Unfinished business: Assessing the spiritual needs of hospice clients. *American Journal of Hospice and Palliative Care, 12*(2), 30–37.

Durienz, B., Luyten, P., Snauwaert, B., & Hutsebaut, D. (2002). The importance of religiosity and values in predicting political attitudes: Evidence for the continuing importance of religiosity in Flanders (Belgium). *Mental Health, Religion, and Culture, 5*(1), 35–54.

El Haase, J., Britt, T., Copward, D.D., Leidy, N.K., & Penn, P.E. (1992). Simultaneous concept analysis of spiritual perspective, hope, acceptance, and self-transcendence. *Image, 24*(2), 141–147.

Fahlberg, L., Wolfer, J., & Fahlberg, L.A. (1992). Personal crisis: Growth or pathology? *Health Promotion, 7*(1), 45–52.

Fehring, R.J., Brennan, P.F., & Keller, M.L. (1987). Psychological and spiritual well-being in college students. *Research in Nursing and Health, 10*, 391–398.

Freeman, D.R. (2001). The relationship between spiritual development and ethnicity in violent men. *Social Thought, 20*(1/2), 95–107.

Fry, P.S. (2000). Religious involvement, spirituality and personal meaning for life: Existential predictors of psychological wellbeing in community-residing and institutional care elders. *Aging and Mental Health, 4*(4), 375–387.

Hover-Kramer, D. (1989). Creating a context for self-healing: The transpersonal perspective. *Holistic Nursing Practice, 3*(3), 27–34.

Labun, E. (1988). Spiritual care: An element in nursing care planning. *Journal of Advanced Nursing, 13*(3), 314–320.

Maltby, J., & Day, L. (2002). Religious experience, religious orientation and schizotypy. *Mental Health, Religion and Culture, 5*(2), 163–174.

Mansen, T.J. (1993). The spiritual dimension of individuals: Conceptual development. *Nursing Diagnosis, 4*(4), 140–147.

Mayer, J. (1992). Wholly responsible for a part, or partly responsible for a whole? The concept of spiritual care in nursing. *Second Opinion, 17*(3), 26–55.

Mickley, J.R., Soeken, K., & Belcher, A. (1992) Spiritual well-being, religiousness and hope among women with breast cancer. *Image: Journal of Nursing Scholarship, 24*(4), 267–336.

Moberg, D.O. (1984). Subjective measures of spiritual well-being. *Review of Religious Research, 25*(4), 351–364.

Nagai-Jacobson, M.G., & Burkhardt, M.A. (1989). Spirituality: Cornerstone of holistic nursing practice. *Holistic Nursing Practice, 3*(3), 18–26.

Narayanasamy, A. (1996). Spiritual care of chronically ill patients. *British Journal of Nursing, 5*(7), 411–416.

Pullen, L., Modrcin-Talbott, M.A., West, W.R., & Muenchen, R. (1999). Spiritual high vs high on spirits: Is religiosity related to adolescent alcohol and drug abuse? *Journal of Psychiatric and Mental Health Nursing, 6*, 3–8.

Reed, P. (1987). Spirituality and well-being in terminally ill hospitalized adults. *Research in Nursing and Health, 15*, 349–357.

Reed, P.G. (1991). Preferences for spiritually related nursing interventions among terminally ill and on terminally ill hospitalized adults and well adults. *Applied Nursing Research, 4*(3), 122–128.

Reed, P.G. (1992). An emerging paradigm for the investigation of spirituality in nursing. *Research in Nursing and Health, 15*, 349–357.

Siddle, R., Haddock, G., Tarrier, N., & Faragher, E.B. (2002). The validation of a religiosity measure for individuals with schizophrenia. *Mental Health, Religion and Culture, 5*(3), 267–284.

Stolley, J.M., Buckwalter, K.C., & Koenig, H.G. (1999). Prayer and religious coping for caregivers of persons with Alzheimer's disease and related disorders. *American Journal of Alzheimer's Disease, 14*(3), 181–191.

Thomas, S.A. (1989). Spirituality: An essential dimension in the treatment of hypertension. *Holistic Nursing Practice, 3*(3), 47–55.

Watson, J. (1994). A frog, a rock, a ritual: Myth, mystery, and metaphors for an ecocaring cosmology in a universe that is turning over. In E.A. Schuster, & C.L. Brown (eds), *Exploring our environmental connections*. New York: National League for Nursing, pp. 17–39.

Whitfield, W. (2002). Research in religion and mental health: Naming of parts – some reflections. *International Journal of Psychiatric Nursing Research, 8*(1), 891–896.

Risk for Impaired **Religiosity** (00170)
(2004, LOE 2.1)

Domain 10: Life Principles
Class 3: Value/Belief/Action Congruence

Definition At risk for an impaired ability to exercise reliance on religious beliefs and/or participate in rituals of a particular faith tradition

Risk Factors

Developmental

- Life transitions

Environmental

- Barriers to practicing religion
- Lack of transportation

Physical

- Hospitalization
- Illness
- Pain

Psychological

- Depression
- Ineffective caregiving
- Ineffective coping
- Ineffective support
- Lack of security

Sociocultural

- Cultural barrier to practicing religion
- Lack of social interaction
- Social isolation

Spiritual

- Suffering

References

Bellingham, R., Cohen, B., Jones, T., Spaniol, L. (1989). Connectedness: Some skills for spiritual health. *American Journal of Health Promotion*, 4(1), 18–24.

Bergan, A., & McConatha, J.T. (2000). Religiosity and life satisfaction. *Activities, Adaptation and Aging*, 24(3), 23–34.

Besthorn, F.H. (2001). Transpersonal psychology and deep ecological philosophy: Exploring linkages and applications for social work. *Social Thought*, 20(1/2), 23–44.

10. Life Principles

Burkhardt, M.A. (1989). Spirituality: An analysis of the concept. *Holistic Nursing Practice*, 3(3), 69–77.

Burkhardt, M.A. (1994). Environmental connections and reawakened spirit. In E.A. Schuster, & C.L. Brown (eds), *Exploring our environmental connections*. New York: National League for Nursing, pp. 287–306.

Burkhart, L., & Solari-Twadell, P.A. (2001). Spirituality and religiousness: Differentiating the diagnosis through a review of the nursing literature. *Nursing Diagnosis: International Journal of Nursing Language and Classification*, 12(2), 45–54.

Carroll, M.M. (2001). Conceptual models of spirituality. *Social Thought*, 20(1/2), 5–21.

Carson, V.B., Winkelstein, M., Soeken, K., & Bruinins, M. (1986). The effect of didactic teaching on spiritual attitudes. *Image: Journal of Nursing Scholarship*, 18(4), 161–164.

Charnes, L.S., & Moore, P.S. (1992). Meeting patients' spiritual needs. The Jewish perspective. *Holistic Nursing Practice*, 6(3), 64–72.

Chatters, L.M., Taylor, R.J., & Lincoln, K.D. (2001). Advances in the measurement of religiosity among older African Americans: Implications for health and mental health researchers. *Journal of Mental Health and Aging*, 7(1), 181–200.

Dudley, J.R., Smith, C., & Millison, M.B. (1995). Unfinished business: Assessing the spiritual needs of hospice clients. *American Journal of Hospice and Palliative Care*, 12(2), 30–37.

Durienz, B., Luyten, P., Snauwaert, B., & Hutsebaut, D. (2002). The importance of religiosity and values in predicting political attitudes: Evidence for the continuing importance of religiosity in Flanders (Belgium). *Mental Health, Religion, and Culture*, 5(1), 35–54.

El Haase, J., Britt, T., Copward, D.D., Leidy, N.K., & Penn, P.E. (1992). Simultaneous concept analysis of spiritual perspective, hope, acceptance, and self-transcendence. *Image*, 24(2), 141–147.

Fahlberg, L., Wolfer, J., & Fahlberg, L.A. (1992). Personal crisis: Growth or pathology? *Health Promotion*, 7(1), 45–52.

Fehring, R.J., Brennan, P.F., & Keller, M.L. (1987). Psychological and spiritual well-being in college students. *Research in Nursing and Health*, 10, 391–398.

Freeman, D.R. (2001). The relationship between spiritual development and ethnicity in violent men. *Social Thought*, 20(1/2), 95–107.

Fry, P.S. (2000). Religious involvement, spirituality and personal meaning for life: Existential predictors of psychological wellbeing in community-residing and institutional care elders. *Aging and Mental Health*, 4(4), 375–387.

Hover-Kramer, D. (1989). Creating a context for self-healing: The transpersonal perspective. *Holistic Nursing Practice*, 3(3), 27–34.

Labun, E. (1988). Spiritual care: An element in nursing care planning. *Journal of Advanced Nursing*, 13(3), 314–320.

Maltby, J., & Day, L. (2002). Religious experience, religious orientation and schizotypy. *Mental Health, Religion and Culture*, 5(2), 163–174.

Mansen, T.J. (1993). The spiritual dimension of individuals: Conceptual development. *Nursing Diagnosis*, 4(4), 140–147.

Mayer, J. (1992). Wholly responsible for a part, or partly responsible for a whole? The concept of spiritual care in nursing. *Second Opinion*, 17(3), 26–55.

Mickley, J.R., Soeken, K., & Belcher, A. (1992) Spiritual well-being, religiousness and hope among women with breast cancer. *Image: Journal of Nursing Scholarship*, 24(4), 267–336.

Moberg, D.O. (1984). Subjective measures of spiritual well-being. *Review of Religious Research*, 25(4), 351–364.

Nagai-Jacobson, M.G., & Burkhardt, M.A. (1989). Spirituality: Cornerstone of holistic nursing practice. *Holistic Nursing Practice*, 3(3), 18–26.

Narayanasamy, A. (1996). Spiritual care of chronically ill patients. *British Journal of Nursing*, 5(7), 411–416.

Pullen, L., Modrcin-Talbott, M.A., West, W.R., & Muenchen, R. (1999). Spiritual high vs high on spirits: Is religiosity related to adolescent alcohol and drug abuse? *Journal of Psychiatric and Mental Health Nursing*, 6, 3–8.

Reed, P. (1987). Spirituality and well-being in terminally ill hospitalized adults. *Research in Nursing and Health*, 15, 349–357.

Reed, P.G. (1991). Preferences for spiritually related nursing interventions among terminally ill and on terminally ill hospitalized adults and well adults. *Applied Nursing Research*, 4(3), 122–128.

Reed, P.G. (1992). An emerging paradigm for the investigation of spirituality in nursing. *Research in Nursing and Health*, 15, 349–357.

Siddle, R., Haddock, G., Tarrier, N., & Faragher, E.B. (2002). The validation of a religiosity measure for individuals with schizophrenia. *Mental Health, Religion and Culture*, 5(3), 267–284.

Stolley, J.M., Buckwalter, K.C., & Koenig, H.G. (1999). Prayer and religious coping for caregivers of persons with Alzheimer's disease and related disorders. *American Journal of Alzheimer's Disease*, 14(3), 181–191.

Thomas, S.A. (1989). Spirituality: An essential dimension in the treatment of hypertension. *Holistic Nursing Practice*, 3(3), 47–55.

Watson, J. (1994). A frog, a rock, a ritual: Myth, mystery, and metaphors for an ecocaring cosmology in a universe that is turning over. In E.A. Schuster, & C.L. Brown (eds), *Exploring our environmental connections*, New York: National League for Nursing, pp. 17–39.

Whitfield, W. (2002). Research in religion and mental health: Naming of parts – some reflections. *International Journal of Psychiatric Nursing Research*, 8(1), 891–896.

10. Life Principles

Spiritual Distress (00066)

(1978, 2002, LOE 2.1)

Domain 10: Life Principles
Class 3: Value/Belief/Action Congruence

Definition Impaired ability to experience and integrate meaning and purpose in life through connectedness with self, others, art, music, literature, nature, and/or a power greater than oneself

Defining Characteristics

Connections to Self

- Anger
- Expresses lack of acceptance
- Expresses lack of courage
- Expresses lack of hope
- Expresses lack of love
- Expresses lack of meaning in life
- Expresses lack of purpose in life
- Expresses lack of self-forgiveness
- Expresses lack of serenity (e.g., peace)
- Guilt
- Ineffective coping

Connections with Others

- Expresses alienation
- Refuses interactions with significant others
- Refuses interactions with spiritual leaders
- Verbalizes being separated from support system

Connections with Art, Music, Literature, and Nature

- Disinterest in nature
- Disinterest in reading spiritual literature
- Inability to express previous state of creativity (e.g., singing/listening to music/writing)

Connections with Power Greater than Self

- Expresses anger toward power greater than self
- Expresses feeling abandoned
- Expresses hopelessness
- Expresses suffering
- Inability for introspection
- Inability to experience the transcendent
- Inability to participate in religious activities
- Inability to pray
- Requests to see a spiritual leader
- Sudden changes in spiritual practices

Related Factors

- Active dying
- Anxiety
- Chronic illness
- Death
- Life change

- Loneliness
- Pain
- Self-alienation
- Social alienation
- Sociocultural deprivation

Risk for Spiritual Distress (00067)
(1998, 2004, LOE 2.1)

Domain 10: Life Principles
Class 3: Value/Belief/Action Congruence

Definition
At risk for an impaired ability to experience and integrate meaning and purpose in life through connectedness with self, others, art, music, literature, nature, and/or a power greater than oneself

Risk Factors

Developmental

- Life changes

Environmental

- Environmental changes
- Natural disasters

Physical

- Chronic illness
- Physical illness
- Substance abuse

Psychosocial

- Anxiety
- Blocks to experiencing love
- Change in religious rituals
- Change in spiritual practices
- Cultural conflict
- Depression
- Inability to forgive
- Loss
- Low self-esteem
- Poor relationships
- Racial conflict
- Separated support systems
- Stress

References

Bellingham, R., Cohen, B., Jones, T., Spaniol, L. (1989). Connectedness: Some skills for spiritual health. *American Journal of Health Promotion*, 4(1), 18–24.

Bergan, A., & McConatha, J.T. (2000). Religiosity and life satisfaction. *Activities, Adaptation and Aging*, 24(3), 23–34.

Besthorn, F.H. (2001). Transpersonal psychology and deep ecological philosophy: Exploring linkages and applications for social work. *Social Thought*, 20(1/2), 23–44.

Burkhardt, M.A. (1989). Spirituality: An analysis of the concept. *Holistic Nursing Practice*, 3(3), 69–77.

Burkhardt, M.A. (1994). Environmental connections and reawakened spirit. In E.A. Schuster, & C.L. Brown (eds), *Exploring our environmental connections*. New York: National League for Nursing, pp. 287–306.

Burkhart, L., & Solari-Twadell, P.A. (2001). Spirituality and religiousness: Differentiating the diagnosis through a review of the nursing literature. *Nursing Diagnosis: International Journal of Nursing Language and Classification, 12*(2), 45–54.

Carroll, M.M. (2001). Conceptual models of spirituality. *Social Thought, 20*(1/2), 5–21.

Carson, V.B., Winkelstein, M., Soeken, K., & Bruinins, M. (1986). The effect of didactic teaching on spiritual attitudes. *Image: Journal of Nursing Scholarship, 18*(4), 161–164.

Cavendish, R., Luise, B., Bauer, M., Gallo, M.A., Horne, K., Medefindt, J., & Russo, D. (2001). Recognizing opportunities for spiritual enhancement in young adults. *Nursing Diagnosis: International Journal of Nursing Language and Classification, 12*(3), 77-91.

Dudley, J.R., Smith, C., & Millison, M.B. (1995). Unfinished business: Assessing the spiritual needs of hospice clients. *American Journal of Hospice and Palliative Care, 12*(2), 30–37.

El Haase, J., Britt, T., Copward, D.D., Leidy, N.K., & Penn, P.E. (1992). Simultaneous concept analysis of spiritual perspective, hope, acceptance, and self-transcendence. *Image, 24*(2), 141–147.

Fahlberg, L., Wolfer, J., & Fahlberg, L.A. (1992). Personal crisis: Growth or pathology? *Health Promotion, 7*(1), 45–52.

Fehring, R.J., Brennan, P.F., & Keller, M.L. (1987). Psychological and spiritual well-being in college students. *Research in Nursing and Health, 10*, 391–398.

Freeman, D.R. (2001). The relationship between spiritual development and ethnicity in violent men. *Social Thought, 20*(1/2), 95–107.

Fry, P.S. (2000). Religious involvement, spirituality and personal meaning for life: Existential predictors of psychological wellbeing in community-residing and institutional care elders. *Aging and Mental Health, 4*(4), 375–387.

Hover-Kramer, D. (1989). Creating a context for self-healing: The transpersonal perspective. *Holistic Nursing Practice, 3*(3), 27–34.

Labun, E. (1988). Spiritual care: An element in nursing care planning. *Journal of Advanced Nursing, 13*(3), 314–320.

Mansen, T.J. (1993). The spiritual dimension of individuals: Conceptual development. *Nursing Diagnosis, 4*(4), 140–147.

Mayer, J. (1992). Wholly responsible for a part, or partly responsible for a whole? The concept of spiritual care in nursing. *Second Opinion, 17*(3), 26–55.

Moberg, D.O. (1984). Subjective measures of spiritual well-being. *Review of Religious Research, 25*(4), 351–364.

Nagai-Jacobson, M.G., & Burkhardt, M.A. (1989). Spirituality: Cornerstone of holistic nursing practice. *Holistic Nursing Practice, 3*(3), 18–26.

Narayanasamy, A. (1996). Spiritual care of chronically ill patients. *British Journal of Nursing, 5*(7), 411–416.

Reed, P. (1987). Spirituality and well-being in terminally ill hospitalized adults. *Research in Nursing and Health, 15*, 349–357.

Reed, P.G. (1991). Preferences for spiritually related nursing interventions among terminally ill and on terminally ill hospitalized adults and well adults. *Applied Nursing Research, 4*(3), 122–128.

Reed, P.G. (1992). An emerging paradigm for the investigation of spirituality in nursing. *Research in Nursing and Health, 15*, 349–357.

Thomas, S.A. (1989). Spirituality: An essential dimension in the treatment of hypertension. *Holistic Nursing Practice, 3*(3), 47–55.

Watson, J. (1994). A frog, a rock, a ritual: Myth, mystery, and metaphors for an ecocaring cosmology in a universe that is turning over. In E.A. Schuster, & C.L. Brown (eds.), *Exploring our environmental connections.* New York: National League for Nursing, pp. 17–39.

10. Life Principles

Domain 11
Safety/Protection

NANDA International Nursing Diagnoses: Definitions & Classification 2012–2014, First Edition.
Edited by T. Heather Herdman.
© 2012 NANDA International. Published 2012 by Blackwell Publishing Ltd.

Domain 11: Safety/Protection
Class 1: Infection

Definition At risk for being invaded by pathogenic organisms

Risk Factors

- Chronic disease
  - Diabetes mellitus
  - Obesity
- Deficient knowledge to avoid exposure to pathogens
- Inadequate primary defenses
  - Altered peristalsis
  - Broken skin (e.g., intravenous catheter placement, invasive procedures)
  - Change in pH of secretions
  - Decrease in ciliary action
  - Premature rupture of amniotic membranes
  - Prolonged rupture of amniotic membranes
  - Smoking
  - Stasis of body fluids
  - Traumatized tissue (e.g., trauma, tissue destruction)
- Inadequate secondary defenses
  - Decreased hemoglobin

- Immunosuppression (e.g., inadequate acquired immunity; pharmaceutical agents including immunosuppressants, steroids, monoclonal antibodies, immunomodulators)
  - Leukopenia
  - Suppressed inflammatory response
- Inadequate vaccination
- Increased environmental exposure to pathogens
  - Outbreaks
- Invasive procedures
- Malnutrition

References

Alexander, M. (ed.). (2006). Infusion Nursing: Standards of Practice [Special issue]. *Journal of Infusion Nursing, 29*(1S).

Allen, U., & Green, M. (2010). Prevention and treatment of infectious complications after solid organ transplantation in children. *Pediatric Clinics of North America, 57*, 459–479.

Ata, A., Lee, J., Bestle, S.L., Desemone, J., & Stain, S.C. (2010). Postoperative hyperglycemia and surgical site infection in general surgery patients. *Archives of Surgery, 145*, 858–864.

Ata, A., Valerian, B.T., Lee, E.C., Bestle, S.L., Elmendorf, S.L., & Stain, S.C. (2010). The effect of diabetes mellitus on surgical site infections after colorectal and non colorectal general surgical operations. *American Surgeon, 76*, 697–702.

Balentine, C.J., Wilks, J., Robinson, C., Marshall, C., Anaya, D., Albo, D., & Berger, D.H. (2010). Obesity increases wound complications in rectal cancer surgery. *Journal of Surgical Research, 163*(1), 35–39.

Bentsi-Enchill, A.D., Halperin, S.A., Scott, J., Maclsaac, K., & Duclos, P. (1997). Estimates of the effectiveness of the whole-cell pertussis vaccine from an outbreak in an immunized population. *Vaccine, 15*, 301–306.

Bleasdale, S.C., Trick, W.E., Gonzales, I.M., Lyles, R.D., Hayden, M.K., & Weinstein, R.A. (2007). Effectiveness of chlorhexidine bathing to reduce catheter-associated bloodstream infections in medical intensive care unit patients. *Archives of Internal Medicine, 167*, 2073–2079.

Bochicchio, G.V., Bochicchio, K.M., Joshi, M., Ilathi, O., & Scalea, T.M. (2010). Acute glucose elevation is highly predictive of infection and outcome in critically injured trauma patients. *Annals of Surgery, 252*, 597–602.

Bouza, E., Muñoz, P., López-Rodríguez, J., Jesús Pérez, M., Rincón, C., Martin Rabadán, P., Sánchez, C., & Bastida, P. M. (2003). A needleless closed system device (CLAVE) protects from intravascular catheter tip and hub colonization: A prospective randomized study. *Journal of Hospital Infection, 54*, 279–287.

Chee, Y.H., Teoh, K.H., Sabnis, B.M., Ballantyne, J.A., & Brenkel, I.J. (2010). Total hip replacement in morbidly obese patients with osteoarthritis: results of a prospectively matched study. *Journal of Bone and Joint Surgery Br, 92*, 1066–1071.

Chen, S., Anderson, M.V., Cheng, W.K., & Wongworawat, M.D. (2009). Diabetes associated with increased surgical site infections in spinal arthrodesis. *Clinical Orthopaedics and Related Research, 467*, 1670–1673.

Claridge, J.A., Sawyer, R.G., Schulman, A.M., McLemore, E.C., & Young, J.S. (2002). Blood transfusions correlate with infections in trauma patients in a dose-dependent manner. *American Surgeon, 68*, 566–572.

Cousens, S., Blencowe, H., Gravett, M., & Lawn, J. (2010). Antibiotic for pre-term pre-labour rupture of membranes: Prevention of neonatal deaths due to complications of pre-term birth and infection. *International Journal of Epidemiology, 39*, 134–143.

Cuellar-Rodriguez, J., & Sierra-Madero, J.G. (2005). Infections in solid organ transplant recipients. *Revista de Investigacion Clinica, 57*, 368–380.

Cunningham-Rundles, S., McNeeley, D.F., & Moon, A. (2005). Mechanisms of nutrient modulation of the immune response. *Journal of Allergy and Clinical Immunology, 115*, 1119–1128.

Dorner, T.E., Schwarz, F., Kranz, A., Freidl, W., Reider, A., & Gisinger, C. (2010). Body mass index and the risk of infections in institutionalized geriatric patients. *British Journal of Nutrition, 103*, 1830–1835.

Dossett, L.A., Dageforde, L.A., Swenson, B.R., Metzger, R., Bonatti, H., Sawyer, R.G., & May, A.K. (2009). Obesity and site-specific nosocomial infection risk in the intensive care unit. *Surgical Infections, 10*, 137–142.

Falagas, M.E., & Kompoti, M. (2006). Obesity and infection. *Lancet Infectious Diseases, 6*, 438–446.

Food and Drug Administration (2001). Important drug warning (Remicade). Retrieved from http://www.fda.gov/Safety/MedWatch/SafetyInformation/SafetyAlertsforHumanMedicalProducts/ucm172751.htm.

Food and Drug Administration (2006). FDA approves resumed marketing of Tysabri under a special distribution program. Retrieved from http://www.fda.gov/NewsEvents/Newsroom/PressAnnouncements/2006/ucm108662.htm.

Free Dictionary (2009). Infection. Retrieved from http://medical-dictionary.thefreedictionary.com/infection.

Gea-Banacloche, J.C., & Weinberg, G.A. (2007). Monoclonal antibody therapeutics and risk for infection. *Pediatric Infectious Disease Journal, 26*, 1049–1052.

Giles, K.A., Hamdan, A.D., Pomposelli, F.B., Wyers, M.C., Siracuse, J.J., & Schermerhorn, M.L. (2010). Body mass index: Surgical site infections and mortality after lower extremity bypass from the National Surgical Quality Improvement Program 2005–2007. *Annals of Vascular Surgery, 24*, 48–56.

Gomez, R., Romero, R., Nien, J.K., Medina, L., Carstens, M., Kim, Y.M. et al. (2007). Antibiotic administration to patients with preterm premature rupture of membranes does not eradicate intra-amniotic infection. *Journal of Maternal Fetal and Neonatal Medicine, 20*, 167–173.

Gravante, G., Araco, A., Sorge, R., Araco, F., Delogu, D., & Cervelli, V. (2007). Wound infections in post-bariatric patients undergoing body contouring abdominoplasty: The role of smoking. *Obesity Surgery, 17*, 1325–1331.

Gravante, G., Araco, A., Sorge, R., Araco, F., Delogu, D., & Cervelli, V. (2008). Wound infections in body contouring mastopexy with breast reduction after laparoscopic adjustable gastric banding: The role of smoking. *Obesity Surgery, 18*, 721–727.

Greco, J.A. III, Castaldo, E.T., Nanney, L.B., Wu, Y.C., Donahue, R., Wendel, J.J. et al. (2008). Autologous breast reconstruction: The Vanderbilt experience (1998 to 2005) of independent predictors of displeasing outcomes. *Journal of the American College of Surgeons, 207*(1), 49–56.

Greenberg, J.D., Reed, G., Kremer, J.M., Tindall, E., Kavanaugh, A., Zheng, C. et al.; CORRONA Investigators. (2010). Association of methotrexate and tumour necrosis factor antagonists with risk of infectious outcomes including opportunistic infections in the CORRONA registry. *Annals of the Rheumatic Diseases, 69*, 380–386.

Ho, L.C., Wang, H.H., Chiang, C.K., Hung, K.Y., & Wu, K.D. (2010). Malnutrition-inflammation scores independently determined cardiovascular and infection risk in peritoneal dialysis patients. *Blood Purification, 29,* 308–316.

Itani, K.M., Jensen, E.H., Finn, T.S., Tomassini, J.E., & Abramson, M.A. (2008). Effect of body mass index and ertapenem versus cefotetan prophylaxis on surgical site infection in elective colorectal surgery. *Surgical Infections, 9,* 131–137.

Jamsen, E., Nevalainen, P., Kalliovalkama, J., & Moilanen, T. (2010). Preoperative hyperglycemia predicts infected total knee replacement. *European Journal of Internal Medicine, 21,* 196–201.

Kamar, N., Milioto, O., Puissant-Lubrano, B., Esposito, L., Pierre, M.C., Mohamed, A.O. et al. (2010). Incidence and predictive factors for infectious disease after rituximab therapy in kidney transplant patients. *American Journal of Transplantation, 10,* 89–98.

Kurpad, A.V. (2006). The requirements of protein and amino acid during acute and chronic infections. *Indian Journal of Medical Research, 124,* 129–148.

Kyaw, M.H., Holmes, E.M., Toolis, F., Wayne, B., Chalmers, J., Jones, I.G. & Campbell, H. (2006). Evaluation of severe infection and survival after splenectomy. *American Journal of Medicine, 119,* 276.e1–7.

Len, O., & Pahissa, A. (2007). Donor-transmitted infections. *Enfermedades Infecciosas y Microbiologia Clinica, 25,* 204–212.

Lynch, R.J., Ranney, D.N., Shijie, C., Lee, D.S., Samala, N., & Englesbe, M.J. (2009). Obesity, surgical site infection, and outcome following renal transplantation. *Annals of Surgery, 250,* 1014–1020.

McMillan, M., & Davis, J.S. (2010). Acute hospital admission for sepsis: An important but under-utilized opportunity for smoking cessation interventions. *Australian and New Zealand Journal of Public Health, 34,* 432–433.

Malinzak, R.A., Ritter, M.A., Berend, M.E., Meding, J.B., Olberding, E.M., & Davis, K.E. (2009). Morbidly obese, diabetic, younger, and unilateral joint arthroplasty patients have elevated total joint arthroplasty infection rates. *Journal of Arthroplasty, 24*(6), 84–88.

Martin-Peña, A., Cordero, E., Fijo, J., Sánchez-Moreno, A., Martin-Govantes, J., Torrubia, F., & Cisneros, J. (2009). Prospective study of infectious complications in a cohort of pediatric renal transplant recipients. *Pediatric Transplantation, 13,* 457–463.

Mayr, F.B., Yende, S., Linde-Zwirble, W.T., Peck-Palmer, O.M., Barnato, A.E., Weissfeld, L.A., & Angus, D.C. (2010). Infection rate and acute organ dysfunction risk as explanations for racial differences in severe sepsis. *JAMA, 303,* 2495–2503.

Medscape (2004). Nutritional support and the surgical patient: Plasma proteins. Retrieved from http://www.medscape.com/viewarticle/474066_6.

Morelon, E., & Touraine, J.L. (2007). Infectious complications due to immunosuppression in organ transplant patients. *Revue du Praticien, 57,* 1677–1686.

Offner, P.J., Moore, E.E., Biffl, W.L., Johnson, J.L., & Silliman, C.C. (2002). Increased rate of infection associated with transfusion of old blood after severe injury. *Archives of Surgery, 137,* 711–716.

Oguz, Y., Bulucu, F., Oktenli, C., Doganci, L., & Vural, A. (2002). Infectious complications in 135 Turkish renal transplant patients. *Central European Journal of Public Health, 10,* 153–156.

Olsen, M.A., Nepple, J.J., Riew, K.D., Lenke, L.G., Bridwell, K.H., Mayfield, J., & Fraser, V.J. (2008). Risk factors for surgical site infection following orthopaedic spinal operations. *Journal of Bone and Joint Surgery Am, 90,* 62–69.

Oltean, M., Herlenius, G., Gabel, M., Friman, V., & Olausson, M. (2006). Infectious complications after multivisceral transplantation in adults. *Transplantation Proceedings, 38,* 2683–2685.

Phaneuf, M. (2008). Clinical judgement – an essential tool in the nursing profession. Retrieved from www.infiressources.ca/.../Clinical_Judgement–An_Essential_Tool_in_the_Nursing_Profession.pdf.

Prielipp, R.C., & Sherertz, R.J. (2003). Skin: The first battlefield. *Anesthesia and Analgesia, 97,* 933–935.

Rupp, M.E., Jourdan, M.D., Tyner, L.K., Iwen, P.C., & Anderson, J.R. (2007). Outbreak of bloodstream infections temporally associated with the use of an intravascular positive displacement needleless valve. *Clinical Infectious Diseases, 44,* 1408–1414.

Schilling, S., Doellman, D., Hutchinson, N., & Jacobs, B. (2006). The impact of needleless connector device design on central venous catheter occlusion in children: A prospective, controlled trial. *Journal of Parenteral and Enteral Nutrition, 30*(2), 85–90.

Serrano, P.E., Khuder, S.A., & Fath, J.J. (2010). Obesity as a risk factor for nosocomial infections in trauma patients. *Journal of the American College of Surgeons, 211,* 61–67.

Sharma, M., Fakih, M.G., Berriel-Cass, D., Meisner, S., Saravolatz, S., & Khatib, R. (2009). Harvest surgical site infection following coronary artery bypass grafting: Risk factors, microbiology, and outcomes. *American Journal of Infection Control, 37,* 653–657.

Shepherd, R.W., Turmelle, Y., Nadler, M., Lowell, J.A., Narkewicz, M.R., McDiarmid, S.V. et al.; SPLIT Research Group. (2008). Risk factors for rejection and infection in pediatric liver transplantation. *American Journal of Transplantation, 8*, 396–403.

Smith, R.L., Chong, T.W., Hedrick, T.L., Hughes, M.G., Evans, H.L., McElearney, S.T. et al. (2007). Does body mass index affect infection-related outcomes in the intensive care unit? *Surgical Infections, 8*, 581–588.

Sommerer, C., Konstandin, M., Dengler, T., Schmidt, J., Meuer, S., Zeier, M., & Giese, T. (2006). Pharmacodynamic monitoring of cyclosporine in renal allograft recipients shows a quantitative relationship between immunosuppression and the occurrence of recurrent infections and malignancies. *Transplantation, 82*, 1280–1285.

Spinkler-Vesel, A., Bengmark, S., Vovk, I., Cerovic, O., & Kompan, L. (2007). Symbiotics, prebiotics, glutamine, or peptide in early enteral nutrition: A randomized study in trauma patients. *Journal of Parenteral and Enteral Nutrition, 31*, 119–126.

Towfigh, S., Chen, F., Katkhouda, N., Kelso, R., Sohn, H., Berne, T.V., & Mason, R.J. (2008). Obesity should not influence the management of appendicitis. *Surgical Endoscopy, 22*, 2601–2605.

Tuggle, D.W., Kuhn, M.A., Jones, S.K., Garza, J.J., & Skinner, S. (2008). Hyperglycemia and infections in pediatric trauma patients. *American Surgeon, 73*, 195–198.

Tyburski, J.G., Wilson, R.F., Warsow, K.M., & McCreadie, S. (1998). A trial of ciprofloxacin and metronidazole vs. gentamicin and metronidazole for penetrating abdominal trauma. *Archives of Surgery, 133*, 1289–1296.

Tyburski, J.G., Dente, C.J., Wilson, R.F., Shanti, C., Steffes, C.P., & Carlin, A. (2001). Infectious complications following duodenal and/or pancreatic trauma. *American Surgeon, 67*, 227–230.

University of Illinois at Chicago (2010). Lesson 1. Introduction to epidemiology. Retrieved from, http://www.uic.edu/uic/search.shtml?cx=009511351313755808885%3Adkx-7mlm6ni&cof=FORID%3A11&ie=UTF-8&q=epidemeologic+triad&sa=#1257.

Veenema, T.G., & Toke, J. (2006). Early detection and surveillance for biopreparedness and emerging infectious disease. *Online Journal of Issues in Nursing, 11*. Retrieved from http://www.nursingworld.org/MainMenuCategories/ANAMarketplace/ANAPeriodicals/OJIN/TableofContents/Volume112006/No1Jan06/tpc29_2c16059.aspx.

Veroux, M., Giuffrida, G., Corona, D., Gagliano, M., Scriffignano, V., Vizcarra, D. et al. (2008). Infective complications in renal allograft recipients: Epidemiology and outcomes. *Transplantation Proceedings, 40*, 1873–1876.

Waisbren, E., Rosen, H., Bader, A.M., Lipsitz, S.R., Rogers, S.O., & Eriksson, E. (2010). Percent body fat and prediction of surgical site infection. *Journal of the American College of Surgeons, 210*, 381–389.

Wang, Z., Tobler, S., Roayaei, J., & Eick, A. (2009). Live attenuated or inactivated influenza vaccines and medical encounters for respiratory illnesses among US military personnel. *JAMA, 301*, 945–953.

Weng, J., Brown, C.V., Rhee, P., Salim, A., Chan, L., Demetriades, D., & Velmahos, G.C. (2005). White blood cell and platelet counts can be used to differentiate between infection and the normal response after splenectomy for trauma: Prospective validation. *Journal of Trauma, 59*, 1076–1080.

Wukich, D.K., Lowery, N.J., McMillen, R.L., & Frykberg, R.G. (2010). Postoperative infection rates in foot and ankle surgery: A comparison of patients with and without diabetes mellitus. *Journal of Bone and Joint Surgery, 92*, 287–295.

11. Safety/Protection

Ineffective Airway Clearance (00031)
(1980, 1996, 1998)

Domain 11: Safety/Protection
Class 2: Physical Injury

Definition Inability to clear secretions or obstructions from the respiratory tract to maintain a clear airway

Defining Characteristics

- Absent cough
- Adventitious breath sounds
- Changes in respiratory rate
- Changes in respiratory rhythm
- Cyanosis
- Difficulty vocalizing
- Diminished breath sounds
- Dyspnea
- Excessive sputum
- Ineffective cough
- Orthopnea
- Restlessness
- Wide-eyed

Related Factors

Environmental

- Second-hand smoke
- Smoke inhalation
- Smoking

Obstructed Airway

- Airway spasm
- Excessive mucus
- Exudate in the alveoli
- Foreign body in airway
- Presence of artificial airway
- Retained secretions
- Secretions in the bronchi

Physiological

- Allergic airways
- Asthma
- Chronic obstructive pulmonary disease
- Hyperplasia of the bronchial walls
- Infection
- Neuromuscular dysfunction

11. Safety/Protection

Risk for Aspiration (00039)
(1988)

Domain 11: Safety/Protection
Class 2: Physical Injury

Definition At risk for entry of gastrointestinal secretions, oropharyngeal secretions, solids, or fluids into the tracheobronchial passages

Risk Factors

- Decreased gastrointestinal motility
- Delayed gastric emptying
- Depressed cough
- Depressed gag reflex
- Facial surgery
- Facial trauma
- Gastrointestinal tubes
- Impaired swallowing
- Incompetent lower esophageal sphincter
- Increased gastric residual
- Increased intragastric pressure
- Neck surgery
- Neck trauma
- Oral surgery
- Oral trauma
- Presence of endotracheal tube
- Presence of tracheostomy tube
- Reduced level of consciousness
- Situations hindering elevation of upper body
- Treatment-related side effects (e.g., pharmaceutical agents)
- Tube feedings
- Wired jaws

Risk for Bleeding (00206)
(2008, LOE 2.1)

Domain 11: Safety/Protection
Class 2: Physical Injury

Definition At risk for a decrease in blood volume that may compromise health

Risk Factors

- Aneurysm
- Circumcision
- Deficient knowledge
- Disseminated intravascular coagulopathy
- History of falls
- Gastrointestinal disorders (e.g., gastric ulcer disease, polyps, varices)
- Impaired liver function (e.g., cirrhosis, hepatitis)
- Inherent coagulopathies (e.g., thrombocytopenia)
- Postpartum complications (e.g., uterine atony, retained placenta)
- Pregnancy-related complications (e.g., placenta previa, molar pregnancy, placenta abruptio [placental abruption])
- Trauma
- Treatment-related side effects (e.g., surgery, medications, administration of platelet-deficient blood products, chemotherapy)

References

Brozenec, S.A. (2007). Hepatic problems. In F.D. Monahan, J.K. Sands, M. Neighbors, J.F. Marek, & C.J. Green-Nigro (eds), *Phipp's medical-surgical nursing: Health and illness perspectives* (8th ed.). St. Louis, MO: Mosby Elsevier, pp. 1315–1350.

Deitch, E.A., & Dayal, S.D. (2006). Intensive care unit management of the trauma patient. *Critical Care Medicine*, 34(9), 2294–2301, 2309.

Erickson, J., & Field, R. (2007). Cancer. In F.D. Monahan, J.K. Sands, M. Neighbors, J.F. Marek, & C.J. Green-Nigro (eds), *Phipp's medical-surgical nursing: Health and illness perspectives* (8th ed.). St. Louis, MO: Mosby Elsevier, pp. 510–564.

Garrigues, A.L. (2007). Hematologic problems. In F.D. Monahan, J.K. Sands, M. Neighbors, J.F. Marek, & C.J. Green-Nigro (eds), *Phipp's medical-surgical nursing: Health and illness perspectives* (8th ed.). St. Louis, MO: Mosby Elsevier, pp. 908–942.

Kleinpill, R. (2007). Supporting independence in hospitalized elders in acute care. *Critical Care Nursing Clinics of North America*, 19(3), 247–252.

Lowdermilk, D., & Perry, S. (2006). *Maternity nursing* (7th ed.). St. Louis, MO: Mosby Elsevier, pp. 599–601.

Marek, J., & Boehnlein, M. (2007). Postoperative nursing. In F.D. Monahan, J.K. Sands, M. Neighbors, J.F. Marek, & C.J. Green-Nigro (eds), *Phipp's medical-surgical nursing: Health and illness perspectives* (8th ed.). St. Louis, MO: Mosby Elsevier, pp. 302–332.

Mattson, S., & Smith, J. (eds.). (2004). *Core curriculum for maternal-newborn nursing* (3rd ed.). St. Louis, MO: Elsevier Saunders.

Maxwell-Thompson, C., & Reid, K. (2007). Vascular problems. In F.D. Monahan, J.K. Sands, M. Neighbors, J.F. Marek, & C.J. Green-Nigro (eds), *Phipp's medical-surgical nursing: Health and illness perspectives* (8th ed.). St. Louis, MO: Mosby Elsevier, pp. 857–896.

Sands, J.K. (2007). Stomach and duodenal problems. In F.D. Monahan, J.K. Sands, M. Neighbors, J.F. Marek, & C.J. Green-Nigro (eds), *Phipp's medical-surgical nursing: Health and illness perspectives* (8th ed.). St. Louis, MO: Mosby Elsevier, pp. 1204–1237.

Warshaw, M. (2007). Male reproductive problems. In F.D. Monahan, J.K. Sands, M. Neighbors, J.F. Marek, & C.J. Green-Nigro (eds), *Phipp's medical-surgical nursing: Health and illness perspectives* (8th ed.). St. Louis, MO: Mosby Elsevier, pp. 1721–1749.

Impaired Dentition (00048)
(1998)

Domain 11: Safety/Protection
Class 2: Physical Injury

Definition Disruption in tooth development/eruption patterns or structural integrity of individual teeth

Defining Characteristics

- Abraded teeth
- Absent teeth
- Asymmetrical facial expression
- Crown caries
- Erosion of enamel
- Excessive calculus
- Excessive plaque
- Halitosis
- Incomplete eruption for age (primary or permanent teeth)
- Loose teeth
- Malocclusion
- Missing teeth
- Premature loss of primary teeth
- Root caries
- Tooth enamel discoloration
- Tooth fracture(s)
- Tooth misalignment
- Toothache
- Worn-down teeth

Related Factors

- Barriers to self-care
- Bruxism
- Chronic use of coffee
- Chronic use of red wine
- Chronic use of tea
- Chronic use of tobacco
- Chronic vomiting
- Deficient knowledge regarding dental health
- Dietary habits
- Economically disadvantaged
- Excessive intake of fluorides
- Excessive use of abrasive cleaning agents
- Genetic predisposition
- Ineffective oral hygiene
- Lack of access to professional care
- Nutritional deficits
- Selected prescription medications
- Sensitivity to cold
- Sensitivity to heat

Risk for Dry Eye (00219)
(2010, LOE 2.1)

Domain 11: Safety/Protection
Class 2: Physical Injury

Definition At risk for eye discomfort or damage to the cornea and conjunctiva due to reduced quantity or quality of tears to moisten the eye

Risk Factors

- Aging
- Autoimmune diseases (rheumatoid arthritis, diabetes mellitus, thyroid disease, gout, osteoporosis, etc.)
- Contact lenses
- Environmental factors (air-conditioning, excessive wind, sunlight exposure, air pollution, low humidity)
- Female gender
- History of allergy
- Hormones
- Lifestyle (e.g., smoking, caffeine use, prolonged reading)
- Mechanical ventilation therapy
- Neurological lesions with sensory or motor reflex loss (lagophthalmos, lack of spontaneous blink reflex due to decreased consciousness and other medical conditions)
- Ocular surface damage
- Place of living
- Treatment-related side effects (e.g., pharmaceutical agents such as angiotensin-converting enzyme inhibitors, antihistamines, diuretics, steroids, antidepressants, tranquilizers, analgesics, sedatives, neuromuscular blockage agents; surgical operations)
- Vitamin A deficiency

References

Bron, A.J. (1997). The Doyne lecture. Reflections on the tears. *Eye, 11*(Pt 5), 583–602.

Cortese, D., Capp, L., & McKinley, S. (1995). Moisture chamber versus lubrication for the prevention of corneal epithelial breakdown. *American Journal of Critical Care, 4*(6):, 425–428.

Cuddihy, P.J., & Whittet, H. (2005). Eye observation and corneal protection during endonasal surgery. *Journal of Laryngology and Otology, 119*(7), 556–557.

Cunningham, C., & Gould, D. (1998). Eye care for the sedated patient undergoing mechanical ventilation: The use of evidence-based care. *International Journal of Nursing Studies, 35*(1–2), 32–40.

Dawson, D. (2005). Development of a new eye care guideline for critically ill patients. *Intensive and Critical Care Nursing, 21*(2), 119–122.

Ezra, D.G., Healy, M., & Coombes, A. (2005). Assessment of corneal epitheliopathy in the critically ill. *Intensive Care Medicine, 31*(2), 313.

Ezra, D.G., Lewis, G., Healy, M., & Coombs, A. (2005). Preventing exposure keratopathy in the critically ill: A prospective study comparing eye care regimes. *British Journal of Ophthalmology, 89*(8), 1068–1069.

Ezra, D.G., Chan, M.P., Solebo, L., Malik, A.P., Crane, E., Coombes, A., & Healy, M. (2009) Randomised trial comparing ocular lubricants and polyacrylamide hydrogel dressings in the prevention of exposure keratopathy in the critically ill. *Intensive Care Medicine, 35*(3), 455–461.

Germano, E.M., Mello, M.J.G., Sena, D.F., Correia, J.B., & Amorim, M.M. (2009). Incidence and risk factors of corneal epithelial defects in mechanically ventilated children. *Critical Care Medicine, 37*(3), 1097–1100.

Hernandez, E., & Mannis, M. (1997). Superficial keratopathy in intensive care unit patients. *American Journal of Ophthalmology*, 124(2), 212–216.

Imanaka, H., Taenaka, N., Nakamura, J., Aoyama, K., & Hosotani, H. (1997). Ocular surface disorders in the critically ill. *Anesthesia and Analgesia*, 85(2), 343–346.

Joyce, N. (2002). Eye care for the intensive care patient: A systemic review. *Best Practice*, 6(1), 1–6. Joanna Briggs Institute for Evidence Based Nursing and Midwifery, North Terrace, South Australia.

Kanski, J.J. (2007). *Clinical ophthalmology: A systemic approach* (6th ed.). London, UK: Butterworth-Heinemann.

Kocacal, E., & Eşer, İ. (2008). [A significant problem in intensive care patient: Eye complications – medical education]. *Turkiye Klinikleri Journal of Medical Science*, 28(2), 193–197.

Kocacal, E.G., Eşer, İ., & Eğrilmez, S. (2008). [Comparison of the effectiveness of polyethylene cover versus carbomer drops to prevent damage due to dry eye in the critically ill]. 3rd EfCCNa Congress and 27th Aniarti Congress Book: *Influencing critical care nursing in Europe*. Florence, Italy.

Koroloff, N., Boots, R., Lipman, J., Thomas, P., Rickard, C., & Coyer, F. (2004). A randomized controlled study of the efficacy of hypromellose and lacri-lube combination versus polyethylene/cling wrap to prevent corneal epithelial breakdown in the semiconscious intensive care patient. *Intensive Care Medicine*, 30(6), 1122–1126.

Latkany, R. (2008). Dry eyes: Etiology and management. *Current Opinion in Ophthalmology*, 19(4), 287–291.

Latkany, R.L., Lock, B., & Speaker, M. (2006). Nocturnal lagophthalmos: An overview and classification. *Ocular Surface*, 4(1), 44–53.

Lenart, S.B., & Garrity, J.A. (2000). Eye care for patients receiving neuromuscular blocking agents or propofol during mechanical ventilation. *American Journal of Critical Care*, 9(3), 188–191.

Lin, P., Cheng, C., Hsu, W. et al. (2005). Association between symptoms and signs of dry eye among an elderly Chinese population in Taiwan: The Shihpai eye study. *Investigative Ophthalmology and Visual Science*, 46(5), 1593–1598.

Mercieca, F., Suresh, P., Morton, A., & Tullo, A. (1999). Ocular surface disease in intensive care unit patients. *Eye*, 13(2), 231–236.

Moss, S.E., Klein, R., & Klein, B.E.K. (2000). Prevalence of and risk factors for dry eye syndrome. *Archives of Ophthalmology*, 118(9), 1264–1268.

Moss, S.E., Klein, R., & Klein, B.E.K. (2004). Incidence of dry eye in an older population. *Archives of Ophthalmology*, 122(3), 369–373.

Nelson, J.D., Helmes, H., Fiscella, R., Southwell, Y., & Hirsch, J.D. (2000). A new look at dry eye disease and its treatment. *Advances in Therapy*, 17(2), 84–93.

Parkin, B., & Cook, S. (2000). A clear view: The way forward for eye care on ICU. *Intensive Care Medicine*, 26(2), 155–156.

Rao, S.N. (2008). Progression: The new approach to dry eye. *Review of Ophthalmology*. Retrieved from http://www.revophth.com/index.asp?page=1_14035.htm.

Rosenberg, J.B., & Eisen, L.A. (2008). Eye care in the intensive care unit: Narrative review and meta-analysis. *Critical Care Medicine*, 36(12), 3151–3155.

Sahai, A., & Malik, P. (2005). Dry eye: prevalence and attributable risk factors in a hospital-based population. *Indian Journal of Ophthalmology*, 53(2), 87–91.

Schiffman, R.M., Walt, J.G., Jacobsen, G., Doyle, J.J., Lebovics, G., & Sumner, W. (2003). Utility assessment among patients with dry eye disease. *Ophthalmology*, 110(7), 1412–1419.

Sendecka, M., Baryluk, A., & Polz-Dacewicz, M. (2004). [Prevalence and risk factors of dry eye sydrome]. *Przegląd Epidemiologiczny*, 58(1), 227–233.

Sivasankar, S., Jasper, S., Simon, S., Jacob, P., John, G., & Raju, R. (2006). Eye care in ICU. *Indian Journal of Critical Care Medicine*, 10(1), 11–14.

So, H.M., Lee, C.C., Leung, A.K., Lim, J.M., Chan, C.S., & Yan, W.W. (2008). Comparing the effectiveness of polyethylene covers with lanolin eye ointment to prevent corneal abrasions in critically ill patients: A randomized controlled study. *International Journal of Nursing Studies*, 45(11), 1565–1571.

Suresh, P., Mercieca, F., Morton, A., & Tullo, A.B. (2000). Eye care for the critically ill. *Intensive Care Medicine*, 26(2), 162–166.

Thomas, E., Hay, E.M., Hajeer, A., & Silman, A.J. (1998). Sjogren's syndrome: A community based study of prevalence and impact. *Rheumatology*, 37(10), 1069–1076.

Risk for Falls (00155)
(2000)

Domain 11: Safety/Protection
Class 2: Physical Injury

Definition At risk for increased susceptibility to falling that may cause physical harm

Risk Factors

Adults

- Age 65 or older
- History of falls
- Lives alone
- Lower limb prosthesis
- Use of assistive devices (e.g., walker, cane)
- Wheelchair use

Children

- Age 2 or younger
- Bed located near window
- Lack of automobile restraints
- Lack of gate on stairs
- Lack of parental supervision
- Lack of window guard
- Male gender when <1 year of age
- Unattended infant on elevated surface (e.g., bed, changing table)

Cognitive

- Diminished mental status

Environment

- Cluttered environment
- Dimly lit room
- Lacks antislip material in bath
- Lacks antislip material in shower
- Restraints
- Throw rugs
- Unfamiliar room
- Weather conditions (e.g., wet floors, ice)

Medications

- Alcohol use
- Angiotensin-converting enzyme inhibitors
- Antianxiety agents
- Antihypertensive agents
- Diuretics
- Hypnotics
- Narcotics/opiates
- Tranquilizers
- Tricyclic antidepressants

Physiological

- Acute illness
- Anemia
- Arthritis
- Decreased lower extremity strength
- Diarrhea
- Difficulty with gait
- Faintness when extending neck
- Faintness when turning neck
- Foot problems
- Hearing difficulties
- Impaired balance
- Impaired physical mobility
- Incontinence
- Neoplasms (i.e., fatigue/limited mobility)
- Neuropathy
- Orthostatic hypotension
- Postoperative conditions
- Postprandial blood sugar changes
- Proprioceptive deficits
- Sleeplessness
- Urinary urgency
- Vascular disease
- Visual difficulties

Risk for Injury (00035)
(1978)

Domain 11: Safety/Protection
Class 2: Physical Injury

Definition At risk for injury as a result of environmental conditions interacting with the individual's adaptive and defensive resources

Risk Factors

External

- Biological (e.g., immunization level of community, microorganism)
- Chemical (e.g., poisons, pollutants, drugs, pharmaceutical agents, alcohol, nicotine, preservatives, cosmetics, dyes)
- Human (e.g., nosocomial agents, staffing patterns, or cognitive, affective, psychomotor factors)
- Mode of transport
- Nutritional (e.g., vitamins, food types)
- Physical (e.g., design, structure, and arrangement of community, building, and/or equipment)

Internal

- Abnormal blood profile (e.g., leukocytosis/leukopenia, altered clotting factors, thrombocytopenia, sickle cell, thalassemia, decreased hemoglobin)
- Biochemical dysfunction
- Developmental age (physiological, psychosocial)
- Effector dysfunction
- Immune/autoimmune dysfunction
- Integrative dysfunction
- Malnutrition
- Physical (e.g., broken skin, altered mobility)
- Psychological (affective orientation)
- Sensory dysfunction
- Tissue hypoxia

Impaired Oral Mucous Membrane (00045)
(1982, 1998)

Domain 11: Safety/Protection
Class 2: Physical Injury

Definition   Disruption of the lips and/or soft tissue of the oral cavity

Defining Characteristics

- Bleeding
- Bluish masses (e.g., hemangiomas)
- Cheilitis
- Coated tongue
- Desquamation
- Difficult speech
- Difficulty eating
- Difficulty swallowing
- Diminished taste
- Edema
- Enlarged tonsils
- Fissures
- Geographic tongue
- Gingival hyperplasia
- Gingival pallor
- Gingival recession
- Halitosis
- Hyperemia
- Macroplasia
- Mucosal denudation
- Mucosal pallor
- Nodules
- Oral discomfort
- Oral lesions
- Oral pain
- Oral ulcers
- Papules
- Pocketing deeper than 4 mm
- Presence of pathogens
- Purulent drainage
- Purulent exudates
- Red masses (e.g., hemangiomas)
- Reports bad taste in mouth
- Smooth atrophic tongue
- Spongy patches
- Stomatitis
- Vesicles
- White, curd-like exudate
- White patches
- White plaques
- Xerostomia

Related Factors

- Barriers to oral self-care
- Barriers to professional care
- Chemical irritants (e.g., alcohol, tobacco, acidic foods, drugs, regular use of inhalers or other noxious agents)
- Cleft lip
- Cleft palate
- Decreased platelets
- Decreased salivation
- Deficient knowledge of appropriate oral hygiene
- Dehydration
- Depression
- Diminished hormone levels (women)
- Ineffective oral hygiene
- Infection
- Immunocompromised
- Immunosuppressed
- Loss of supportive structures
- Malnutrition
- Mechanical factors (e.g., ill-fitting dentures, braces, tubes [endotracheal/nasogastric], surgery in oral cavity)

- Mouth breathing
- Nil by mouth (NPO) for more than 24 hours
- Stress

- Treatment-related side effects (e.g., chemotherapy, pharmaceutical agents, radiation therapy)
- Trauma

Risk for Perioperative Positioning Injury (00087)

(1994, 2006, LOE 2.1)

Domain 11: Safety/Protection
Class 2: Physical Injury

Definition   At risk for inadvertent anatomical and physical changes as a result of posture or equipment used during an invasive/surgical procedure

Risk Factors

- Disorientation
- Edema
- Emaciation
- Immobilization
- Muscle weakness
- Obesity
- Sensory/perceptual disturbances due to anesthesia

References

Ali, A.A., Breslin, D.S., Hardman, H.D., & Martin, G. (2003). Unusual presentation and complication of the prone position for spinal surgery. *Journal of Clinical Anesthesia, 15*(6), 471–473.

Blumenreich, G.A. (1998). Positioning, padding, documentation, and the CRNA. *AANA Journal, 66*(5), 435–438.

Fritzlen, T., Kremer, M., & Biddle, C. (2003). The AANA Foundation Closed Malpractice Claims Study on nerve injuries during anesthesia care. *AANA Journal, 71*(5), 347–352.

Li, W.W., Lee, T.W., & Yim, A.P. (2004). Shoulder function after thoracic surgery. *Thoracic Surgery Clinics, 14*(3), 331–343.

Litwiller, J.P., Wells, R.E., Halliwill, J.R., Carmichael, S.W., & Warner, M.A. (2004). Effect of lithotomy positions on strain of the obturator and lateral femoral cutaneous nerves. *Clinical Anatomy, 17*(1), 45–49.

McEwen, D.R. (1996). Intraoperative positioning of surgical patients. *AORN Journal, 63*(6), 1058–1063, 1066–1075, 1077–1082.

Murphy, E.K. (2004). Negligence cases concerning positioning injuries. *AORN Journal, 80*(2), 311–312, 314.

Risk for Peripheral Neurovascular Dysfunction (00086)
(1992)

Domain 11: Safety/Protection
Class 2: Physical Injury

Definition   At risk for disruption in the circulation, sensation, or motion of an extremity

Risk Factors

- Burns
- Fractures
- Immobilization
- Mechanical compression (e.g., tourniquet, cane, cast, brace, dressing, restraint)
- Orthopedic surgery
- Trauma
- Vascular obstruction

Risk for Shock (00205)
(2008, LOE 2.1)

Domain 11: Safety/Protection
Class 2: Physical Injury

Definition   At risk for an inadequate blood flow to the body's tissues, which may lead to life-threatening cellular dysfunction

Risk Factors

- Hypotension
- Hypovolemia
- Hypoxemia
- Hypoxia
- Infection
- Sepsis
- Systemic inflammatory response syndrome

References

Bridges, E.J., & Dukes, M.S. (2005). Cardiovascular aspects of septic shock: Pathophysiology, monitoring, and treatment. *Critical Care Nurse*, 25(2), 14–16, 18–20, 22–24.

Goodrich, C. (2006). Endpoints of resuscitation: What should we be monitoring? *AACN Advanced Critical Care*, 17(3), 306–316.

Goodrich, D. (2006). Continuous central venous oximetry monitoring. *Critical Care Nursing Clinics*, 18(2), 203–209.

O'Donnell, J.M., & N'acul, F. (eds) (2001). *Surgical intensive care medicine*. Boston: Kluwer Academic.

Swearingen, P.L., & Hicks Keen, J. (eds) (2001). *Manual of critical care nursing: Nursing interventions and collaborative management* (4th ed.). St. Louis, MO: Mosby.

Impaired Skin Integrity (00046)
(1975, 1998)

Domain 11: Safety/Protection
Class 2: Physical Injury

Definition Altered epidermis and/or dermis

Defining Characteristics

- Destruction of skin layers
- Disruption of skin surface
- Invasion of body structures

Related Factors

External

- Chemical substance
- Extremes of age
- Humidity
- Hyperthermia
- Hypothermia
- Mechanical factors (e.g., shearing forces, pressure, restraint)
- Moisture
- Pharmaceutical agents
- Physical immobilization
- Radiation

Internal

- Changes in fluid status
- Changes in pigmentation
- Changes in turgor
- Developmental factors
- Imbalanced nutritional state (e.g., obesity, emaciation)
- Immunological deficit
- Impaired circulation
- Impaired metabolic state
- Impaired sensation
- Skeletal prominence

Risk for Impaired Skin Integrity (00047)*
(1975, 1998, 2010)

Domain 11: Safety/Protection
Class 2: Physical Injury

Definition   At risk for alteration in epidermis and/or dermis

Risk Factors

External

- Chemical substance
- Excretions
- Extremes of age
- Humidity
- Hyperthermia
- Hypothermia

- Mechanical factors (e.g., shearing forces, pressure, restraint)
- Moisture
- Physical immobilization
- Radiation
- Secretions

Internal

- Changes in pigmentation
- Changes in skin turgor
- Developmental factors
- Imbalanced nutritional state (e.g., obesity, emaciation)
- Immunological factors

- Impaired circulation
- Impaired metabolic state
- Impaired sensation
- Medications
- Psychogenetic factors
- Skeletal prominence

Note: risk should be determined by use of a standardized risk assessment tool.

Risk for Sudden Infant Death Syndrome (00156)
(2002, LOE 3.3)

Domain 11: Safety/Protection
Class 2: Physical Injury

Definition At risk for sudden death of an infant under 1 year of age

Risk Factors

Modifiable

- Delayed prenatal care
- Infant overheating
- Infant overwrapping
- Infant placed in prone position to sleep
- Infant placed in side-lying position to sleep
- Lack of prenatal care
- Postnatal infant smoke exposure
- Prenatal infant smoke exposure
- Soft underlayment (loose articles in the sleep environment)

Potentially Modifiable

- Low birth weight
- Prematurity
- Young maternal age

Nonmodifiable

- Ethnicity (e.g., African–American or Native American)
- Infant age of 2–4 months
- Male gender
- Seasonality of sudden infant death syndrome deaths (e.g., winter and fall months)

Risk for Suffocation (00036)

(1980)

Domain 11: Safety/Protection
Class 2: Physical Injury

Definition   At risk of accidental suffocation (inadequate air available for inhalation)

Risk Factors

External

- Children unattended in water
- Discarding refrigerators without removing doors
- Eating large mouthfuls of food
- Hanging a pacifier around infant's neck
- Household gas leaks
- Inserting small objects into airway
- Low-strung clothesline
- Pillow in infant's crib
- Playing with plastic bags
- Propped bottle in infant's crib
- Smoking in bed
- Fuel-burning heaters not vented to outside
- Vehicle warming in closed garage

Internal

- Cognitive difficulties
- Deficient knowledge regarding safe situations
- Deficient knowledge regarding safety precautions
- Disease process
- Emotional difficulties
- Injury process
- Reduced motor abilities
- Reduced olfactory sensation

Delayed Surgical Recovery (00100)
(1998, 2006, LOE 2.1)

Domain 11: Safety/Protection
Class 2: Physical Injury

Definition
Extension of the number of postoperative days required to initiate and perform activities that maintain life, health, and well-being

Defining Characteristics

- Difficulty in moving about
- Evidence of interrupted healing of surgical area (e.g., red, indurated, draining, immobilized)
- Fatigue
- Loss of appetite with nausea
- Loss of appetite without nausea
- Perception that more time is needed to recover
- Postpones resumption of work/employment activities
- Report of discomfort
- Report of pain
- Requires help to complete self-care

Related Factors

- Extensive surgical procedure
- Obesity
- Pain
- Postoperative surgical site infection
- Preoperative expectations
- Prolonged surgical procedure

References

Bruggeman, N., Turner, N., Dahm, D., Voll, A., Hoskin, T., Jacofsky, D., & Haidukewych, G. (2004). Wound complications after open Achilles tendon repair: An analysis of risk factors. *Clinical Orthopedics and Related Research, 427,* 63–66.

Burger, J., Luijendijk, R., Hop, W., Halm, J., Verdaasdonk, E., & Jeekel, J. (2004). Long-term follow-up of a randomized controlled trial of suture versus mesh repair of incisional hernia. *Annals of Surgery, 240*(4), 578–583.

Callesen, T. (2003). Inguinal hernia repair: Anaesthesia, pain and convalescence. *Danish Medical Bulletin, 50*(3), 203–218.

Chung, F. (1995). Recovery pattern and home-readiness after ambulatory surgery. *Anesthesia and Analgesia, 80*(5), 896–902.

Fallis, W., & Scurrah, D. (2001). Outpatient laparoscopic cholecystectomy: Home visit versus telephone follow-up. *Canadian Journal of Surgery, 44*(1), 39–44.

Harrington, G., Russo, P., Spelman, D. et al. (2004). Surgical-site infection rates and risk factor analysis in coronary artery bypass graft surgery. *Infection Control and Hospital Epidemiology, 25*(6), 472–476.

Hollington, P., Toogood, G., & Padbury, R. (1999). A prospective randomized trial of day-stay only versus overnight-stay laparoscopic cholecystectomy. *Australia and New Zealand Journal of Surgery, 69*(12), 841–843.

Horvath, K.J. (2003). Postoperative recovery at home after ambulatory gynecologic laparoscopic surgery. *Journal of Perianesthesia Nursing, 18*(5), 324–334.

Jibodh, S., Gurkan, I., & Wenz, J. (2004). In-hospital outcome and resource use in hip arthroplasty: Influence of body mass. *Orthopedics, 27*(6), 594–601.

Kabon, B., Nagele, A., Reddy, D. et al. (2004). Obesity decreases perioperative tissue oxygenation. *Anesthesiology, 100*(2), 274–280.

Kleinbeck, S.V. (2000). Self-reported at-home postoperative recovery: Postdischarge Surgery Recovery (PSR) Scale. *Research in Nursing and Health*, *23*(6), 461–472.

Kotiniemi, L., Ryhanen, P., Valanne, J., Jokela, R., Mustonen, A., & Poukkula, E. (1997). Postoperative symptoms at home following day-case surgery in children: A multicentre survey of 551 children. *Anaesthesia*, *52*(10), 963–969.

Kuo, C., Wang, S., Yu, W., Chang, M., Liu, C., & Chen, T. (2004). Postoperative spinal deep wound infection: A six-year review of 3230 selective procedures. *Journal of the Chinese Medical Association*, *67*(8), 398–402.

Lehmann, H., Fleisher, L., Lam, J., Frink, B., & Bass, E. (1999). Patient preferences for early discharge after laparoscopic cholecystectomy. *Anesthesia and Analgesia*, *88*(6), 1280–1285.

Levy, B., Rosson, J., & Blake, A. (2004). MRSA in patients presenting with femoral fractures. *Surgeon*, *2*(3), 171–172.

Lofgren, M., Poromaa, I., Stjerndahl, J., & Renstrom, B. (2004). Postoperative infections and antibiotic prophylaxis for hysterectomy in Sweden: A study by the Swedish National Register for Gynecologic Surgery. *Acta Obstetrica et Gynecologica Scandinavica*, *83*(12), 1202–1207.

Morales, C.H., Villegas, M.I., Villavicencio, R., González, G., Pérez, L.F., Peña, A.M., & Vanegas, L.E. (2004). Intra-abdominal infection in patients with abdominal trauma. *Archives of Surgery*, *9*(12), 1278–1285.

Mortenson, M.M., Schneider, P.D., Khatri, V.P., Stevenson, T.R., Whetzel, T.P., Sommerhaug, E.J., Goodnight, J.E., & Bold, R.J. (2004). Immediate breast reconstruction after mastectomy increases wound complications: However, initiation of adjuvant chemotherapy is not delayed. *Archives of Surgery*, *139*(9), 988–991.

Muschik, M., Luck, W., & Schlenzka, D. (2004). Implant removal for late-developing infection alter instrumented posterior spinal fusion for scoliosis: Reinstrumentation reduces loss of correction. A retrospective analysis of 45 cases. *European Spine Journal*, *13*(7), 645–651.

Nguyen, N., Nguyen, C., Stevens, C., Steward, E., & Paya, M. (2004). The efficacy of fibrin sealant in prevention of anastomotic leak after laparoscopic gastric bypass. *Journal of Surgical Research*, *122*(2), 218–224.

Phillips, C., Kiyak, H., Bloomquist, D., & Turvey, T. (2004). Perceptions of recovery and satisfaction in the short term after orthognathic surgery. *Journal of Oral Maxillofacial Surgery*, *62*(5), 535–544.

Smith, R., Bohl, J., McElearney, S., Friel, C., Barclay, M., Sawyer, R., & Foley, E. (2004). Wound infection after elective colorectal resection. *Annals of Surgery*, *239*(5), 599–605.

Watt-Watson, J., Chung, F., Chan, V., & McGillion, M. (2004). Pain management following discharge after ambulatory same-day surgery. *Journal of Nursing Management*, *12*(3), 153–161.

Young, J., & O'Connell, B. (2001). Recovery following laparoscopic cholecystectomy in either a 23 hour or an 8 hour facility. *Journal of Quality Clinical Practice*, *21*(1–2), 2–7.

Zalon, M. (2004). Correlates of recovery among older adults after major abdominal surgery. *Nursing Research*, *53*(2), 99–106.

Risk for Thermal Injury (00220)
(2010, LOE 2.1)

Domain 11: Safety/Protection
Class 2: Physical Injury

Definition At risk for damage to skin and mucous membranes due to extreme temperatures

Risk Factors

- Cognitive impairment (e.g. dementia, psychoses)
- Developmental level (infants, aged)
- Exposure to extreme temperatures
- Fatigue
- Inadequate supervision
- Inattentiveness
- Intoxication (alcohol, drug)
- Lack of knowledge (patient, caregiver)
- Lack of protective clothing (e.g. flame-retardant sleepwear, gloves, ear covering)
- Neuromuscular impairment (e.g. stroke, amyotrophic lateral sclerosis, multiple sclerosis)
- Neuropathy
- Smoking
- Treatment-related side effects (e.g., pharmaceutical agents)
- Unsafe environment

References

Centers for Disease Control. (2006). *Injury fact book 2006.* Retrieved from http://www.cdc.gov/ncipc/fact_book/factbook.htm.

Christoffel, T., & Gallagher, S.S. (2006). *Injury prevention and public health* (2nd ed.). Sudbury, MA: Jones & Bartlett.

DiGuiseppi, C., Edwards, P., Godward, C., Roberts, I., & Wade, A. (2000). Urban residential fire and flame injuries: A population based study. *Injury Prevention, 6*(4), 250–254.

Horan, M.A., & Little, R.A. (eds). (1998). *Injury in the aging.* Cambridge: Cambridge University Press.

Murray, R.B., Zentner, J.P., & Yakimo, R. (2009). *Health promotion strategies through the life span* (8th ed.). Upper Saddle River, NJ: Pearson.

Pickett, W., Streight, S., Simpson, K., & Brison, R.J. (2003). Injuries experienced by infant children: A population based epidemiological analysis. *Pediatrics, 111*(4), 365–370.

Sommers, M.S. (2006). Injury as a global phenomenon of concern in nursing science. *Image: Journal of Nursing Scholarship, 38*(4), 314–320.

Impaired Tissue Integrity (00044)
(1986, 1998)

Domain 11: Safety/Protection
Class 2: Physical Injury

Definition Damage to mucous membrane, corneal, integumentary, or subcutaneous tissues

Defining Characteristics

- Damaged tissue (e.g., cornea, mucous membrane, integumentary, subcutaneous)
- Destroyed tissue

Related Factors

- Altered circulation
- Chemical irritants
- Deficient fluid volume
- Deficient knowledge
- Excess fluid volume
- Impaired physical mobility
- Mechanical factors (e.g., pressure, shear, friction)
- Nutritional factors (e.g., deficit or excess)
- Radiation
- Temperature extremes

Risk for Trauma (00038)
(1980)

Domain 11: Safety/Protection
Class 2: Physical Injury

Definition At risk of accidental tissue injury (e.g., wound, burn, fracture)

Risk Factors

External

- Accessibility of guns
- Bathing in very hot water (e.g., unsupervised bathing of young children)
- Children playing with dangerous objects
- Children riding in the front seat in car
- Contact with corrosives
- Contact with intense cold
- Contact with rapidly moving machinery
- Defective appliances
- Delayed lighting of gas appliances
- Driving a mechanically unsafe vehicle
- Driving at excessive speeds
- Driving while intoxicated
- Driving without necessary visual aids
- Entering unlighted rooms
- Experimenting with chemicals
- Exposure to dangerous machinery
- Faulty electrical plugs
- Flammable children's clothing
- Flammable children's toys
- Frayed wires
- Grease waste collected on stoves
- High beds
- High-crime neighborhood
- Inadequate stair rails
- Inadequately stored combustibles (e.g., matches, oily rags)
- Inadequately stored corrosives (e.g., lye)
- Inappropriate call-for-aid mechanisms for bed-bound client
- Knives stored uncovered
- Lack of gate at top of stairs
- Lack of protection from heat source
- Lacks antislip material in bath
- Lacks antislip material in shower
- Large icicles hanging from roof
- Misuse of necessary headgear
- Misuse of seat restraints
- Nonuse of seat restraints
- Obstructed passageways
- Overexposure to radiation
- Overloaded electrical outlets
- Overloaded fuse boxes
- Physical proximity to vehicle pathways (e.g., driveways, lanes, railroad tracks)
- Playing with explosives
- Pot handles facing toward front of stove
- Potential igniting of gas leaks
- Slippery floors (e.g., wet or highly waxed)
- Smoking in bed
- Smoking near oxygen
- Struggling with restraints
- Throw rugs
- Unanchored electric wires
- Unsafe road
- Unsafe walkways
- Unsafe window protection in homes with young children
- Use of cracked dishware
- Use of unsteady chairs
- Use of unsteady ladders
- Wearing flowing clothes around open flame

Internal

- Balancing difficulties
- Cognitive difficulties
- Deficient knowledge regarding safe procedures
- Deficient knowledge regarding safety precautions
- Economically disadvantaged
- Emotional difficulties
- History of previous trauma
- Poor vision
- Reduced hand–eye coordination
- Reduced muscle coordination
- Reduced sensation
- Weakness

Risk for Vascular Trauma (00213)
(2008, LOE 2.1)

Domain 11: Safety/Protection
Class 2: Physical Injury

Definition
At risk for damage to a vein and its surrounding tissues related to the presence of a catheter and/or infused solutions

Risk Factors

- Catheter type
- Catheter width
- Impaired ability to visualize the insertion site
- Inadequate catheter fixation
- Infusion rate

- Insertion site
- Length of insertion time
- Nature of solution (e.g., concentration, chemical irritant, temperature, pH)

References

Adami N.P., Gutiérrez M.G.R., da Fonseca S.M., & de Almeida, E.P.M. (2005). Risk management of extravasation of cytostatic drugs at the adult chemotherapy outpatient clinic of a university hospital. *Journal of Clinical Nursing*, 14(7), 876–882.

Arreguy-Sena, C. (2002). *A trajetória de construção e validação dos diagnósticos de enfermagem: Trauma Vascular e Risco para Trauma Vascular*. [Tese] Ribeirão Preto: Escola de Enfermagem de Ribeirão Preto-USP.

Arreguy-Sena, C., & de Carvalho, E.C. (2003). Punção venosa periférica: Análise dos critérios adotados por uma equipe de enfermagem para avaliar e remover um dispositivo endovenoso. *Escola Anna Nery Revista de Enfermagem*, 7, 351–360.

Phillips, L. (2005). *Manual of IV Therapeutics* (4th ed.). Philadelphia, PA: Davis.

Polimeno, N., Hara, M., Appezzato, L., Fernandes, V., Cintra, L., & Hara, C. (1995) Incidência e caracterização da tromboflebite superficial (TFS) pós-venóclise em Hospital Universitário. *Jornal Brasileiro de Medicina*, 69, 196–204.

Risk for Other-Directed Violence (00138)

(1980, 1996)

Domain 11: Safety/Protection
Class 3: Violence

Definition   At risk for behaviors in which an individual demonstrates that he or she can be physically, emotionally, and/or sexually harmful to others

Risk Factors

- Availability of weapon(s)
- Body language (e.g., rigid posture, clenching of fists and jaw, hyperactivity, pacing, breathlessness, threatening stances)
- Cognitive impairment (e.g., learning disabilities, attention deficit disorder, decreased intellectual functioning)
- Cruelty to animals
- Firesetting
- History of childhood abuse
- History of indirect violence (e.g., tearing off clothes, ripping objects off walls, writing on walls, urinating on floor, defecating on floor, stamping feet, temper tantrum, running in corridors, yelling, throwing objects, breaking a window, slamming doors, sexual advances)
- History of other-directed violence (e.g., hitting someone, kicking someone, spitting at someone, scratching someone, throwing objects at someone, biting someone, attempted rape, rape, sexual molestation, urinating/defecating on a person)
- History of substance abuse
- History of threats of violence (e.g., verbal threats against property, verbal threats against person, social threats, cursing, threatening notes/letters, threatening gestures, sexual threats)
- History of violent antisocial behavior (e.g., stealing, insistent borrowing, insistent demands for privileges, insistent interruption of meetings, refusal to eat, refusal to take medication, ignoring instructions)
- History of witnessing family violence
- Impulsivity
- Motor vehicle offenses (e.g., frequent traffic violations, use of a motor vehicle to release anger)
- Neurological impairment (e.g., positive EEG, computed tomography, or magnetic resonance imaging scan, neurological findings, head trauma, seizure disorders)
- Pathological intoxication
- Perinatal complications
- Prenatal complications
- Psychotic symptomatology (e.g., auditory, visual, command hallucinations; paranoid delusions; loose, rambling, or illogical thought processes)
- Suicidal behavior

11. Safety/Protection

Risk for Self-Directed Violence (00140)
(1994)

Domain 11: Safety/Protection
Class 3: Violence

Definition At risk for behaviors in which an individual demonstrates that he or she can be physically, emotionally, and/or sexually harmful to self

Risk Factors

- Age 15–19
- Age 45 or older
- Behavioral cues (e.g., writing forlorn love notes, directing angry messages at a significant other who has rejected the person, giving away personal items, taking out a large life insurance policy)
- Conflictual interpersonal relationships
- Emotional problems (e.g., hopelessness, despair, increased anxiety, panic, anger, hostility)
- Employment problems (e.g., unemployed, recent job loss/failure)
- Engagement in autoerotic sexual acts
- Family background (e.g., chaotic or conflictual, history of suicide)
- History of multiple suicide attempts
- Lack of personal resources (e.g., poor achievement, poor insight, affect unavailable and poorly controlled)
- Lack of social resources (e.g., poor rapport, socially isolated, unresponsive family)
- Marital status (single, widowed, divorced)
- Mental health problems (e.g., severe depression, psychosis, severe personality disorder, alcoholism or drug abuse)
- Occupation (executive, administrator/owner of business, professional, semi-skilled worker)
- Physical health problems (e.g., hypochondriasis, chronic or terminal illness)
- Sexual orientation (bisexual [active], homosexual [inactive])
- Suicidal ideation
- Suicidal plan
- Verbal cues (e.g., talking about death, "better off without me," asking questions about lethal dosages of drugs)

Self-Mutilation (00151)
(2000)

Domain 11: Safety/Protection
Class 3: Violence

Definition Deliberate self-injurious behavior causing tissue damage with the intent of causing nonfatal injury to attain relief of tension

Defining Characteristics

- Abrading
- Biting
- Constricting a body part
- Cuts on body
- Hitting
- Ingestion of harmful substances
- Inhalation of harmful substances
- Insertion of object into body orifice
- Picking at wounds
- Scratches on body
- Self-inflicted burns
- Severing

Related Factors

- Adolescence
- Autistic individual
- Battered child
- Borderline personality disorder
- Character disorder
- Childhood illness
- Childhood sexual abuse
- Childhood surgery
- Depersonalization
- Developmentally delayed individual
- Dissociation
- Disturbed body image
- Disturbed interpersonal relationships
- Eating disorders
- Emotional disorder
- Family divorce
- Family history of self-destructive behaviors
- Family substance abuse
- Feels threatened with loss of significant relationship
- History of inability to plan solutions
- History of inability to see long-term consequences
- History of self-directed violence
- Impulsivity
- Inability to express tension verbally
- Incarceration
- Ineffective coping
- Irresistible urge to cut self
- Irresistible urge for self-directed violence
- Isolation from peers
- Labile behavior
- Lack of family confidant
- Living in nontraditional setting (e.g., foster, group, or institutional care)
- Low self-esteem
- Mounting tension that is intolerable
- Need for quick reduction of stress
- Peers who self-mutilate
- Perfectionism
- Poor communication between parent and adolescent
- Psychotic state (e.g., command hallucinations)
- Reports negative feelings (e.g., depression, rejection, self-hatred, separation anxiety, guilt, depersonalization)

- Sexual identity crisis
- Substance abuse
- Unstable body image
- Unstable self-esteem
- Use of manipulation to obtain nurturing relationship with others
- Violence between parental figures

Risk for Self-Mutilation (00139)
(1992, 2000)

Domain 11: Safety/Protection
Class 3: Violence

Definition At risk for deliberate self-injurious behavior causing tissue damage with the intent of causing nonfatal injury to attain relief of tension

Risk Factors

- Adolescence
- Autistic individuals
- Battered child
- Borderline personality disorders
- Character disorders
- Childhood illness
- Childhood sexual abuse
- Childhood surgery
- Depersonalization
- Developmentally delayed individuals
- Dissociation
- Disturbed body image
- Disturbed interpersonal relationships
- Eating disorders
- Emotional disorder
- Family divorce
- Family history of self-destructive behaviors
- Family substance abuse
- Feels threatened with loss of significant relationship
- History of inability to plan solutions
- History of inability to see long-term consequences
- History of self-directed violence
- Impulsivity
- Inability to express tension verbally
- Inadequate coping
- Incarceration
- Irresistible urge for self-directed violence
- Isolation from peers
- Living in nontraditional setting (e.g., foster, group, or institutional care)
- Loss of control over problem-solving situations
- Loss of significant relationship(s)
- Low self-esteem
- Mounting tension that is intolerable
- Need for quick reduction of stress
- Peers who self-mutilate
- Perfectionism
- Psychotic state (e.g., command hallucinations)
- Reports negative feelings (e.g., depression, rejection, self-hatred, separation anxiety, guilt)
- Sexual identity crisis
- Substance abuse
- Unstable self-esteem
- Use of manipulation to obtain nurturing relationship with others
- Violence between parental figures

Risk for Suicide (00150)
(2000)

Domain 11: Safety/Protection
Class 3: Violence

Definition At risk for self-inflicted, life-threatening injury

Risk Factors

Behavioral

- Buying a gun
- Changing a will
- Giving away possessions
- History of prior suicide attempt
- Impulsiveness
- Making a will
- Marked changes in attitude
- Marked changes in behavior
- Marked changes in school performance
- Stockpiling medicines
- Sudden euphoric recovery from major depression

Demographic

- Age (e.g., elderly people, young adult males, adolescents)
- Divorced
- Male gender
- Race (e.g., white, Native American)
- Widowed

Physical

- Chronic pain
- Physical illness
- Terminal illness

Psychological

- Childhood abuse
- Family history of suicide
- Guilt
- Homosexual youth
- Psychiatric disorder
- Psychiatric illness
- Substance abuse

Situational

- Adolescents living in nontraditional settings (e.g., juvenile detention center, prison, half-way house, group home)
- Economically disadvantaged
- Institutionalization
- Living alone
- Loss of autonomy
- Loss of independence
- Presence of gun in home
- Relocation
- Retired

Social

- Cluster suicides
- Disciplinary problems
- Disrupted family life
- Grieving
- Helplessness
- Hopelessness
- Legal problems
- Loneliness
- Loss of important relationship
- Poor support systems
- Social isolation

Verbal

- States desire to die
- Threats of killing oneself

Contamination (00181)

(2006, LOE 2.1)

Domain 11: Safety/Protection
Class 4: Environmental Hazards

Definition Exposure to environmental contaminants in doses sufficient to cause adverse health effects

Defining Characteristics

Defining characteristics are dependent on the causative agent. Agents cause a variety of individual organ responses as well as systemic responses.

Pesticides[1]

- Dermatological effects of pesticide exposure
- Gastrointestinal effects of pesticide exposure
- Neurological effects of pesticide exposure
- Pulmonary effects of pesticide exposure
- Renal effects of pesticide exposure

Chemicals[2]

- Dermatological effects of chemical exposure
- Gastrointestinal effects of chemical exposure
- Immunological effects of chemical exposure
- Neurological effects of chemical exposure
- Pulmonary effects of chemical exposure
- Renal effects of chemical exposure

Biologics[3]

- Dermatological effects of exposure to biologics
- Gastrointestinal effects of exposure to biologics
- Neurological effects of exposure to biologics
- Pulmonary effects of exposure to biologics
- Renal effects of exposure to biologics

[1]Major categories of pesticides: insecticides, herbicides, fungicides, antimicrobials, rodenticides; major pesticides: organophosphates, carbamates, organochlorines, pyrethrum, arsenic, glycophosphates, bipyridyls, chlorophenoxy compounds.
[2]Major chemical agents: petroleum-based agents, anticholinesterase type I agents act on proximal tracheobronchial portion of the respiratory tract; type II agents act on alveoli; type III agents produce systemic effects.
[3]Toxins from living organisms (bacteria, viruses, fungi).

Pollution[4]

- Neurological effects of pollution exposure

- Pulmonary effects of pollution exposure

Waste[5]

- Dermatological effects of waste exposure
- Gastrointestinal effects of waste exposure

- Hepatic effects of waste exposure
- Pulmonary effects of waste exposure

Radiation

- External exposure through direct contact with radioactive material
- Genetic effects of radiation exposure
- Immunological effects of radiation exposure

- Neurological effects of radiation exposure
- Oncological effects of radiation exposure

Related Factors

External

- Chemical contamination of food
- Chemical contamination of water
- Economically disadvantaged (increases potential for multiple exposure, lack of access to healthcare, poor diet)
- Exposure through ingestion of radioactive material (e.g., food/ water contamination)
- Exposure to bioterrorism
- Exposure to disaster (natural or man-made)
- Exposure to radiation (occupation in radiology, employment in nuclear industries and electrical generating plants, living near nuclear industries and/or electrical generating plants)

- Flaking, peeling paint in presence of young children
- Flaking, peeling plaster in presence of young children
- Flooring surface (carpeted surfaces hold contaminant residue more than hard floor surfaces)
- Geographical area (living in area where high levels of contaminants exist)
- Household hygiene practices
- Inadequate municipal services (trash removal, sewage treatment facilities)
- Inappropriate use of protective clothing
- Lack of breakdown of contaminants once indoors (breakdown is inhibited without sun and rain exposure)

---

[4]Major locations: air, water, soil; major agents: asbestos, radon, tobacco, heavy metal, lead, noise, exhaust fumes.

[5]Categories of waste: trash, raw sewage, industrial waste.

- Lack of protective clothing
- Lacquer in poorly ventilated areas
- Lacquer without effective protection
- Paint in poorly ventilated areas
- Paint without effective protection
- Personal hygiene practices
- Playing in outdoor areas where environmental contaminants are used

- Presence of atmospheric pollutants
- Unprotected contact with chemicals (e.g., arsenic)
- Unprotected contact with heavy metals (e.g., chromium, lead)
- Use of environmental contaminants in the home (e.g., pesticides, chemicals, environmental tobacco smoke)

Internal

- Age (children <5 years, older adults)
- Concomitant exposures
- Developmental characteristics of children
- Female gender
- Gestational age during exposure

- Nutritional factors (e.g., obesity, vitamin and mineral deficiencies)
- Pre-existing disease states
- Pregnancy
- Previous exposures
- Smoking

References

Baker, J.E.L. (1992). Primary, secondary, and tertiary prevention in reducing pesticide related illness in farmers. *Journal of Community Health Nursing, 9*(4), 245–253.

Berkowitz, G.S., Obel, J., Deych, E., Lapinski, R., Godbold, J., & Liu, Z. (2003). Exposure to indoor pesticides during pregnancy in a multiethnic, urban cohort. *Environmental Health Perspectives, 111*(1), 79–84.

Brender, J., Suarez, L., Hendricks, K., Baetz, R.A., & Larsen, R. (2002). Parental occupation and neural tube defect-affected pregnancies among Mexican Americans. *Journal of Occupational and Environmental Medicine, 44*(7), 650–656.

Butterfield, P.G. (2002). Upstream reflections on environmental health: An abbreviated history and framework for action. *Advances in Nursing Science, 25*(1), 32–49.

Center for Disease Control and Prevention (2004). Agency for Toxic Substances and Disease Registry. Retrieved from http://www.atsdr.cdc.gov.

Center for Disease Control and Prevention (2005). *Third national report on human exposure to environmental chemicals: Executive summary.* NCEH Publication 05–0725. Atlanta, GA: Center for Disease Control and Prevention.

Chalupka, S.M. (2001a). Essentials of environmental health. Enhancing your occupational health nursing practice. Part I. *American Association of Occupational Health Nurses or Nursing, 49*(3), 137–154.

Chalupka, S.M. (2001b). Essentials of environmental health. Enhancing your occupational health nursing practice. Part II. *American Association of Occupational Health Nurses or Nursing, 49*(4), 194–213.

Children's Environmental Health Network. (2004). Resource guide on children's environmental health. Retrieved from http://www.cehn.org.

Children's Environmental Health Network. (2005). Training manual on pediatric environmental health: Putting it into practice. Retrieved from http://www.cehn.org.

Diaz, J.D.M., Lopez, M.A., & Campbell, P. (1999). Voluntary ingestion of organophosphate insecticide by a young farmer. *Journal of Emergency Nursing, 25*(4), 266–268.

Dixon, J.K., & Dixon, J.P. (2002). An integrative model for environmental health research. *Advances in Nursing Science, 24*(3), 43–57.

Environmental Protection Agency, (2004). Understanding radiation health effects. Retrieved from http://www.epa.gov.

Etzel, R., & Balk, S. (1999). *Handbook of pediatric environmental health.* Elk Grove, IL: American Academy of Pediatrics.

Gerrard, C.E. (1998). Farmer's occupational health: Cause for concern, cause for action. *Journal of Advanced Nursing, 28*(1), 155–163.

Goldman, L.R., Shannon, M.W., & the Committee on Environmental Health. (2001). Technical report. Mercury in the environment: Implications for physicians. *Pediatrics, 108*(1), 197–205.

King, C., & Harber, P. (1998). Community environmental health concerns and the nursing process: Four environmental health nursing care plans. *American Association of Occupational Health Nursing Journal, 46*(1), 20–27.

Larsson, L.S., & Butterfield, P. (2002). Mapping the future of environmental health and nursing: Strategies for integrating national competencies into nursing practice. *Public Health Nursing, 19*(4), 301–308.

McCauley, L.A., Michaels, S., Rothlein, J., Muniz, J., Lasarev, M., & Ebbert, C. (2003). Pesticide exposure and self-reported home hygiene: Practices in agricultural families. *American Association of Occupational Health Nurses or Nursing, 51*(3), 113–119.

Massey-Stokes, M., & Lanning, B. (2002). Childhood cancer and environmental toxins: The debate continues. *Family and Community Health, 24*(4), 27–38.

Meeker, B.J., Curruth, A., & Holland, C.B. (2002). Health hazards and preventive measures of farm women: Emerging issues. *AAOHN, 50*(7), 307–314.

Melum, M.F. (2001). Organophosphate toxicity. *American Journal of Nursing, 101*(5), 57–58.

Rice, R. (1999). Environmental threats in the home: Home care nursing perspectives. *Geriatric Nursing, 20*(6), 332–336.

Schneider, D., & Freeman, N. (2001). Children's environmental health risks: A state of the art conference. *Archives of Environmental Health, 56*(2), 103–110.

Silbergeld, E.K., & Flaws, J.A. (2002). Environmental exposures and women's health. *Clinical Obstetrics and Gynecology, 45*(4), 1119–1128.

Thornton, J.W., McCally, M., & Houlihan, J. (2002). Biomonitoring of industrial pollutants: Health and policy implications of the chemical body burden. *Public Health Reports, 117*(4), 315–323.

11. Safety/Protection

Risk for Contamination (00180)

(2006, LOE 2.1)

Domain 11: Safety/Protection
Class 4: Environmental Hazards

Definition At risk for exposure to environmental contaminants in doses sufficient to cause adverse health effects

Risk Factors

External

- Chemical contamination of food
- Chemical contamination of water
- Economically disadvantaged (increases potential for multiple exposure, lack of access to healthcare, poor diet)
- Exposure to bioterrorism
- Exposure to disaster (natural or man-made)
- Exposure to radiation (occupation in radiography, employment in nuclear industries and electrical generating plants, living near nuclear industries and/or electrical generating plants)
- Flaking, peeling paint in presence of young children
- Flaking, peeling plaster in presence of young children
- Flooring surface (carpeted surfaces hold contaminant residue more than hard floor surfaces)
- Geographical area (living in area where high levels of contaminants exist)
- Household hygiene practices
- Inadequate municipal services (e.g., trash removal, sewage treatment facilities)
- Inappropriate use of protective clothing
- Lack of breakdown of contaminants once indoors (breakdown is inhibited without sun and rain exposure)
- Lack of protective clothing
- Lacquer in poorly ventilated areas
- Lacquer without effective protection
- Paint, lacquer, etc. in poorly ventilated areas
- Paint, lacquer, etc. without effective protection
- Personal hygiene practices
- Playing in outdoor areas where environmental contaminants are used
- Presence of atmospheric pollutants
- Unprotected contact with chemicals (e.g., arsenic)
- Unprotected contact with heavy metals (e.g., chromium, lead)
- Use of environmental contaminants in the home (e.g., pesticides, chemicals, environmental tobacco smoke)

Internal

- Age (children <5 years, older adults)
- Concomitant exposures
- Developmental characteristics of children
- Female gender
- Gestational age during exposure
- Nutritional factors (e.g., obesity, vitamin and mineral deficiencies)
- Pre-existing disease states
- Pregnancy
- Previous exposures
- Smoking

References

Baker, J.E.L. (1992). Primary, secondary, and tertiary prevention in reducing pesticide related illness in farmers. *Journal of Community Health Nursing*, 9(4), 245–253.

Berkowitz, G.S., Obel, J., Deych, E., Lapinski, R., Godbold, J., & Liu, Z. (2003). Exposure to indoor pesticides during pregnancy in a multiethnic, urban cohort. *Environmental Health Perspectives*, 111(1), 79–84.

Brender, J., Suarez, L., Hendricks, K., Baetz, R.A., & Larsen, R. (2002). Parental occupation and neural tube defect-affected pregnancies among Mexican Americans. *Journal of Occupational and Environmental Medicine*, 44(7), 650–656.

Butterfield, P.G. (2002). Upstream reflections on environmental health: An abbreviated history and framework for action. *Advances in Nursing Science*, 25(1), 32–49.

Center for Disease Control and Prevention (2004). Agency for Toxic Substances and Disease Registry. Retrieved from http://www.atsdr.cdc.gov.

Center for Disease Control and Prevention (2005). *Third national report on human exposure to environmental chemicals: Executive summary*. NCEH Publication 05–0725. Atlanta, GA: Center for Disease Control and Prevention.

Chalupka, S.M. (2001a). Essentials of environmental health. Enhancing your occupational health nursing practice. Part I. *American Association of Occupational Health Nurses or Nursing*, 49(3), 137–154.

Chalupka, S.M. (2001b). Essentials of environmental health. Enhancing your occupational health nursing practice. Part II. *American Association of Occupational Health Nurses or Nursing*, 49(4), 194–213.

Children's Environmental Health Network. (2004). Resource guide on children's environmental health. Retrieved from http://www.cehn.org.

Children's Environmental Health Network. (2005). Training manual on pediatric environmental health: Putting it into practice. Retrieved from http://www.cehn.org.

Diaz, J.D.M., Lopez, M.A., & Campbell, P. (1999). Voluntary ingestion of organophosphate insecticide by a young farmer. *Journal of Emergency Nursing*, 25(4), 266–268.

Dixon, J.K., & Dixon, J.P. (2002). An integrative model for environmental health research. *Advances in Nursing Science*, 24(3), 43–57.

Environmental Protection Agency, (2004). Understanding radiation health effects. Retrieved from http://www.epa.gov.

Etzel, R., & Balk, S. (1999). *Handbook of pediatric environmental health*. Elk Grove, IL: American Academy of Pediatrics.

Gerrard, C.E. (1998). Farmer's occupational health: Cause for concern, cause for action. *Journal of Advanced Nursing*, 28(1), 155–163.

Goldman, L.R., Shannon, M.W., & the Committee on Environmental Health. (2001). Technical report. Mercury in the environment: Implications for physicians. *Pediatrics*, 108(1), 197–205.

King, C., & Harber, P. (1998). Community environmental health concerns and the nursing process: Four environmental health nursing care plans. *American Association of Occupational Health Nursing Journal*, 46(1), 20–27.

Larsson, L.S., & Butterfield, P. (2002). Mapping the future of environmental health and nursing: strategies for integrating national competencies into nursing practice. *Public Health Nursing*, 19(4), 301–308.

McCauley, L.A., Michaels, S., Rothlein, J., Muniz, J., Lasarev, M., & Ebbert, C. (2003). Pesticide exposure and self-reported home hygiene: Practices in agricultural families. *American Association of Occupational Health Nurses or Nursing*, 51(3), 113–119.

Massey-Stokes, M., & Lanning, B. (2002). Childhood cancer and environmental toxins: The debate continues. *Family and Community Health*, 24(4), 27–38.

Meeker, B.J., Curruth, A., & Holland, C.B. (2002). Health hazards and preventive measures of farm women: Emerging issues. *AAOHN*, 50(7), 307–314.

Melum, M.F. (2001). Organophosphate toxicity. *American Journal of Nursing*, 101(5), 57–58.

Rice, R. (1999). Environmental threats in the home: Home care nursing perspectives. *Geriatric Nursing*, 20(6), 332–336.

Schneider, D., & Freeman, N. (2001). Children's environmental health risks: A state of the art conference. *Archives of Environmental Health*, 56(2), 103–110.

Silbergeld, E.K., & Flaws, J.A. (2002). Environmental exposures and women's health. *Clinical Obstetrics and Gynecology*, 45(4), 1119–1128.

Thornton, J.W., McCally, M., & Houlihan, J. (2002). Biomonitoring of industrial pollutants: Health and policy implications of the chemical body burden. *Public Health Reports*, 117(4), 315–323.

11. Safety/Protection

Risk for Poisoning (00037)
(1980, 2006, LOE 2.1)

Domain 11: Safety/Protection
Class 4: Environmental Hazards

Definition At risk of accidental exposure to, or ingestion of, drugs or dangerous products in sufficient doses that may compromise health

Risk Factors

External

- Availability of illicit drugs potentially contaminated by poisonous additives
- Dangerous products placed within reach of children
- Dangerous products placed within reach of confused individuals
- Large supplies of pharmaceutical agents in house
- Pharmaceutical agents stored in unlocked cabinets accessible to children
- Pharmaceutical agents stored in unlocked cabinets accessible to confused individuals

Internal

- Cognitive difficulties
- Deficient knowledge regarding pharmaceutical agents
- Deficient knowledge regarding poisoning prevention
- Emotional difficulties
- Lack of proper precaution
- Reduced vision
- Reports occupational setting is without adequate safeguards

Reference

Center for Disease Control and Prevention (2005). *Third national report on human exposure to environmental chemicals: Executive summary.* NCEH Publication 05–0725. Atlanta, GA: Center for Disease Control and Prevention.

Risk for Adverse Reaction to Iodinated Contrast Media (00218)

(2010, LOE 2.1)

Domain 11: Safety Protection
Class 5: Defensive Processes

Definition
At risk for any noxious or unintended reaction associated with the use of iodinated contrast media that can occur within seven (7) days after contrast agent injection

Risk Factors

- Anxiety
- Concurrent use of medications (e.g., beta-blockers, interleukin-2, metformin, nephrotoxic medications)
- Dehydration
- Extremes of age
- Fragile veins (e.g., prior or actual chemotherapy treatment or radiation in the limb to be injected, multiple attempts to obtain intravenous access, indwelling intravenous lines in place for more than 24 hours, previous axillary lymph node dissection in the limb to be injected, distal intravenous access sites: hand, wrist, foot, ankle)
- Generalized debilitation
- History of allergies
- History of previous adverse effect from iodinated contrast media
- Physical and chemical properties of the contrast media (e.g., iodine concentration, viscosity, high osmolality, ion toxicity)
- Unconsciousness
- Underlying disease (e.g., heart disease, pulmonary disease, blood dyscrasias, endocrine disease, renal disease, pheochromocytoma, autoimmune disease)

References

American College of Radiology. (2008). *Manual on contrast media* (version 6). Reston, VA: Author.

Bellin, M., Jakobsen, J., Tomassin, I., Thomsen, H.S., & Morcos, S.K. (2002). Contrast medium extravasation injury: Guidelines for prevention and management. *European Radiology, 12*(11), 2807–2812.

Bettmann, M.A. (2004). Frequently asked questions: Iodinated contrast agents. *Radiographics, 24* (Special Issue), S3–S10.

Brockow, K., Christiansen, C., Kanny, G., Clément, O., Barbaud, A., Bircher, A. et al.; ENDA EAACI Interest Group on Drug Hypersensitivity. (2005). Management of hypersensitivity reactions to iodinated contrast media. *Allergy, 60*(2), 150–158.

Cohan, R.H., Ellis, J.H., & Garner, W.L. (1996). Extravasation of radiographic contrast material: Recognition, prevention, and treatment. *Radiology, 200*(3), 593–604.

Costa, N. (2004). Understanding contrast media. *Journal of Infusion Nursing, 27*(5), 302–312.

European Society of Urogenital Radiology. (2007). *ESUR Guidelines on contrast media* (version 6). Heidelberg: Springer-Verlag.

Hash, R.B. (1999). Intravascular radiographic contrast media: Issues for family physicians. *Journal of the American Board of Family Practice, 12*(1), 32–42.

Juchem, B.C., & Dall'Agnol, C.M. (2007). Immediate adverse reactions to intravenous iodinated contrast media in computed tomography. *Revista Latino-Americana de Enfermagem, 15*(1), 78–83.

Juchem, B.C., Dall'Agnol, C.M., & Magalhães, A.M.M. (2004). Contraste iodado em tomografia computadorizada: Prevenção de reações adversas. *Revista Brasileira de Enfermagem, 57*(1), 57–61.

Katayama, H., Yamaguchi, K., Kozuka, T., Takashima, T., Seez, P., & Matsuura, K. (1990). Adverse reactions to ionic and nonionic contrast media: A report from the Japanese Committee on the Safety of Contrast Media. *Radiology, 175*(3), 621–628.

Maddox, T.G. (2002). Adverse reactions to contrast material: Recognition, prevention, and treatment. *American Family Physician, 66*(7), 1229–1234.

Namasivayam, S., Kalra, M.K., Torres, W.E., & Small, W.C. (2006). Adverse reactions to intravenous iodinated contrast media: A primer for radiologists. *Emergency Radiology, 12*(5), 210–215.

Reddan, D. (2007). Patients at high risk of adverse events from intravenous contrast media after computed tomography examination. *European Journal of Radiology, 62*(1), 26–32.

Riedl, M.A., & Casillas, A.M. (2003). Adverse drug reactions: Types and treatment options. *American Family Physician, 68*(9), 1781–1790.

Schild, H.H., Kuhl, C.K., Hübner-Steiner, U., Böhm, I., & Speck, U. (2006). Adverse events after unenhanced and monomeric and dimeric contrast-enhanced CT: A prospective randomized controlled trial. *Radiology, 240*(1), 56–64.

Siddiqi, N.H. (2008). Contrast medium reactions, recognition and treatment. *Emedicine.* Retrieved from http://www.emedicine.com/Radio/topic864.htm.

Singh, J., & Daftary, A. (2008). Iodinated contrast media and their adverse reactions. *Journal of Nuclear Medicine Technology, 36*(2), 69–74.

Stacul, F. (2007). Managing the risk associated with use of contrast media for computed tomography. *European Journal of Radiology, 62*(1), 33–37.

Thomsen, H.S., & Morcos, S. K. (2004). Management of acute adverse reactions to contrast media. *European Radiology, 14*(3), 476–481.

Valls, C., Andía, E., Sánchez, A., & Moreno, V. (2003). Selective use of low-osmolality contrast media in computed tomography. *European Radiology, 13*(8), 2000–2005.

Vervloet, D., & Durham, S. (1998). Adverse reactions to drugs. *British Medical Journal, 316*(7143), 1511–1514.

Webb, J.A., Stacul, F., Thompsen, H.S., & Morcos, S.K. (2003) Late adverse reactions to intravascular iodinated contrast media. *European Radiology, 13*(1), 181–184.

Widmark, J.M. (2007). Imaging-related medications: A class overview. *Proceedings (Baylor University Medical Center), 20*(4), 408–417.

11. Safety/Protection

Latex Allergy Response (00041)

(1998, 2006, LOE 2.1)

Domain 11: Safety/Protection
Class 5: Defensive Processes

Definition A hypersensitive reaction to natural latex rubber products

Defining Characteristics

Life-threatening reactions occurring in the first hour after exposure to latex protein

- Bronchospasm
- Cardiac arrest
- Contact urticaria progressing to generalized symptoms
- Dyspnea
- Edema of the lips
- Edema of the throat

- Edema of the tongue
- Edema of the uvula
- Hypotension
- Respiratory arrest
- Syncope
- Tightness in chest
- Wheezing

Orofacial Characteristics

- Edema of eyelids
- Edema of the sclerae
- Erythema of the eyes
- Facial erythema
- Facial itching
- Itching of the eyes

- Nasal congestion
- Nasal erythema
- Nasal itching
- Oral itching
- Rhinorrhea
- Tearing of the eyes

Gastrointestinal Characteristics

- Abdominal pain

- Nausea

Generalized Characteristics

- Flushing
- Generalized discomfort
- Generalized edema

- Increasing complaint of total body warmth
- Restlessness

Type IV reactions occurring 1 hour or more after exposure to latex protein

- Discomfort reaction to additives such as thiurams and carbamates
- Eczema

- Irritation
- Redness

Related Factors

- Hypersensitivity to natural latex
  rubber protein

References

American Society of Anesthesiologists (2005). *Natural rubber latex allergy: Considerations for anesthesiologists. A practice guideline.* Park Ridge, IL: American Society of Anesthesiologists.

Association of Perioperative Registered Nurses. (2004). AORN latex guideline. In *AORN standards, recommended practices and guidelines.* Denver, CO: AORN, pp. 103–118.

Kelly, K.J. (2000). Latex allergy: Where do we go from here? *Canadian Journal of Allergy and Clinical Immunology, 5*(8), 337–340.

Sussman, G.L. (2000) Latex allergy: An overview. *Canadian Journal of Allergy and Clinical Immunology, 5*(8), 317–321.

Swanson, M.C., & Olson, D.Q. (2000). Latex allergen affinity for starch powders applied to natural rubber gloves and released as an aerosol. *Canadian Journal of Allergy and Clinical Immunology, 5*(8), 328–336.

Risk for Allergy Response (00217)

(2010, LOE 2.1)

Domain 11: Safety/Protection
Class 5: Defensive Processes

Definition
Risk of an exaggerated immune response or reaction to substances

Risk Factors

- Chemical products (e.g., bleach, cosmetics)
- Dander
- Environmental substances (e.g., mold, dust, pollen)
- Foods (e.g., peanuts, shellfish, mushrooms)
- Insect stings
- Pharmaceutical agents (e.g., penicillins)
- Repeated exposure to environmental substances

References

Alexiou, C., Kau, R.J., Luppa, P., & Arnold, W. (1998). Allergic reactions after systemic administration of glucocorticosteroid therapy. *Archives of Otolaryngology – Head and Neck Surgery, 124*(11), 1260–1264.

de Andrade, E.D., Ranali, J., Volpato, M.C., & de Oliveira, M.M. (2000). Allergic reaction after rubber dam placement. *Journal of Endodontics, 26*(3), 182–183.

Diaz, J.H. (2005). Syndromic diagnosis and management of confirmed mushroom poisonings. *Critical Care Medicine, 33*(2), 427–436.

Ellis, A.K., & Day, J.H. (2005). Clinical reactivity to insect stings. *Current Opinion in Allergy and Clinical Immunology, 5*(4), 349–354.

Friedlaender, M.H. (2004). Objective measurement of allergic reactions in the eye. *Current Opinion in Allergy and Clinical Immunology, 4*(5), 447–453.

Gomes, E.R., & Demoly, P. (2005). Epidemiology of hypersensitivity drug reactions. *Current Opinion in Allergy and Clinical Immunology, 5*(4), 309–316.

Haberman, M.L. (1978). Malignant hyperthermia. An allergic reaction to thioridazine therapy. *Archives of Internal Medicine, 138*(5), 800–801.

Hansen, I., Klimek, L., Mosges, R., & Hormann, K. (2004). Mediators of inflammation in the early and the late phase of allergic rhinitis. *Current Opinion in Allergy and Clinical Immunology, 4*(3), 159–163.

Hathaway, L.R. (2005). Anaphylaxis. *LPN, 1*(3), 38–39.

Huby, R.D., Dearman, R.J., & Kimber, I. (2000). Why are some proteins allergens? *Toxicological Sciences, 55*(2), 235–246.

Leung, D.Y.M., Boguniewicz, M., Howell, M.D., Nomura, I., & Hamid, Q.A. (2004). New insights into atopic dermatitis. *Journal of Clinical Investigation, 113*(5), 651–657.

McKevith, B., & Theobald, H. (2005). Common food allergies. *Nursing Standard, 19*(29), 39–42.

Merrill, D.B., William, G., & Goff, D.C. (2005). Adverse cardiac effects associated with clozapine. *Journal of Clinical Psychopharmacology, 25*(1), 32–41.

Nowak-Wegrzyn, A., Conover-Walker, M., & Wood, R.A. (2001). Food-allergic reactions in schools and preschools. *Archives of Pediatric and Adolescent Medicine, 155*, 790–795.

Reisman, R.E. (2005). Unusual reactions to insect stings. *Current Opinion in Allergy and Clinical Immunology, 5*, 355–358.

Shovlin, J.P., & Corso, M.P. (2005). Ocular allergy: Recognizing, treating, and avoiding. *Contemporary Optometry, 3*(3), 1–7.

Weir, E. (2005). Sushi, nematodes, and allergies. *Canadian Medical Association Journal, 172*(3), 329.

11. Safety/Protection

Risk for Latex Allergy Response (00042)
(1998, 2006, LOE 2.1)

Domain 11: Safety/Protection
Class 5: Defensive Processes

Definition Risk of hypersensitivity to natural latex rubber products that may compromise health

Risk Factors

- Allergies to avocados
- Allergies to bananas
- Allergies to chestnuts
- Allergies to kiwis
- Allergies to poinsettia plants
- Allergies to tropical fruits
- History of allergies

- History of asthma
- History of reactions to latex
- Multiple surgical procedures, especially beginning in infancy
- Professions with daily exposure to latex

References

American Society of Anesthesiologists (2005). *Natural rubber latex allergy: Considerations for anesthesiologists. A practice guideline*. Park Ridge, IL: American Society of Anesthesiologists.

Association of Perioperative Registered Nurses. (2004). AORN latex guideline. In *AORN standards, recommended practices and guidelines*. Denver, CO: AORN, pp. 103–118.

Kelly, K.J. (2000). Latex allergy: Where do we go from here? *Canadian Journal of Allergy and Clinical Immunology*, 5(8), 337–340.

Sussman, G.L. (2000) Latex allergy: An overview. *Canadian Journal of Allergy and Clinical Immunology*, 5(8), 317–321.

Swanson, M.C., & Olson, D.Q. (2000). Latex allergen affinity for starch powders applied to natural rubber gloves and released as an aerosol. *Canadian Journal of Allergy and Clinical Immunology*, 5(8), 328–336.

Risk for Imbalanced Body Temperature (00005)
(1986, 2000)

Domain 11: Safety/Protection
Class 6: Thermoregulation

Definition At risk for failure to maintain body temperature within normal range

Risk Factors

- Altered metabolic rate
- Dehydration
- Exposure to extremes of environmental temperature
- Extremes of age
- Extremes of weight
- Illness affecting temperature regulation
- Inactivity
- Inappropriate clothing for environmental temperature
- Pharmaceutical agents causing vasoconstriction
- Pharmaceutical agents causing vasodilation
- Sedation
- Trauma affecting temperature regulation
- Vigorous activity

Hyperthermia (00007)
(1986)

Domain 11: Safety/Protection
Class 6: Thermoregulation

Definition   Body temperature elevated above normal range

Defining Characteristics

- Convulsions
- Flushed skin
- Increase in body temperature above normal range
- Seizures
- Skin warm to touch
- Tachycardia
- Tachypnea

Related Factors

- Anesthesia
- Decreased perspiration
- Dehydration
- Exposure to hot environment
- Illness
- Inappropriate clothing
- Increased metabolic rate
- Pharmaceutical agents
- Trauma
- Vigorous activity

Hypothermia (00006)
(1986, 1988)

Domain 11: Safety/Protection
Class 6: Thermoregulation

Definition   Body temperature below normal range

Defining Characteristics

- Body temperature below normal range
- Cool skin
- Cyanotic nail beds
- Hypertension
- Pallor
- Piloerection
- Shivering
- Slow capillary refill
- Tachycardia

Related Factors

- Aging
- Consumption of alcohol
- Damage to hypothalamus
- Decreased ability to shiver
- Decreased metabolic rate
- Evaporation from skin in cool environment
- Exposure to cool environment
- Illness
- Inactivity
- Inadequate clothing
- Malnutrition
- Pharmaceutical agents
- Trauma

Ineffective Thermoregulation (00008)
(1986)

Domain 11: Safety/Protection
Class 6: Thermoregulation

Definition Temperature fluctuation between hypothermia and hyperthermia

Defining Characteristics

- Cyanotic nail beds
- Fluctuations in body temperature above and below the normal range
- Flushed skin
- Hypertension
- Increase in body temperature above normal range
- Increased respiratory rate
- Mild shivering
- Moderate pallor
- Piloerection
- Reduction in body temperature below normal range
- Seizures
- Skin cool to touch
- Skin warm to touch
- Slow capillary refill
- Tachycardia

Related Factors

- Extremes of age
- Fluctuating environmental temperature
- Illness
- Trauma

Domain 12
Comfort

NANDA International Nursing Diagnoses: Definitions & Classification 2012–2014, First Edition.
Edited by T. Heather Herdman.
© 2012 NANDA International. Published 2012 by Blackwell Publishing Ltd.

Impaired Comfort (00214)
(2008, 2010, LOE 2.1)

Domain 12: Comfort
Class 1: Physical Comfort
Class 2: Environmental Comfort
Class 3: Social Comfort

Definition Perceived lack of ease, relief, and transcendence in physical, psychospiritual, environmental, cultural, and social dimensions

Defining Characteristics

- Anxiety
- Crying
- Disturbed sleep pattern
- Fear
- Inability to relax
- Irritability
- Moaning
- Reports being cold
- Reports being hot
- Reports being uncomfortable
- Reports distressing symptoms
- Reports hunger
- Reports itching
- Reports lack of contentment in situation
- Reports lack of ease in situation
- Restlessness
- Sighing

Related Factors

- Illness-related symptoms
- Insufficient resources (e.g., financial, social support)
- Lack of environmental control
- Lack of privacy
- Lack of situational control
- Noxious environmental stimuli
- Treatment-related side effects (e.g., medication, radiation)

References

Cameron, B.L. (1993). The nature of comfort to hospitalized medical surgical patients. *Journal of Advanced Nursing, 18*(3), 424–436.

Honkus, V. (2003). Sleep deprivation in critical care units. *Critical Care Nursing Quarterly, 26*(3), 179–189.

Jenny, J., & Logan, J. (1996). Caring and comfort metaphors used by patients in critical care. *Image: Journal of Nursing Scholarship, 28*(4), 349–352.

Kolcaba, K. (1992). The concept of comfort in an environmental framework. *Journal of Gerontological Nursing, 18*(6), 33–38.

Kolcaba, K. (2003). *Comfort theory and practice: A vision for holistic health care and research.* New York: Springer.

Kolcaba, K., & Fox, C. (1999). The effects of guided imagery on comfort of women with early-stage breast cancer going through radiation therapy. *Oncology Nursing Forum, 26*(1), 67–71.

Kolcaba, K., Schirm, V., & Steiner, R. (2006). Effects of hand massage on comfort of nursing home residents. *Geriatric Nursing, 27*(2), 85–91.

Minden, P. (2005). The importance of words: Suggesting comfort rather than pain. *Holistic nursing practice, 19*(6), 267–271.

Schoener, C. (1996). The comfort and discomfort of infertility. *JOGNN, 25*(2), 167–172.

Taylor, B. (1992). Relieving pain through ordinariness in nursing: A phenomenological account of a comforting nurse-patient encounter. *Advances in Nursing Science, 15*(1), 33–43.

Wilson, L. (2002). An investigation of the relationships of perceived nurse caring, social support and emotion-focused coping to comfort in hospitalized medical patients. *Dissertation Abstracts International.* UMI No. AA13043623.

Walker, A. (2002). Safety and comfort work of nurses glimpsed through patient narratives. *International Journal of Nursing Practice, 8*(1), 42–48.

12. Comfort

Readiness for Enhanced Comfort (00183)
(2006, LOE 2.1)

Domain 12: Comfort
Class 1: Physical Comfort
Class 2: Environmental Comfort
Class 3: Social Comfort

Definition A pattern of ease, relief, and transcendence in physical, psychospiritual, environmental, and/or social dimensions that is sufficient for well-being and can be strengthened

Defining Characteristics

- Expresses desire to enhance comfort
- Expresses desire to enhance feeling of contentment
- Expresses desire to enhance relaxation
- Expresses desire to enhance resolution of complaints

References

Arruda, E., Larson, P., & Meleis, A. (1992). Immigrant Hispanic cancer patients' views. *Cancer Nursing, 15*(6), 387–395.

Cameron, B.L. (1993). The nature of comfort to hospitalized medical surgical patients. *Journal of Advanced Nursing, 18*(3), 424–436.

Duggleby, W., & Berry, P. (2005). Transitions in shifting goals of care for palliative patients and their families. *Clinical Journal of Oncology Nursing, 9*(4), 425–428.

Gropper, E.I. (1992). Promoting health by promoting comfort. *Nursing Forum, 27*(2), 5–8.

Jenny, J., & Logan, J. (1996). Caring and comfort metaphors used by patients in critical care. *Image: Journal of Nursing Scholarship, 28*(4), 349–352.

Kolcaba, K. (1991). A taxonomic structure for the concept comfort. *Image: Journal of Nursing Scholarship, 23*(4), 237–240.

Kolcaba, K. (1992). Holistic comfort: Operationalizing the construct as a nurse-sensitive outcome. *Advances in Nursing Science, 15*(1), 1–10.

Kolcaba, K. (1994). A theory of holistic comfort for nursing. *Journal of Advanced Nursing, 19*(6), 1178–1184.

Kolcaba, K., & Kolcaba, R. (1991). An analysis of the concept of comfort. *Journal of Advanced Nursing, 16*(11), 1301–1310.

Malinowski, A., & Stamler, L.L. (2002). Comfort: Exploration of the concept in nursing. *Journal of Advanced Nursing, 39*(6), 599–606.

Mitchell, G.J., & Pilkington, F.B. (2000). Comfort-discomfort with ambiguity: Flight and freedom in nursing practice. *Nursing Science Quarterly, 13*(1), 31–36.

Morse, J.M. (2000). On comfort and comforting. *American Journal of Nursing, 100*(9), 34–38.

Morse, J.M., Bottoroff, J.L., & Hutchinson, S. (1994). The phenomenology of comfort. *Journal of Advanced Nursing, 20*(1), 189–195.

12. Comfort

Nausea (00134)
(1998, 2002, 2010, LOE 2.1)

Domain 12: Comfort
Class 1: Physical Comfort

Definition A subjective phenomenon of an unpleasant feeling in the back of the throat and stomach that may or may not result in vomiting

Defining Characteristics

- Aversion toward food
- Gagging sensation
- Increased salivation
- Increased swallowing
- Reports nausea
- Reports sour taste in mouth

Related Factors

Biophysical

- Biochemical disorders (e.g., uremia, diabetic ketoacidosis)
- Esophageal disease
- Gastric distension
- Gastric irritation
- Increased intracranial pressure
- Intra-abdominal tumors
- Labyrinthitis
- Liver capsule stretch
- Localized tumors (e.g., acoustic neuroma, primary or secondary brain tumors, bone metastases at base of skull)
- Ménière's disease
- Meningitis
- Motion sickness
- Pain
- Pancreatic disease
- Pregnancy
- Splenetic capsule stretch
- Toxins (e.g., tumor-produced peptides, abnormal metabolites due to cancer)

Situational

- Anxiety
- Fear
- Noxious odors
- Noxious taste
- Pain
- Psychological factors
- Unpleasant visual stimulation

Treatment

- Gastric distension
- Gastric irritation
- Pharmaceutical agents

References

Fessele, K.S. (1996). Managing the multiple causes of nausea and vomiting in the patient with cancer. *Oncology Nursing Forum, 23*(9), 1409–1418.

Finley, J. (2000). Management of cancer cachexia. *AACN Clinical Issues, 11*(4), 590–603.

Grant, M. (1987). Nausea, vomiting, and anorexia. *Seminars in Oncology Nursing, 3*(4), 277–286.

Hogan, C.M. (1990). Advances in the management of nausea and vomiting. *Nursing Clinics of North America, 25*(2), 475–497.

Hogan, C.M., & Grant, M. (1997). Physiologic mechanisms of nausea and vomiting in patients with cancer. *Oncology Nursing Forum, 24*(7), 8–12.

Larson, P., Halliburton, P., & Di Julio, J. (1993). Nausea, vomiting, and retching. In V. Carrier-Kohlman, A.M. Lindsey, & C.M. West (eds), *Pathophysiological phenomena in nursing human responses to illness.* Philadelphia, PA: WB Saunders, pp. 371–394.

Lichter, I. (1993). Which antiemetic? *Journal of Palliative Care, 9*(1), 42–50.

Metz, A., & Hebbard, G. (2007). Nausea and vomiting in adults – a diagnostic approach. *Australian Family Physician, 36*(9), 688–692.

Nachman, J.A. (1993). Postoperative nausea and vomiting. *Current Reviews for Post-Anesthesia Care Nurses, 15*(5), 39–44.

Rousseau, P. (1995). Antiemetic therapy in adults with terminal disease: A brief review. *American Journal of Hospice and Palliative Care,* Jan/Feb, 13–18.

Tang, J.H.C. (1998). *Management of chemotherapy-induced nausea: Relaxation therapy.* Unpublished research report, University of Iowa, Iowa City, Iowa.

Taylor, J.P. (1994). Validation of altered comfort: Nausea as experienced by patients receiving chemotherapy. In R.M. Carroll-Johnson, & M. Paquette (eds), *Classification of nursing diagnoses: Proceedings of the Tenth Conference.* Philadelphia, PA: JB Lippincott, pp. 206–207.

Acute Pain (00132)
(1996)

Domain 12: Comfort
Class 1: Physical Comfort

Definition Unpleasant sensory and emotional experience arising from actual or potential tissue damage or described in terms of such damage (International Association for the Study of Pain); sudden or slow onset of any intensity from mild to severe with an anticipated or predictable end and a duration of <6 months

Defining Characteristics

- Changes in appetite
- Changes in blood pressure
- Changes in heart rate
- Changes in respiratory rate
- Coded report (e.g., use of pain scale)
- Diaphoresis
- Distraction behavior (e.g., pacing, seeking out other people and/or activities, repetitive activities)
- Expressive behavior (e.g., restlessness, moaning, crying, vigilance, irritability, sighing)
- Facial mask (e.g., eyes lack luster, beaten look, fixed or scattered movement, grimace)
- Guarding behavior
- Narrowed focus (e.g., altered time perception, impaired thought processes, reduced interaction with people and environment)
- Observed evidence of pain
- Positioning to avoid pain
- Protective gestures
- Pupillary dilation
- Reports pain
- Self-focus
- Sleep pattern disturbance

Related Factors

- Injury agents (e.g., biological, chemical, physical, psychological)

Chronic Pain (00133)
(1986, 1996)

Domain 12: Comfort
Class 1: Physical Comfort

Definition Unpleasant sensory and emotional experience arising from actual or potential tissue damage or described in terms of such damage (International Association for the Study of Pain); sudden or slow onset of any intensity from mild to severe, constant or recurring without an anticipated or predictable end and with a duration of >6 months

Defining Characteristics

- Altered ability to continue previous activities
- Anorexia
- Atrophy of involved muscle group
- Changes in sleep pattern
- Coded report (e.g., use of pain scale)
- Depression
- Facial mask (e.g. eyes lack luster, beaten look, fixed or scattered movement, grimace)
- Fatigue
- Fear of reinjury
- Guarding behavior
- Irritability
- Observed protective behavior
- Reduced interaction with people
- Reports pain
- Restlessness
- Self-focusing
- Sympathetic mediated responses (e.g., temperature, cold, changes of body position, hypersensitivity)

Related Factors

- Chronic physical disability
- Chronic psychosocial disability

12. Comfort

Social Isolation (00053)

(1982)

Domain 12: Comfort
Class 3: Social Comfort

Definition Aloneness experienced by the individual and perceived as imposed by others and as a negative or threatening state

Defining Characteristics

Objective

- Absence of supportive significant other(s)
- Developmentally inappropriate behaviors
- Dull affect
- Evidence of handicap (e.g., physical, mental)
- Exists in a subculture
- Illness
- Meaningless actions
- No eye contact
- Preoccupation with own thoughts
- Projects hostility
- Repetitive actions
- Sad affect
- Seeks to be alone
- Shows behavior unaccepted by dominant cultural group
- Uncommunicative
- Withdrawn

Subjective

- Developmentally inappropriate interests
- Experiences feelings of differences from others
- Inability to meet expectations of others
- Insecurity in public
- Reports feelings of aloneness imposed by others
- Reports feelings of rejection
- Reports inadequate purpose in life
- Reports values unacceptable to the dominant cultural group

Related Factors

- Alterations in mental status
- Alterations in physical appearance
- Altered state of wellness
- Factors contributing to the absence of satisfying personal relationships (e.g., delay in accomplishing developmental tasks)
- Immature interests
- Inability to engage in satisfying personal relationships
- Inadequate personal resources
- Unaccepted social behavior
- Unaccepted social values

Domain 13
Growth/Development

NANDA International Nursing Diagnoses: Definitions & Classification 2012–2014, First Edition.
Edited by T. Heather Herdman.
© 2012 NANDA International. Published 2012 by Blackwell Publishing Ltd.

Risk for Disproportionate Growth (00113)
(1998)

Domain 13: Growth/Development
Class 1: Growth

Definition At risk for growth above the 97th percentile or below the 3rd percentile for age, crossing two percentile channels

Risk Factors

Caregiver

- Abuse
- Learning difficulties (mental handicap)
- Mental illness
- Severe learning disability

Environmental

- Deprivation
- Economically disadvantaged
- Lead poisoning
- Natural disasters
- Teratogen
- Violence

Individual

- Anorexia
- Caregiver's maladaptive feeding behaviors
- Chronic illness
- Individual maladaptive feeding behaviors
- Infection
- Insatiable appetite
- Malnutrition
- Prematurity
- Substance abuse

Prenatal

- Congenital disorders
- Genetic disorders
- Maternal infection
- Maternal nutrition
- Multiple gestation
- Substance abuse
- Teratogen exposure

Delayed Growth and Development* (00111)
(1986)

Domain 13: Growth/Development
Class 1: Growth
Class 2: Development

Definition   Deviations from age-group norms

Defining Characteristics

- Altered physical growth
- Decreased response time
- Delay in performing skills typical of age group
- Difficulty in performing skills typical of age group
- Flat affect
- Inability to perform self-care activities appropriate for age
- Inability to perform self-control activities appropriate for age
- Listlessness

Related Factors

- Effects of physical disability
- Environmental deficiencies
- Inadequate caretaking
- Inconsistent responsiveness
- Indifference
- Multiple caretakers
- Prescribed dependence
- Separation from significant others
- Stimulation deficiencies

This diagnosis will retire from the NANDA-I Taxonomy in the 2015–2017 edition unless additional work is completed to separate the diagnostic foci of (1) growth, and (2) development into separate diagnostic concepts.

484 *Domain 13: Growth/Development*

Risk for Delayed Development (00112)
(1998)

Domain 13: Growth/Development
Class 2: Development

Definition At risk for delay of 25% or more in one or more of the areas of social or self-regulatory behavior, or in cognitive, language, gross or fine motor skills

Risk Factors

Prenatal

- Economically disadvantaged
- Endocrine disorders
- Genetic disorders
- Illiteracy
- Inadequate nutrition
- Inadequate prenatal care
- Infections
- Lack of prenatal care
- Late prenatal care
- Maternal age <15 years
- Maternal age >35 years
- Substance abuse
- Unplanned pregnancy
- Unwanted pregnancy

Individual

- Adopted child
- Behavior disorders
- Brain damage (e.g., hemorrhage in postnatal period, shaken baby, abuse, accident)
- Chronic illness
- Congenital disorders
- Failure to thrive
- Foster child
- Frequent otitis media
- Genetic disorders
- Hearing impairment
- Inadequate nutrition
- Lead poisoning
- Natural disasters
- Positive drug screen(s)
- Prematurity
- Seizures
- Substance abuse
- Technology dependent
- Treatment-related side effects (e.g., chemotherapy, radiation therapy, pharmaceutical agents)
- Vision impairment

Environmental

- Economically disadvantaged
- Violence

Caregiver

- Abuse
- Learning disabilities
- Mental illness
- Severe learning disability

Nursing Diagnoses Retired from the NANDA-I Taxonomy 2009–2014

NANDA International Nursing Diagnoses: Definitions & Classification 2012–2014, First Edition.
Edited by T. Heather Herdman.
© 2012 NANDA International. Published 2012 by Blackwell Publishing Ltd.

One diagnosis that was retired during the 2009–2011 cycle was inadvertently omitted from the chapter on Retired Diagnoses in that text. It is included here to enable individuals to review it and determine whether it might be returned to the Taxonomy with revision. The lack of related factors was the primary reason for the removal of this diagnosis from the Taxonomy.

Health-seeking Behaviors (00084) – Retired 2009–2011
(1988)

Domain 1: Health Promotion
Class 2: Health Management

Definition Active seeking (by a person in stable health) of ways to alter personal health habits and/or the environment in order to move toward a higher level of health

Defining Characteristics

- Demonstrated lack of knowledge about health-promotion behaviors
- Expressed concern about current environmental conditions on health status
- Expressed desire to seek a higher level of wellness
- Observed unfamiliarity with wellness community resources
- States unfamiliarity with wellness community resources

Related Factors

- *To be developed*

Only one diagnosis is being retired from the NANDA-I Taxonomy in this 2012–2014 edition. It was noted in the 2009–2011 edition that this diagnosis would be retired unless significant work was done to bring it to a level of evidence (LOE) of 2.1 or higher. Specifically, this diagnosis requires a break-out of focus areas within it into separate diagnoses (e.g., Visual Sensory Perception Deficit, Auditory Sensory Perception Deficit, etc.). Unfortunately, no work was completed on this diagnosis and therefore the diagnosis has been retired. The Diagnosis Development Committee (DDC) would be very willing to review new diagnoses related to these focus areas in the future, and to encourages nurses to work on these concepts and submit them through the DDC submission process.

Disturbed Sensory Perception (Specify: Visual, Auditory, Kinesthetic, Gustatory, Tactile, Olfactory) (00122) – Retired 2012–2014
(1978, 1980, 1998)

Domain 5: Perception/Cognition
Class 3: Sensation/Perception

Definition   Change in the amount or patterning of incoming stimuli accompanied by a diminished, exaggerated, distorted, or impaired response to such stimuli

Defining Characteristics

- Change in behavior pattern
- Change in problem-solving abilities
- Change in sensory acuity
- Change in usual response to stimuli
- Disorientation
- Hallucinations

- Impaired communication
- Irritability
- Poor concentration
- Restlessness
- Sensory distortions

Related Factors

- Altered sensory integration
- Altered sensory reception
- Altered sensory transmission
- Biochemical imbalance

- Electrolyte imbalance
- Excessive environmental stimuli
- Insufficient environmental stimuli
- Psychological stress

The following chart provides a list of all diagnoses removed from the NANDA-I Taxonomy since 2009, and the rationale for that removal. As with the diagnosis being removed during this edition, it is hoped that nurses will consider the appropriateness of these diagnoses and, if felt to be appropriate, further develop these concepts and resubmit them to NANDA-I so that they might be returned to the Taxonomy in an updated manner in the future. The full diagnoses that were removed from the Taxonomy in the previous edition (2009–2011) can be found within that text (*Part 4: Nursing diagnoses retired from the NANDA-I taxonomy, 2009–2011*).

Year removed	Diagnosis	Rationale
2009–2011	**Health-seeking Behaviors**	Lacked related factors and needed to be updated to reflect the current level of scientific knowledge
2009–2011	Total Urinary **Incontinence**	Concept required differentiation from other incontinence diagnoses, and needed to be updated to reflect the current level of scientific knowledge
2009–2011	**Rape-Trauma Syndrome**: Compound Reaction	Shared the same definition as the diagnosis, Rape-Trauma Syndrome: Silent Reaction; lacked related factors
2009–2011	**Rape-Trauma Syndrome**: Silent Reaction	Shared the same definition as the diagnosis, Rape-Trauma Syndrome: Compound Reaction; lacked related factors
2009–2011	Effective **Therapeutic Regimen Management**	Lacked related factors and needed to be updated to reflect the current level of scientific knowledge
2009–2011	Ineffective Community **Therapeutic Regimen Management**	Lacked related factors and needed to be updated to reflect the current level of scientific knowledge
2009–2011	Disturbed **Thought Processes**	Lacked related factors and needed to be updated to reflect the current level of scientific knowledge
2012–2014	Disturbed **Sensory Perception** (Specify: Visual, Auditory, Kinesthetic, Gustatory, Tactile, Olfactory)	Focus areas within the diagnosis should be separated into individual concepts (e.g., Visual Sensory Perception Deficit, Auditory Sensory Perception Deficit, etc.), with defining characteristics and related factors specific to each focus clearly identified

Finally, one actual diagnosis is slated for removal from the Taxonomy during the next cycle if work is not conducted to separate the diagnostic foci contained in the diagnosis label. The diagnosis, *Delayed Growth and Development* (00111), includes two diagnostic foci: growth, and development. It is important to separate these foci into two distinct diagnoses to decrease confusion and to improve diagnostic accuracy.

In addition, one syndrome diagnosis will be removed from the taxonomy during the next cycle if work is not conducted to bring it into line with the new definition of syndrome diagnoses. This definition requires that two or more nursing diagnoses must be used as defining characteristics. This diagnosis is, *Impaired Environmental Interpretation Syndrome* (00127).

Part 4
NANDA International
2012–2014

NANDA International Nursing Diagnoses: Definitions & Classification 2012–2014, First Edition.
Edited by T. Heather Herdman.
© 2012 NANDA International. Published 2012 by Blackwell Publishing Ltd.

NANDA International Think Tank Meeting

In October 2009, the NANDA International Board of Directors convened a 2-day Think Tank meeting in Chicago, which included face-to-face dialogue, teleconferencing/videoconferencing, and survey responses from renowned researchers, educators, administrators, and informaticists working with NANDA-I terminology from 24 different countries. Experts from Brazil, Japan, Nigeria, Norway, Peru, Switzerland, the United Kingdom, and the United States participated in the face-to-face and teleconference/videoconference meetings. Additionally, responses to a survey distributed prior to the meeting were received from 86 individuals representing 16 additional countries, and included 44 members and 42 nonmembers. The purpose of the Think Tank was to address several issues with which the Diagnosis Development Committee (DDC) was grappling, including the appropriateness of physiological diagnoses in a nursing diagnosis taxonomy, translation issues, and how to address diagnoses that might not be globally appropriate due to differences in the scope of nursing practice around the world.

Comments on the value of NANDA-I were frequently cited in the survey responses and interviews. This value included: that NANDA-I provides an evidence-based standardized language that helps to define and describe the focus of the profession of nursing; that it enables computerization of nursing judgment in a consistent way; that it enables research on concepts of importance to nursing practice; and that a well-defined standardized language facilitates intra- and interdisciplinary collaboration. The importance of linkages to defined, evidence-based nursing outcomes and interventions was also repeatedly mentioned (predominantly with reference to the Nursing Outcomes Classification and the Nursing Intervention Classification).

The following statements were agreed upon unanimously at the Think Tank meeting.

Issues Related to the DDC

It was decided that any time an actual diagnosis submission was accepted, the DDC should determine if a risk diagnosis and/or health-promotion diagnosis should also be considered. A decision was made to change the submission form to help submitters think through this possibility and to provide the risk factors for a risk diagnosis, and the defining characteristics for a health-promotion diagnosis, with the initial submission of an actual diagnosis.

Submitters sometimes submit "letters of intent" to the DDC when they are considering development of new diagnoses. Therefore, the DDC will develop guidelines providing what information would be most helpful for the committee to make a determination as to the appropriateness of a candidate diagnosis, in order to provide support for submitters in terms of whether or not to pursue development

NANDA International Nursing Diagnoses: Definitions & Classification 2012–2014, First Edition.
Edited by T. Heather Herdman.
© 2012 NANDA International. Published 2012 by Blackwell Publishing Ltd.

of this new diagnosis. This information will be provided on the NANDA-I website and within the submission form.

Nursing diagnoses exist at different levels of granularity; it was identified that there are instances in which more broad diagnoses may be more appropriate, as well as instances in which specific diagnoses may be more appropriate. The decision regarding granularity will be made in terms of which level of specificity will provide better clinical direction for intervention.

It is not the intention of NANDA-I to rename medical diagnoses to explain nursing judgments. There was a strong feeling that medical diagnoses do not always capture holistic human responses, so it is possible that alternative terms may be needed to add conceptual meaning where the medical diagnosis does not capture the complete response. It may be appropriate to interpret medical diagnoses within a nursing context, using the same terms as our medical colleagues, but with a different focus that captures the phenomena of concern to nursing practice. An example of one of these diagnoses that may need to be changed as a result of this discussion is that of *Decreased Intracranial Adaptive Capacity*. It is believed that this will also increase the clarity of interdepartmental communication. Likewise, the discussion and work that evolved from this meeting will lead to review of many current diagnoses, such as *Risk for Peripheral Neurovascular Dysfunction*.

If a condition is an event that can be reversed or ameliorated, it is appropriate for the event itself to be a nursing diagnosis. If all that can be done is to deal with the sequelae of the event, it is a matter of intervention but would not require a nursing diagnosis. For example, a nurse cannot reverse or ameliorate a fall, but she can prevent a fall from occurring. Therefore, NANDA-I would not accept an actual diagnosis, *Fall*, but it is appropriate to include the risk diagnosis, *Risk for Falls*.

Globalization of the Taxonomy

Diverse needs related to the conceptual language of nursing exist among nurses based on geography, economic climate, practice setting, culture, specialty, etc. There are also diverse needs unique to nurses' skills, competence, and the scope of practice and standards where they practice their profession. As an international organization, we value this diversity and are clear that we must broaden our taxonomy to allow for nursing concepts that meet the needs of nurses across the world for nursing terminology appropriate to their practice.

Not every nursing diagnosis within the NANDA-I Taxonomy is appropriate for every nurse in practice – nor has it ever been. Nursing diagnoses do not capture all of nurses' work. Nursing's work is very diverse, and nursing diagnoses represent many of the clinical judgments made by the nurse.

Some of the diagnoses are specialty-specific, and would not necessarily be used by all nurses in clinical practice. There are diagnoses within the Taxonomy that may be outside the scope or standards of nursing practice governing a particular geographical area in which a nurse practices. These diagnoses would, in these instances, not be appropriate for practice, and should not be used if they lie outside the scope or standards of nursing practice for a particular geographical region. However, it is appropriate for these diagnoses to remain in the Taxonomy because it represents clinical judgments made by nurses around the world, and not just those made in a particular region or country. Every nurse should be aware of, and work within, the standards and scope of practice within which he or she is licensed to practice. However, it is also important for all nurses to be aware of the areas of nursing practice that exist globally, as this informs discussion and may over time support the broadening of nursing practice across other countries.

Issues for Future Discussion and Research

It was determined that it is necessary to define "human response" to assist nurses as well as the DDC in verifying that a new diagnosis submission does indeed meet the definition of a nursing diagnosis. The relationship between etiology and intervention was also identified as requiring better explanation and emphasis.

NANDA International Position Statements

From time to time, the NANDA-I Board of Directors provides position statements as a result of requests from members or users of the NANDA-I Taxonomy. Currently, there are two position statements (updated in October 2010 by NANDA-I Board of Directors): one addresses the use of the NANDA-I Taxonomy as an assessment framework, and the other addresses the structure of the nursing diagnosis statement when included in a care plan. NANDA-I publishes these statements in an attempt to prevent others from interpreting NANDA-I's stance on important issues, and to prevent misunderstandings or misinterpretations.

NANDA-I Position Statement 1: The Use of Taxonomy II as an Assessment Framework

Nursing assessments provide the starting point for determining nursing diagnoses. It is vital that a recognized nursing assessment framework is used in practice to identify the patient's* problems, risks, and outcomes for enhancing health.

NANDA-I does not endorse one single assessment method or tool. The use of an evidence-based nursing framework such as Gordon's Functional Health Pattern Assessment should guide assessment that supports nurses in determination of NANDA-I nursing diagnoses.

For accurate determination of nursing diagnoses, a useful, evidence-based assessment framework is best practice.

NANDA-I Position Statement 2: The Structure of the Nursing Diagnosis Statement when Included in a Care Plan

NANDA-I believes that the structure of a nursing diagnosis as a statement including the diagnosis label and the related factors as exhibited by defining characteristics is best clinical practice, and may be an effective teaching strategy.

The accuracy of the nursing diagnosis is validated when a nurse is able to clearly identify and link to the defining characteristics, related factors, and/or risk factors found within the patient's* assessment.

While this is recognized as best practice, it may be that some information systems do not provide this opportunity. Nurse leaders and nurse informaticists must work together to ensure that vendor solutions are available that allow the nurse to validate accurate diagnoses through clear identification of the diagnostic statement, related and/or risk factors, and defining characteristics.

*NANDA-I defines patient as "individual, family, group, or community."

NANDA International Nursing Diagnoses: Definitions & Classification 2012–2014, First Edition.
Edited by T. Heather Herdman.
© 2012 NANDA International. Published 2012 by Blackwell Publishing Ltd.

Chapter 8

The Process for Development of an Approved NANDA International Nursing Diagnosis

Leann M. Scroggins

This article is designed to assist in the development of a nursing diagnosis that will meet the inclusion criteria for acceptance into the NANDA-I classification system. It is recommended that the submitter follow the steps below to move through the process. If at any point there are questions, please contact the Chair of the Diagnosis Development Committee (DDC) for assistance and guidance through the NANDA-I website (www.nanda.org).

An additional resource that will facilitate completion of the process is the NANDA-I website: www.nanda.org/DiagnosisDevelopment/DiagnosisSubmission.aspx. Reviewing the following information will provide a good basis on which to begin this important work.

To be accepted for publication and inclusion in NANDA-I Taxonomy II, a nursing diagnosis submission must minimally have a label, definition, defining characteristics or risk factors, related factors (if an actual diagnosis), references to support these diagnostic components, and examples of appropriate interventions and outcomes. The official definition of a nursing diagnosis is "a clinical judgment about individual, family, group, or community experiences/responses to actual or potential health problems/life processes. A nursing diagnosis provides the basis for selection of nursing interventions to achieve outcomes for which the nurse has accountability" (NANDA-I Think Tank Meeting, 2009).

NANDA-I uses a multiaxial approach in the creation of diagnoses. When creating a diagnosis it is essential to consider all seven axes (see Figure 1.1).

Axis 1: The Diagnostic Focus

The diagnostic focus is the principal element or the fundamental and essential part, the root, of the diagnostic concept. It describes the "human response" that is the core of the diagnosis.

The diagnostic focus may consist of one or more nouns. When more than one noun is used (e.g., *Activity Intolerance*), each one contributes a unique meaning to the diagnostic focus, as if the two were a single noun; the meaning of the combined term, however, is different from when the nouns are stated separately. Frequently, an adjective (e.g., Spiritual) may be used with a noun (e.g., Distress) to denote the diagnostic focus, here *Spiritual Distress*.

NANDA International Nursing Diagnoses: Definitions & Classification 2012–2014, First Edition.
Edited by T. Heather Herdman.
© 2012 NANDA International. Published 2012 by Blackwell Publishing Ltd.

In some cases, the diagnostic focus and the diagnostic concept are one and the same, for example *Nausea*. This occurs when the nursing diagnosis is stated at its most clinically useful level and the separation of the diagnostic focus adds no meaningful level of abstraction.

The following are examples of diagnostic foci. For a complete listing, refer to Chapter 1, Axis 1. Examples of diagnostic concepts in Taxonomy II include:

- Activity intolerance
- Airway clearance
- Grieving
- Hope
- Memory
- Pain
- Parenting.

Axis 2: Subject of the Diagnosis

The subject of the diagnosis is defined as the person(s) for whom a nursing diagnosis is determined. The values in Axis 2 are individual, family, group, and community, representing the NANDA-I definition of "patient":

- *Individual*: a single human being distinct from others, a person.
- *Family*: two or more people having continuous or sustained relationships, perceiving reciprocal obligations, sensing common meaning, and sharing certain obligations toward others; related by blood and/or choice.
- *Group*: a number of people with shared characteristics.
- *Community*: a group of people living in the same locale under the same governance. Examples include neighborhoods and cities.

Axis 3: Judgment

A judgment is a descriptor or modifier that limits or specifies the meaning of the diagnostic focus. The diagnostic focus together with the nurse's judgment about it forms the diagnosis. The judgment limits or specifies meaning to the diagnostic focus. For a complete listing of descriptors and modifiers, refer to Chapter 1, Axis 3.

Some diagnoses, depending on the level of specificity, do not require a modifier or descriptor. Examples of such diagnoses include *Nausea* and *Fatigue*.

Axis 4: Location

Location describes the parts/regions of the body and/or their related functions – all tissues, organs, anatomical sites, or structures. For a complete listing refer to Chapter 1, Axis 4. Location does not pertain to all diagnoses.

Axis 5: Age

Age refers to the age of the person who is the subject of the diagnosis. For a complete listing refer to Chapter 1, Axis 5.

Axis 6: Time

Time describes the duration of the diagnostic focus found within the diagnostic label. For a complete listing refer to Chapter 1.

Axis 7: Status of the Diagnosis

Status refers to the actuality or potentiality of the diagnosis or the categorization of the diagnosis. NANDA-I has identified the following:

- *Actual nursing diagnosis*: describes human responses to health conditions/life processes that exist in an individual, family, or community. These diagnoses are sometimes referred to as "problem" diagnoses. Requirement for submission: defining characteristics (manifestations, signs, and symptoms) that cluster in patterns of related cues or inferences. An example of an actual diagnosis is *Nausea*.
- *Health-promotion nursing diagnosis*: describes a clinical judgment about a person's, family's, group's, or community's motivation and desire to increase well-being and actualize human health potential as expressed in the readiness to enhance specific health behaviors, and which can be used in any health state. Requirement for submission: defining characteristics. An example of an existing health-promotion diagnosis is *Readiness for Enhanced Hope*. Each label of a health-promotion diagnosis begins with the phrase "Readiness for Enhanced."
- *Risk nursing diagnosis*: a clinical judgment about human experience/responses to health conditions/life processes that have a high probability of developing in a vulnerable individual, family, or community. Requirement for submission: supported by risk factors that contribute to increased vulnerability. An example of a risk diagnosis is *Risk for Impaired Skin Integrity*. Each label of a risk diagnosis begins with the phrase "Risk for."
- *Syndrome*: a clinical judgment describing a specific cluster of nursing diagnoses that occur together, and are best addressed together and through similar interventions. Requirement for submission: two or more nursing diagnoses must be used as defining characteristics. Related factors may be used if they add clarity to the definition.
- *Wellness nursing diagnosis*: *NANDA-I no longer defines a category of nursing diagnosis as a "wellness diagnosis."* It was determined at the NANDA-I Think Tank meeting (2009) that this area of concern was already encompassed within the health-promotion nursing diagnosis category. This diagnosis type and definition will be eliminated from the NANDA-I Taxonomy, and wellness diagnoses will be converted to health-promotion diagnoses.

To begin developing the nursing diagnosis, consider the following:

1. Is this diagnostic focus of your proposed diagnosis a human response? (Axis 1). If yes, then proceed.
2. Is this concept consistent with the definition of a nursing diagnosis? "A nursing diagnosis is a clinical judgment about individual, family, or community responses to actual or potential health problems/life processes. A nursing diagnosis provides the basis for selection of nursing interventions to achieve outcomes for which the nurse has accountability" (NANDA-I Think Tank statement, 2009). If yes, then proceed.
3. Who is the subject of this concept? (Axis 2).
   _____ Individual patient/client
   _____ Family
   _____ Group
   _____ Community
4. Is this diagnostic focus already included in NANDA-I? If so, review the related existing diagnoses currently in the NANDA-I Taxonomy.
   Is the concept currently represented? If there is a similar diagnosis, it may be appropriate to revise the existing diagnosis rather than create a new diagnosis. If this concept is not included as a current NANDA-I diagnosis, it is appropriate to proceed with the development of a new diagnosis.
5. Is a descriptor or a modifier required to accurately identify this concept? (Axis 3).
   If yes, select the appropriate descriptor/modifier (see Chapter 1, Axis 3, for the full list of judgments). Is a descriptor/modifier other than those identified above required for this concept?
   If yes, identify and define the descriptor or modifier that best describes this concept:
   Descriptor/modifier: _____
   Definition: _____
6. Is location (Axis 4) relevant for the diagnostic concept? Examples of current diagnoses requiring location to be specified are *Impaired Skin Integrity* and *Risk for Peripheral Neurovascular Dysfunction*.
   If yes, identify the location: _____
7. Should age (Axis 5) be specified in this diagnostic concept? An example of a current diagnosis requiring age to be specified is *Adult Failure to Thrive*.
   If age should be identified in your diagnostic concept, please identify the appropriate age term: _____
8. Is Axis 6, Time, required to describe this diagnostic concept?
   If yes, select the appropriate term:
   - Acute
   - Chronic
   - Intermittent
   - Continuous
9. Select the appropriate status (Axis 7) for this diagnostic concept (see above for definitions of these terms):
   - Actual diagnosis
   - Health-promotion diagnosis
   - Risk diagnosis
   - Syndrome diagnosis

It is now appropriate to begin creating the new diagnosis. As NANDA-I uses a multiaxial approach in the creation of diagnoses, it is essential to consider all seven axes.

Congratulations! Many steps have been completed in developing this diagnosis, and the diagnostic label may now be identified. Verify that the appropriate axes have been incorporated into your proposed label:

- Diagnostic focus
- Subject of the diagnosis
- Judgment about the diagnosis (descriptor/modifier)
- Location
- Age
- Time
- Status of the diagnosis

State the proposed label here: _____

Label and Definition

The next step in creating this diagnosis is to define the label that has been selected.

Go to the literature, focusing on literature published in the last 5 years. Most of the literature should be nursing, but you may find supporting literature in related fields such as the psychosocial sciences.

It is best to have research-based literature, but if such literature does not exist, nonresearch-based literature may be referenced. The literature must support both the label and the definition. References addressing nursing interventions are not appropriate as supporting references for the label and definition.

The definition must provide a clear, precise description of the label without using the language of the label. The definition gives meaning and helps differentiate this diagnosis from other similar diagnoses. Create the definition here:

_____
_____
_____

Identify the references used to support the label and definition:

_____
_____

Defining Characteristics versus Risk Factors

If this diagnosis is an actual or health-promotion diagnosis, identify the defining characteristics for the diagnosis. If this diagnosis is a risk diagnosis, identify the risk factors for the diagnosis. Select which of the following are appropriate for this diagnosis:

- *Defining characteristics* – observable cues/inferences that cluster as manifestations of an actual or health-promotion diagnosis.

- *Risk factors* – environmental factors and physiological, psychological, genetic, or chemical elements that increase the vulnerability of an individual, family, or community to an unhealthful event. Risk factors are identified for Risk diagnoses.

Defining characteristics or risk factors must be supported by literature. Like the literature supporting the label and definition of this diagnosis, literature supporting each defining characteristic or risk factor should also focus on literature published in the last 5 years. Again, most of the literature should be nursing, but supporting literature in related fields such as the psychosocial sciences may also be used.

It is best to have research-based literature, but if such literature does not exist, nonresearch-based literature may be referenced. The literature must support the defining characteristics or risk factors. References addressing nursing interventions for the proposed diagnosis are not appropriate as supporting references for defining characteristics or risk factors. *The use of textbooks is not appropriate unless no other literature is available* (please indicate this on your submission); *books and articles referencing nursing interventions, nursing diagnoses, or nursing outcomes are also not relevant to the diagnosis submission.*

If this diagnosis is an Actual or Health-Promotion diagnosis, list the defining characteristics in Table 8.1. Following this list of defining characteristics, list and number the references supporting the defining characteristics. Indicate the number of the supporting reference with each defining characteristic.

If the diagnosis is a Risk diagnosis, list the risk factors in Table 8.2. Following the list of risk factors, list and number the references supporting the risk factors. Indicate the number of the supporting reference with each risk factor.

Taxonomy Rules

The following are some "diagnosis construction rules" that apply to attributes of nursing diagnoses, both defining characteristics and risk factors. Check each of

Table 8.1 *Defining characteristics with references*

Defining characteristics	Supporting reference (number from list below)
Defining characteristic #1	Reference #____
Defining characteristic #2	Reference #____
Defining characteristic #3	Reference #____

References:

1.
2.
3.
4.

Table 8.2 *Risk factors*

Risk factors	**Supporting reference (number from list below)**
Risk factor #1	Reference #____
Risk factor #2	Reference #____
Risk factor #3	Reference #____

References:

1.
2.
3.
4.

these rules to make certain the attributes for the proposed diagnosis are stated correctly.

The attributes of a nursing diagnosis may not contain the following stop-words: "i.e.," "and," "&," "or," ":," ";," "/," "( )," or "e.g.,".
The attributes of a nursing diagnosis may not contain quotes.
The number of attributes should be limited to those that actually drive the decision of whether or not the diagnosis exists.

Congratulations! A label, definition, and either defining characteristics or risk factors all supported by literature have now been developed. If the diagnosis is a Health-Promotion or Risk diagnosis, each of the steps necessary to submit your proposal to NANDA-I for inclusion into Taxonomy II has been completed. Please refer to the "Protocol for Submission of Diagnoses" in one of the following references for assistance in the submission process:

NANDA International Nursing Diagnoses: Definitions & Classification 2012–2014
NANDA-I website: www.nanda.org/DiagnosisDevelopment/DiagnosisSubmission.aspx.

Related Factors

If the diagnosis is an *actual* diagnosis, there is, however, still more work to do.

Identify Related Factors

Related factors show a patterned relationship with the nursing diagnosis. Such factors may be described as antecedent to, associated with, related to, contributing

Table 8.3 *Related factors*

Related factors	Supporting reference (number from list below)
Related factor #1	Reference #____
Related factor #2	Reference #____
Related factor #3	Reference #____

References:

1.
2.
3.
4.

to, or abetting. Only actual nursing diagnoses have related factors. Related factors must be supported by literature.

Similar to the literature supporting the label, definition, and defining characteristic or risk factors, the literature supporting related factors should also have been published in the last 5 years. Again, most of the literature should be nursing, but you may find supporting literature in related fields such as the psychosocial sciences.

It is best to have research-based literature, but if such literature does not exist, nonresearch-based literature may be referenced. The literature must support the related factors. References addressing nursing interventions for the proposed diagnosis are not appropriate as supporting references for the related factors.

Please list the Related Factors in Table 8.3 and link the related factor to the supporting reference by identifying the number of the reference(s). Indicate the number of the supporting reference with each related factor.

The following "construction rules" apply to related factors. Check each of these rules to make certain that the related factors are stated correctly.

The related factors of a nursing diagnosis may not contain the following stop-words: "and," "&," "or," ":," ";," "/," "( )," or "e.g.".
The related factors of a nursing diagnosis may not contain quotes.

Congratulations! A label, definition, defining characteristics, and related factors all supported by literature have been created.

All the steps necessary to submit the proposal to NANDA-I for inclusion into Taxonomy II have been completed. Please refer to the "Protocol for Submission of Diagnoses" in one of the following references for assistance in the submission process:

NANDA International Nursing Diagnoses: Definitions & Classification 2012–2014
NANDA-I website: www.nanda.org/DiagnosisDevelopment/DiagnosisSubmission. aspx

References

McCourt, A.E. (1991). Syndromes in nursing: A continuing concern. In R.M. Carrol-Johnson (ed.), *Classification of nursing diagnoses: Proceedings of the ninth conference of North American Nursing Diagnosis Association*. Philadelphia: JB Lippincott, pp. 79–82.

NANDA International. (2007). *Nursing diagnoses: Definitions & classification*, 2007–2008. Philadelphia: NANDA-I. Retrieved from www.nanda.org/DiagnosisDevelopment/DiagnosisSubmission.aspx.

Pender, N.J., Murdaugh, C., & Parsons, M.A. (2006). *Health promotion in nursing practice*, 5th edn. Upper Saddle River, NJ: Pearson/Prentice-Hall.

NANDA International Processes and Procedures

Proposed diagnoses and revisions of diagnoses undergo a systematic review to determine consistency with the established criteria for a nursing diagnosis. All submissions are subsequently staged according to evidence supporting either the level of development or validation.

Diagnoses may be submitted at various levels of development (e.g., label and definition; label, definition, defining characteristics, or risk factors; label, definition, defining characteristics, and related factors). All submissions must include supporting references. Articles used for the submission are to be catalogued in the reference section of the submission form using American Psychological Association (APA) format.

NANDA-I Diagnosis Submission Guidelines are available on the NANDA-I website (www.nanda.org). Diagnoses should be submitted electronically using the form available on the NANDA-I website.

On receipt, the diagnosis will be assigned to a primary reviewer from the Diagnosis Development Committee (DDC). This person will work with the submitter as the DDC reviews for submission.

Full Review Process

New diagnoses go through a *full review process*, which includes the following steps:

1. Review of submission is made by the primary reviewer.
2. Primary reviewer works with the submitter to address changes that need to be made.
3. Submission is forwarded to the full DDC for review.
4. The DDC recommends one of the following:
    (a) approve with no recommendations;
    (b) approve pending follow-up with recommendations (the most frequent DDC decision);
    (c) disapprove.
5. The primary reviewer forwards the DDC recommendations to the submitter and works with the submitter to make the recommended changes.
6. Submissions approved by the DDC are presented to the NANDA-I membership electronically for review and vote. Recommended changes from the membership must be supported by the literature.
7. Once revisions recommended by the membership have been addressed, the submission is then forwarded to the NANDA-I Board of Directors for final approval.

NANDA International Nursing Diagnoses: Definitions & Classification 2012–2014, First Edition.
Edited by T. Heather Herdman.
© 2012 NANDA International. Published 2012 by Blackwell Publishing Ltd.

Diagnoses accepted at the 2.1 level of evidence will be incorporated into both the NANDA-I Taxonomy and the NNN Taxonomy of Nursing Practice, and will be published in the next edition of *NANDA-I Nursing Diagnoses: Definitions and Classification*.

Expedited Review Process

The expedited review process (ERP) is a streamlined process to facilitate the rapid review of proposed revisions of current diagnoses, when those revisions are determined by the DDC to be minor in nature and when they do not alter the original intent of the diagnoses. Examples of such revisions may include:

- editing and clarification of the definition;
- a limited addition or deletion of defining characteristics, risk factors, or related factors.

An ERP includes the following steps:

1. Review of the submission by the primary DDC reviewer.
2. The primary reviewer works with the submitter to address any needed revisions that may need to be made to enable acceptance of the revised diagnosis.
3. The submission is forwarded to the DDC for review.
4. The DDC recommends one of the following:
   (a) approve with no recommendations;
   (b) approve pending follow-up with recommendations (the most frequent DDC decision);
   (c) disapprove.
5. The primary reviewer forwards the DDC recommendations to the submitter and works with the submitter to make the recommended changes.
6. Submissions approved by the DDC are presented to the NANDA-I Board of Directors for final approval. Approval of the proposed revisions is posted on the NANDA-I website.

Submission Process for New Diagnoses

To submit a new diagnosis for consideration by the DDC, follow these steps:

1. Review this edition of *NANDA-I Nursing Diagnoses: Definitions & Classification* and review any potentially related diagnoses in the book. Refer to the NANDA-I Diagnosis Submission Guidelines on the NANDA-I website (www.nanda.org). Follow the guidelines on the NANDA-I website in case they have been updated since publication of this edition of the NANDA-I book.
2. Contact the Chair of the DDC for more specific instructions, guidelines regarding format, criteria for assigning level of evidence, and protocol for submission.
3. Review the "Glossary of Terms" in this edition of *NANDA-I Nursing Diagnoses: Definitions & Classification*.

4. Decide whether your diagnosis is an actual diagnosis, risk diagnosis, or health-promotion diagnosis. The DDC strongly recommends that you consider whether you could submit all three types of diagnosis using the same references. For example, if you were submitting a diagnosis for *Obesity* (an actual diagnosis), please consider including a recommendation for *Risk for Obesity* (a risk diagnosis). Or if you were submitting the diagnosis of *Delayed Development* (an actual diagnosis), please consider including a recommendation for *Risk for Delayed Development* (a risk diagnosis) and *Readiness for Enhanced Development* (a health-promotion diagnosis).

5. Provide a label for the diagnosis, supported by references. Identify the references.

6. Provide a definition for the diagnosis that is supported by references. Identify the references.

7. Identify the defining characteristics or risk factors for the diagnosis. Actual and health-promotion diagnoses have defining characteristics; risk diagnoses have risk factors. To facilitate coding, each defining characteristic and risk factor must contain a single concept rather than multiple concepts. For example, "nausea and vomiting" cannot be listed as a single concept, but rather as two separate concepts ("nausea" and "vomiting").

8. Identify related factors for the actual diagnosis. To facilitate coding, each related factor must contain a single concept rather than multiple concepts. Risk and health-promotion diagnoses do not have related factors. References are required for each related factor and must be identified (see point 9 below).

9. Develop a bibliography, including all the articles referenced. *The reference list must be in APA format.* Number each reference and link the reference to the component(s) of your submission that the reference supports (e.g., definition, defining characteristic, risk factor, or related factor). References from research and/or clinical practice articles related to the concept (*not from textbooks*) should be used to back up each defining characteristic and risk factor. The references should be research-based, if at all possible. If no research-based or nursing references are available, indicate this in your submission.

10. Provide up to three examples of appropriate nursing outcomes and nursing interventions from one of the standardized nursing terminologies (e.g., NOC, NIC) for the diagnosis. Although not components of a diagnosis, interventions and outcomes are requested to delineate the role of nursing in treating the diagnosis, and the accountability of nursing related to the proposed diagnosis.

11. Use the electronic submission process available on the NANDA-I website.

12. You will be notified when your work is received, and will be given an estimate of the time that it will take before you can expect to receive a response from the DDC. Most submissions require some refinement before acceptance into the NANDA-I Taxonomy. You will be assigned a mentor from the DDC to assist you through the process.

13. If you submit your diagnosis in a language other than English, please recognize that the review process will necessarily be lengthened in order to facilitate review by the DDC in the working language of NANDA-I, which is English.

Submission Process for Revising a Current Nursing Diagnosis

To submit a revision of a current diagnosis for consideration by the DDC, follow these steps:

1. Review this edition of *NANDA-I Nursing Diagnoses: Definitions & Classification* and review any potentially related diagnoses in the book. Refer to the NANDA-I Diagnosis Submission Guidelines on the NANDA-I website (www.nanda.org). Follow the guidelines on the NANDA-I website in case they have been updated since publication of this edition of the NANDA-I book.
2. Contact the Chair of the DDC for more specific instructions, guidelines regarding format, criteria for assigning level of evidence, and protocol for submission.
3. Review the "Glossary of Terms" in this edition of *NANDA-I Nursing Diagnoses: Definitions & Classification*.
4. Identify whether the label of the diagnosis requires revision, and revise it as appropriate. The revision must be supported by references, and the references must be identified.
5. Review the definition of the diagnosis to determine if revision is necessary; revise as appropriate. The revision must be supported by references, and the references must be identified.
6. Review the defining characteristics or risk factors for the diagnosis. Actual and health-promotion diagnoses have defining characteristics; risk diagnoses have risk factors. To facilitate coding, each defining characteristic and risk factor must contain a single concept rather than multiple concepts. For example, "nausea and vomiting" cannot be listed as a single concept, but rather as two separate concepts ("nausea" and "vomiting").
7. Review the related factors for the actual diagnosis. To facilitate coding, each related factor must contain a single concept rather than multiple concepts. Risk diagnoses do not have related factors; related factors are not required for health-promotion diagnoses, but may be included if they add clarity to the diagnosis. References are required for each related factor and must be identified (see point 8 below).
8. Develop a bibliography, including all the articles referenced. *The reference list must be in APA format.* Number each reference and link the reference to the component(s) of your submission that the reference supports (e.g., definition, defining characteristic, risk factor, or related factor). References from articles related to the concept (*not from textbooks*) should be used to back up each defining characteristic and risk factor, and must be identified. The references should be research-based, if at all possible. If no research-based or nursing references are available, indicate this in your submission.
9. Use the electronic submission process available on the NANDA-I website.
10. You will be notified when your work is received and will be given an estimate of the time that it will take before you can expect to receive a response from the DDC. Revised diagnoses may undergo a full review process or an expedited review process, depending on the extent of the revisions being proposed. The DDC will make this decision and inform you which process will be followed.

Most submissions require some refinement before acceptance into the NANDA-I Taxonomy. You will be assigned a mentor from the DDC to assist you through the process.

Procedure to Appeal a DDC Decision on Diagnosis Review

If a new or revised diagnosis is reviewed by the DDC and returned to the submitter(s) either for revision or because it is judged not to meet one or more criteria for staging a diagnosis, the submitter(s) may appeal the decision.

If the DDC chooses not to accept a new or revised diagnosis, notification of the lack of approval will be given to the submitter(s) with a detailed rationale. One or more of the following reasons will be explained:

1. Reject diagnosis (e.g., does not meet criteria for the definition of a nursing diagnosis, or does not meet level of evidence criteria).
2. Return – requires substantial revision (e.g., need to make major content changes).
3. Insufficient/old literature support (e.g., failure to reference meta-analyses, concept papers, or current research, or lack of research articles with reliance on textbooks only).
4. Return with editorial changes (e.g., solicit submitter response to DDC rationale and/or revision to submission).

If the submitter(s) choose(s) to appeal the DDC decision, the proposed new or revised diagnosis will be placed on the NANDA-I website (www.nanda.org), and the appeal will be announced in the journal. A period of 90 days after the distribution of the journal will be provided for members to submit evidence supporting, modifying, or rejecting the submission. After the close of 90 days, the DDC will review feedback and submit a second decision to the submitter(s).

If the DDC chooses not to accept a diagnosis after this second review, the submitter(s) will have an opportunity at the biennial conference to present the submission and the rationale for the disagreement with the DDC decision. The presentation will occur in an open session and require evidence-based argument from the submitter(s) and the DDC about the decision. Conference attendees will also have the opportunity to present evidence-based argument supporting, modifying, or rejecting the submission. Following this presentation, the DDC will review all information and forward a decision to the submitter(s) and the NANDA-I Board of Directors.

The NANDA-I Board of Directors will have an opportunity to provide evidence-based argument supporting, modifying, or rejecting submission at two points:

- during the open forum at the biennial conference;
- after the conference in its final review of the DDC recommendations for approval. A decision by the Board to modify or reject the DDC's recommendation must be evidence-based and at the same level of evidence as or higher than the evidence presented by the submitter(s) and/or by the DDC.

NANDA-I Diagnosis Submission: Level of Evidence Criteria

1. Received for Development (Consultation from DDC)

1.1 Label Only

This level is intended primarily for submission by organized groups rather than individuals. The label is clear, stated at a basic level, and supported by literature references, and these are identified. The DDC will consult with the submitter and provide education related to diagnostic development through printed guidelines and workshops. At this stage, the label is categorized as "Received for Development" and identified as such on the NANDA-I website.

1.2 Label and Definition

The label is clear and stated at a basic level. The definition is consistent with the label. The label and definition are distinct from other NANDA-I diagnoses and definitions. The definition differs from the defining characteristics and label, and these components are not included in the definition. At this stage, the diagnosis must be consistent with the current NANDA-I definition of nursing diagnosis (see the "Glossary of Terms"). The label and definition are supported by literature references, and these are identified.

2. Accepted for Publication and Inclusion in the NANDA-I Taxonomy

2.1 Label, Definition, Defining Characteristics or Risk Factors, Related Factors, and References

References are cited for the definition, each defining characteristic or risk factor, and each related factor. In addition, it is required that nursing outcomes and nursing interventions from a standardized nursing terminology (e.g., NOC, NIC) be provided for each diagnosis. If approved, the diagnosis will be forwarded to the Taxonomy Committee for classification within the NANDA-I taxonomy.

2.2 Concept Analysis

The criteria in 2.1 are met. In addition, a narrative review of relevant literature, culminating in a written concept analysis, is required to demonstrate the existence of a substantive body of knowledge underlying the diagnosis. The literature review / concept analysis supports the label and definition, and includes discussion and support of the defining characteristics, risk factors (for risk diagnoses), or related factors (for actual diagnoses).

2.3 Consensus Studies Related to Diagnosis Using Experts

The criteria in 2.1 are met. Studies include those soliciting expert opinion, Delphi, and similar studies of diagnostic components in which nurses are subjects.

3. Clinically Supported (Validation and Testing)

3.1 Literature Synthesis

The criteria in 2.2 are met. The synthesis is in the form of an integrated review of the literature. Search terms/MESH terms used in the review are provided to assist future researchers.

3.2 Clinical Studies Related to Diagnosis, but Not Generalizable to the Population

The criteria in 2.2 are met. The narrative includes a description of studies related to the diagnosis, which includes defining characteristics or risk factors, and related factors. Studies may be qualitative in nature, or quantitative studies using nonrandom samples in which patients are subjects.

3.3 Well-designed Clinical Studies with Small Sample Sizes

The criteria in 2.2 are met. The narrative includes a description of studies related to the diagnosis, which includes defining characteristics or risk factors, and related factors. Random sampling is used in these studies, but the sample size is limited.

3.4 Well-designed Clinical Studies with Random Sample of Sufficient Size to Allow for Generalizability to the Overall Population

The criteria in 2.2 are met. The narrative includes a description of studies related to the diagnosis, which includes defining characteristics or risk factors, and related factors. Random sampling is used in these studies, and the sample size is sufficient to allow for generalizability of results to the overall population.

Glossary of Terms

Nursing Diagnosis

A nursing diagnosis is a clinical judgment about individual, family, or community experiences/responses to actual or potential health problems/life processes. A nursing diagnosis provides the basis for selection of nursing interventions to achieve outcomes for which the nurse has accountability. (Approved at the ninth NANDA Conference; amended in 2009.)

Actual Nursing Diagnosis

Describes human responses to health conditions/life processes that exist in an individual, family, group, or community. These diagnoses are sometimes refered to as "problem" diagnoses.

Requirement for submission: defining characteristics (manifestations, signs, and symptoms) that cluster in patterns of related cues or inferences. Related factors (etiological factors) that are related to, contribute to, or antecedent to the diagnostic focus are also required.

Health-promotion Nursing Diagnosis

A clinical judgment about a person's, family's, group's, or community's motivation and desire to increase well-being and actualize human health potential as expressed in the readiness to enhance specific health behaviors, and which can be used in any health state.

Requirement for submission: defining characteristics.

Risk Nursing Diagnosis

A clinical judgment about human experience/responses to health conditions/life processes that have a high probability of developing in a vulnerable individual, family, group, or community.

Requirement for submission: supported by risk factors that contribute to increased vulnerability.

Syndrome

A clinical judgment describing a specific cluster of nursing diagnoses that occur together, and are best addressed together and through similar interventions.

NANDA International Nursing Diagnoses: Definitions & Classification 2012–2014, First Edition.
Edited by T. Heather Herdman.
© 2012 NANDA International. Published 2012 by Blackwell Publishing Ltd.

Requirement for submission: two or more nursing diagnoses must be used as defining characteristics/risk factors. Related factors may be used if they add clarity to the definition.

Wellness Nursing Diagnosis

NANDA-I no longer defines a category of nursing diagnosis as a "wellness diagnosis." It was determined at the NANDA-I Think Tank meeting in 2009 that this area of concern was already encompassed within the health-promotion nursing diagnosis category. This diagnosis type and definition have been eliminated from the NANDA-I Taxonomy, and wellness diagnoses have been converted to health-promotion diagnoses.

Components of a Nursing Diagnosis

Diagnosis Label

Provides a name for a diagnosis that includes, at a minimum, the diagnostic focus (from Axis 1) and the nursing judgment (from Axis 3). It is a concise term or phrase that represents a pattern of related cues. It may include modifiers.

Definition

Provides a clear, precise description; delineates its meaning and helps differentiate it from similar diagnoses.

Defining Characteristics

Observable cues/inferences that cluster as manifestations of an actual or health-promotion diagnosis.

Risk Factors

Environmental factors and physiological, psychological, genetic, or chemical elements that increase the vulnerability of an individual, family, group, or community to an unhealthy event. Only risk diagnoses have risk factors.

Related Factors

Factors that appear to show some type of patterned relationship with the nursing diagnosis. Such factors may be described as antecedent to, associated with, related to, contributing to, or abetting. Only actual nursing diagnoses and syndromes have related factors.

Definitions for Classification of Nursing Diagnoses

Classification

Systematic arrangement of related phenomena in groups or classes based on characteristics that objects have in common.

Level of Abstraction

Describes the concreteness/abstractness of a concept:

- Very abstract concepts are theoretical, may not be directly measurable, are defined by concrete concepts, are inclusive of concrete concepts, are disassociated from any specific instance, are independent of time and space, have more general descriptors, and may not be clinically useful for planning treatment.
- Concrete concepts are observable and measurable, limited by time and space, constitute a specific category, are more exclusive, name a real thing or class of things, are restricted by nature, and may be clinically useful for planning treatment.

Nomenclature

A system or set of terms or symbols especially in a particular science, discipline, or art; the act or process or an instance of naming (Merriam-Webster, 2009).

Taxonomy

"Classification: especially orderly classification of plants and animals according to their presumed natural relationships"; the word is derived from the root word, taxon – "the name applied to a taxonomic group in a formal system of nomenclature" (Merriam-Webster, 2009).

Reference

Merriam-Webster, Inc. (2009). *Merriam-Webster's Collegiate Dictionary* (11th ed.). Springfield, MA: Merriam-Webster.

NANDA International 2010–2012

NANDA International Board of Directors

President	Dickon Weir-Hughes, EdD, RN, FRSH
President-Elect	Jane M. Brokel, PhD, RN
Treasurer	Anne Perry, EdD, RN, FAAN
Directors	Shigemi Kamitsuru, PhD, RN
	Gail Keenan, PhD, RN
	Maria Müller-Staub, PhD, RN
	Matthias Odenbreit, MNS, RN
	Gunn Von Krogh, MNSc, RN
Executive Director	T. Heather Herdman, PhD, RN

NANDA International Diagnosis Development Committee

Chair	Shigemi Kamitsuru, PhD, RN
Members	Miriam de Abreu Almeida, PhD, RN
	Helen De Graaf, Clinical Nurse Specialist
	Gail Ladwig, MSN, CHTP, RN
	Geraldine Lyte, PhD, RSCN, RN
	Maria Müller-Staub, PhD, RN
	Chie Ogasawara, PhD, MEd, RN
	Anne Perry, EdD, RN, FAAN
	Leann Scroggins, MS, CRRN-A, APRN BC, RN

NANDA International Education & Research Committee

Chair	Maria Müller-Staub, PhD, MNS, EdN, RN
Members	Maria Márcia Bachion, PhD, RN
	Marcelo Chanes, PhD(c), MS, RN
	Anita Collins, PhD, RN
	Fritz Frauenfelder, MNS, RN
	Barbara Krainovich-Miller, EdD, PMHCNS-BC, ANEF, RN FAAN
	Margaret Lunney, PhD, RN
	Mary F. Moorhouse, MSN, CRRN, RN
	Wolter Paans, MSC, RN

NANDA International Nursing Diagnoses: Definitions & Classification 2012–2014, First Edition.
Edited by T. Heather Herdman.
© 2012 NANDA International. Published 2012 by Blackwell Publishing Ltd.

NANDA International Informatics Committee

Chair	Matthias Odenbreit, MNS, RN
Members	Shari Falan, PhD, RN
	Noreen Frisch, PhD, APHN, RN, FAAN
	Gail Keenan, PhD, RN
	Joan Klehr, MPH, RNC

NANDA International Taxonomy Committee

Chair	Gunn Von Krogh, MNSc, RN
Members	Kay C. Avant, PhD, RN, FAAN
	Marta Avena, PhD(c), MSN, RN
	Emilia Campos de Carvalho, PhD, RN
	Marjory Gordon, PhD, RN, FAAN
	T. Heather Herdman, PhD, RN
	Dorothy Jones, EdD, RN, FAAN
	Kimikazu Kashiwagi, MHS, RN
	Carol Soares O'Hearn, PhD, CPRQ, RN
DDC Consultant	Shigemi Kamitsuru, PhD, RN

An Invitation to Join NANDA International

Words are powerful. They allow us to communicate ideas and experiences to others so that they may share our understanding. Nursing diagnoses are an example of a powerful and precise terminology that highlights and renders visible the unique contribution of nursing to global health. Nursing diagnoses communicate the professional judgments that nurses make every day to our patients, our colleagues, members of other disciplines, and the public. They are our words.

NANDA International: A Member-driven Organization

Our Vision

NANDA International will be a global force for the development and use of nursing's standardized diagnostic terminology to improve the healthcare of all people.

Our Mission

To facilitate the development, refinement, dissemination, and use of standardized nursing diagnostic terminology.

- We provide the world's leading evidence-based nursing diagnoses for use in practice and to determine interventions and outcomes.
- We fund research through the NANDA-I Foundation.
- We are a supportive and energetic global network of nurses who are committed to improving the quality of nursing care through evidence-based practice.

Our Purpose

Implementation of nursing diagnosis enhances every aspect of nursing practice, from garnering professional respect to assuring accurate documentation for reimbursement.

NANDA International exists to develop, refine, and promote terminology that accurately reflects nurses' clinical judgments. This unique, evidence-based perspective includes social, psychological, and spiritual dimensions of care.

Our History

NANDA International (NANDA-I; originally known as the North American Nursing Diagnosis Association, founded in 1982) grew out of the National Conference

NANDA International Nursing Diagnoses: Definitions & Classification 2012–2014, First Edition.
Edited by T. Heather Herdman.
© 2012 NANDA International. Published 2012 by Blackwell Publishing Ltd.

Group, a task force established at the First National Conference on the Classification of Nursing Diagnoses, held in St. Louis, Missouri, USA, in 1973. This conference and the ensuing task force ignited interest in the concept of standardizing nursing terminology. In 2002, NANDA was re-launched as NANDA International to reflect increasing worldwide interest in the field of nursing terminology development. Although we no longer use the name "North American Nursing Diagnosis Association," we did maintain "NANDA" within our name because of its international recognition as the leader in nursing diagnostic terminology.

NANDA-I has approved 217 diagnoses for clinical use, testing, and refinement. A dynamic, international process of diagnosis review and classification approves and updates terms and definitions for identified human responses. In collaboration with the Nursing Classification Center at the University of Iowa, USA, NANDA-I has developed a nursing practice taxonomy and class structure. This system allows for the placement of NANDA-I diagnoses in an organizing framework that accommodates interventions and outcomes from the Nursing Interventions Classification (NIC) and the Nursing Outcomes Classification (NOC), thus creating a comprehensive language system capable of documenting nursing care in a standardized manner.

NANDA-I has international networks in Brazil, Colombia, Ecuador, Nigeria–Ghana, and Peru, as well as a German-language group; other country, specialty, and/or language groups interested in forming a NANDA-I Network should contact the Executive Director of NANDA-I at execdir@nanda.org. NANDA-I also has collaborative links with nursing terminology societies around the world such as the Japanese Society of Nursing Diagnoses (JSND), the Association for Common European Nursing Diagnoses, Interventions and Outcomes (ACENDIO), the Asociacíon Española de Nomenclatura, Taxonomia y Diagnóstico de Enfermeria (AENTDE), and the Association Francophone Européenne des Diagnostics Interventions Résultats Infirmiers (AFEDI). Joint membership is available with some of these organizations; contact us to see if a joint membership is available with other organizations related to standardized nursing language to which you belong.

NANDA International's Commitment

NANDA-I is a member-driven, grassroots organization committed to the development of nursing diagnostic terminology. The desired outcome of the Association's work is to provide nurses at all levels and in all areas of practice with a standardized nursing terminology with which to:

- name human responses to actual or potential health problems, and life processes;
- develop, refine, and disseminate evidence-based terminology representing clinical judgments made by professional nurses;
- facilitate study of the phenomena of concern to nurses for the purpose of improving patient care, patient safety, and patient outcomes for which nurses have accountability;
- document care for reimbursement of nursing services;
- contribute to the development of informatics and information standards, ensuring the inclusion of nursing terminology in electronic healthcare records.

Nursing terminology is the key to defining the future of nursing practice and ensuring the knowledge of nursing is represented in the patient record – NANDA-I is the global leader in this effort. Join us and become a part of this exciting process.

Involvement Opportunities

The participation of NANDA-I members is critical to the growth and development of nursing terminology. Many opportunities exist for participation on committees, as well as in the development, use, and refinement of diagnoses, and in research. Opportunities also exist for international liaison work and networking with nursing leaders.

Why Join NANDA-I?

Professional Networking

- Professional relationships are built through serving on committees, attending our biennial conference, and participation in the Nursing Diagnosis Discussion Forum.
- NANDA-I Membership Network Groups connect colleagues within a specific country, region, language, or nursing specialty.
- Professional contribution and achievement are recognized through our Founders, Mentors, Unique Contribution, and Editor's Awards. Research grant awards are offered through the NANDA-I Foundation.

Resources

- Members receive a complimentary subscription to our quarterly journal, *The International Journal of Nursing Terminologies and Classifications* (IJNTC). IJNTC communicates efforts to develop and implement standardized nursing language across the globe.

   NANDA-I News, our quarterly e-newsletter, provides updates on new programs and services, website features, and membership benefits.

   The NANDA-I website offers resources for nursing diagnosis development, refinement, and submission, and NANDA-I taxonomy updates.

Member Benefits

- Members receive discounts on NANDA-I taxonomy publications, including print, electronic, and summary list versions of *NANDA-I Nursing Diagnoses & Classification*.
- We partner with organizations offering products/services of interest to the nursing community, with a price advantage for members. Member discounts apply to our biennial conference and NANDA-I products, such as our T-shirts and tote bags.

- Our Regular Membership fees are based on the World Health Organization's classification of countries. It is our hope this will enable more individuals with interest in the work of NANDA-I to participate in setting the future direction of the organization.

How to Join

Go to www.nanda.org for more information and instructions for membership registration.

Who is Using the NANDA International Taxonomy?

- International Standards Organization compatible
- Health Level 7 International registered
- SNOMED-CT available
- Unified Medical Language System compatible
- American Nurses' Association recognized terminology

The NANDA-I taxonomy is currently available in Bahasa Indonesian, Basque, Chinese, Czech, Dutch, English, Estonian, French, German, Italian, Japanese, Portuguese, Spanish, and Swedish.

  For more information, and to apply for membership online, please visit www.nanda.org.

Index

Note: Page numbers in *italics* refer to figures; those in **bold** to tables.

NANDA International Nursing Diagnoses: Definitions & Classification 2012–2014, First Edition.
Edited by T. Heather Herdman.
© 2012 NANDA International. Published 2012 by Blackwell Publishing Ltd.

self-concept **13–14**, **33**, 279–84
  readiness for enhanced **14**, **33**, **46**, 284
self-directed violence, risk for **27**, **37**, **44**, 56, 112, 448
self-esteem **14**, **33**, 285–90
  chronic low xxxi, **14**, **33**, **46**, 285–6
  risk for chronic low xxvii, **14**, **33**, **46**, 288–9
  risk for situational low **14**, **33**, **46**, 290
  situational low **14**, **33**, **46**, 287
self-health management
  ineffective xxxii, **4**, **29**, **43**, 77, 161–3
  readiness for enhanced **4**, **29**, **43**, 77, 81, 164–6
self-mutilation **27**, **37**, **44**, 449–50
  risk for **27**, **37**, **44**, 451
self-neglect 254–6
self-perception **46**
  domain **13–15**, **33**, 277–92
sensation/perception **12**, **32**, **43**, 490
sensitivity of clinical indicators 117
sensory perception, disturbed xxviii, **12**, **43**, 490–1
sexual dysfunction **18**, **34**, **40**, 58, 114, 323–4
sexual function **17**, **34**, 323–5
sexual identity **34**
sexuality **40**
  domain **17–19**, **34**, 321–31
sexuality pattern, ineffective **18**, **34**, **40**, 114, 325
shock, risk for xxix, **26**, **36**, **41**, 435
short-term memory 71
simulation, clinical 91, 93
skin integrity
  impaired **26**, **36**, **43**, 81, 94, 100, 436, 502
  risk for impaired xxviii, **26**, **36**, **43**, 437, 501
sleep
  deprivation **8**, **31**, **40**, 104, 219
  pattern, disturbed **8**, **31**, **40**, 118, 221
  readiness for enhanced **8**, **31**, **40**, 220
sleep/rest **9**, **31**, **40**, 217–21
SNOMED International 53
social comfort **28**, **38**, 473–5, 480
social interaction, impaired **17**, **34**, **45**, 320
social isolation **28**, **38**, **45**, 58, **112**, 480
sorrow, chronic **23**, **35**, **45**, 379
specificity of clinical indicators 117
spiritual distress **25**, **36**, **40**, 55, 58, 410–11, 499
  risk for **25**, **36**, **40**, 55, 58, 412–13
spiritual well-being, readiness for enhanced **24**, **36**, **40**, 394

spirituality, impaired 117
status of diagnosis 61–2, 501, 502
stress overload **23**, **34**, **45**, 380–2
stress tolerance domain *see* coping/stress tolerance domain
subject of diagnosis 59, 500
subjective data 91, 92
submission of diagnoses 495–6, 499, 502–6, 508–14
  appeals procedure 512
  expedited review process 509
  full review process 508–9
  level of evidence criteria 513–14
  new diagnoses 509–10
  revisions of current diagnoses 511–12
sudden infant death syndrome, risk for **26**, **36**, **47**, 58, 438
suffocation, risk for **26**, **36**, **43**, 58, 439
suicide, risk for **27**, **37**, **44**, 59, 452–3
supportive family role performance 114
surgical recovery, delayed xxix, **26**, **36**, 59, 440–1
swallowing, impaired **6**, **29**, **40**, 103, 178–9
syndrome 62, 501, 502, 515–16
Synergy Model 105

taxonomy
  defined 50, 94, 517
  education 94
  rules 64, 504–5
Taxonomy II, NANDA-I 49–65, 90, 127, 147–8, 523
  construction of a nursing diagnostic concept 62–3, *62–3*
  definitions of axes 55–62
  diagnoses, placement, coding structure and contributors 3, **4–28**, 48
  domains, classes, and diagnoses **29–38**
  education 91, 93–4, 95
  EHRs 101, 103, 105, 107, 109–10, 111
  further development 64
  globalization 496–7
  history of development 49–50
  multiaxial system 53–62, *55*, 499–501, 503
  research 114
  retired diagnoses 487–91
  structure **29–38**, 50–3, *51–2*, 53
  submission of diagnosis *see* submission of diagnoses
  use as an assessment framework 498
Taxonomy Committee 49, 50, 64, 513, 519
technical competencies 74–5